Nutritional Therapy

Featuring the

Core Program
for Diet Revision

Stephen J. Gislason, M.D.

VOLUME 2

OF THE NUTRITIONAL MEDICINE SERIES

PERSONA PUBLICATIONS

Copyright © 1991 Stephen J. Gislason, M.D. & Environmed Research Inc.

Canadian Cataloguing in Publication Data

Gislason, Stephen J., 1943 - Nutritional Therapy featuring the Core
Program for Diet Revision. (Nutritional Medicine Series; v 2)
ISBN 0-9694145-2-8

1. Nutrition 2. Diet Revision Therapy 3. Food Allergy 4. Therapy,
Nutritional 5. Medicine, Nutritional
I. Title. II. Series: Gislason, Stephen J., 1943- Nutritional Medicine
Series; 2.
RM216.G58 1991   615.8'54   C90-091308-8

Nutritional Medicine Series 1991:

Volumes: 1. Nutritional Programming
         2. Nutritional Therapy featuring the
            Core Program for Diet Revision
         3. The Core Diet for Kids, 2nd ed.
         4. Core Program Cooking, 2nd ed.

Published by:

PerSona Publications
a division of Environmed Research Inc.
#1-3661 West 4th Avenue
Vancouver, B.C., Canada, V6R 1P2
Tel (604) 731-5898, (604) 731-9168

Printers: Printed in Canada by Hignell Printing, Winnipeg Man.

ACKNOWLEDGEMENTS

My patients and co-workers have inspired and contributed many of the insights in this work. The Core Program is a therapeutic approach that I did not anticipate in my early medical career, but only discovered after becoming ill with food allergy. Subsequently, working with insightful and considerate patients, I developed the point-of-view manifest in this book. Their observations, kept in daily food-intake and symptom journals, were essential to my understanding of food-illness relationships. The insights and research of many physicians and scientists are also represented in this book. The book, therefore speaks from the vantage point of the collective "we"; many minds, many experiences, all seeking a solution to human illness and suffering.

I have based my understanding of food-illness mechanisms on the work of physicians and scientists that I do not know - the reports of W. A. Hemmings first alerted me to the passage of intact proteins through the intestinal wall and the distribution of these proteins to body tissues, especially the brain. This occurred at a time when I was increasingly symptomatic with food allergy (but did not, at the time, recognize the nature of the illness). My search for answers to my own "strange disease" sent me on a scholar's journey through the medical literature and eventually changed my career. I then discovered the pioneers in the clinical observation of food allergy patterns. The writings of Drs.W. Alvarez, M. Brent Campbell, Fredrick Speer, Theron Randolph, A.H. Rowe, Wm. Rea, Doris Rapp, and Dr. J. Gerrard were helpful early in my investigations, confirming the general validity of my clinical observations; although, many questions about the nature and mechanisms of food allergy remained unanswered. The work and writings of Drs. R. Rienhardt, R.R.A. Coombs, P. McLaughlin, D.J. Atherton, Jonathan Brostroff, Wm. Knicker, R. Pagnelli, Joseph Egger, Claudio Carini, L. Businco, J.A. Bellanti, J.F. Soothill, G. Halpern, John Bienenstock, W. Allen Walker, and their associates have been helpful in explaining the biological mechanisms underlying the diverse expressions of food allergy in my patients. Some of these physicians may be uncomfortable with my emphasis on the importance and prevalence of food allergy. The descriptions and arguments in this book will hopefully support my contentions and awaken a greater interest in food allergy.

I am grateful to Dr. Justin Parr and Dr. David Stinson for their insightful early teachings and the view of medicine as the synthesis of compassion and scientific rigor. David taught clinical physiology, a system's approach to the body, and the importance of the four senses- humor, beauty, rhythm, and awe - in the healing process, years before others had thought of it. Justin introduced me to the human brain and taught medicine as an expression of rational humanism with compassion. Justin is responsible for WIRGO, my most valuable epistemological probe - What Is Really Going On Here?

The friendship and intellectual support of Dr. David M. Low and Barbara Low has been invaluable; they have now taken their considerable talents to Texas and I wish them well. I am specially grateful for the friendship and support of Jack Wise, a long-time friend and gifted artist. Dr. Alan Burton has freely offered his biochemical expertise. My early efforts were encouraged and facilitated by Charles Bates who contributed insights into addiction problems and depression, connected with food allergy. Linda Gomez assisted early in the development of the Core Program and her helpful comments have been preserved in the instructions for the Core Program. Claire Alston supported my early efforts to write about nutritional programming and diet revision as therapy, and has remained a source of intellectual support.

I am grateful to physicians who refer their interesting and challenging patients to teach me more about the intricacies of food allergy: Drs. Tanya Wulff, David Anderson, Eric Young, Jacob Meyerhoff have been particularly interested and supportive; many others deserve my special thanks. Al Fowler has been supportive of my efforts to develop ENFood, an important tool of diet revision technology, and deserves special thanks. Lisa Morrow deserves special thanks for her work on ENF research. Many others have contributed to this work and supported my efforts: Dr. Julianne Conry, Ula Timmermans, Jerry Kinmont, Patrick Couling, Ray Lipovsky, Katherine Johnson, Valerie Giles, Toby Bell all deserve my thanks. I am also grateful to Daniel Fretts for material and moral support and for sharing insights into the experience of food allergy. Special thanks to Jim Bjerring for critical proof-reading of the book. Bruce Wilson has become a valued collaborator and co-worker with valuable personal and scientific insights. Kathleen Ferns also contributed her proof-reading skills. I am entirely to blame for the remaining mistakes and stylistic idiosyncracies. My assistant, Pamela Fajardo has worked consistently on patient-care instructions, book materials, and all the nitty-gritty practical details of publishing and deserves special thanks. Thanks to Hignell Printers for their quality work and friendly support. Kelly Whiteway has kept order when chaos otherwise would have taken-over; my special thanks for helping to send our message into the world, and for special treats. My debt cannot be repaid to all these wonderful people.

Thank You All.

Preface Second Edition

This book is about change. Problems in our food, air and water make us ill. Old and new diseases can be traced to wrong food selection. New problems in foods, altered by manufacturing and processing, and in foods contaminated by agricultural chemicals and atmospheric pollution increase the disease-causing potential of our food supply. Nutritional Therapy is based on recognizing food sources of common diseases and initiating treatment with diet revision.

Food is that part of our environment which we ingest. But now, our numbers are so great and our ability to change the planet so increased, that we will determine what will happen to the biosphere. We have become our own product, for better or worse. We thrive when our habits mesh positively with life-cycles on earth. We fail by becoming ill, despondent and reckless, when our habits thwart the balance of nature. Our awareness of man-made environmental disasters has never been as acute. The world community finally awoke to the environmental crisis in 1989. Time magazine set the media tone by declaring the "Endangered Earth" planet of the year. Major magazines ran specials on the environmental crisis and politicians announced their awareness of the problems and promised to act. Marshall Arisman writing in Omni magazine's environmental special, September 1989, stated:

> "The earth's in serious trouble. We've polluted the very water we drink and bathe in with human sewage and an endless amount of toxic chemicals... Many of our ills are self-inflicted, the sins of selfishness and greed. And that problem has a solution: we can curb our seemingly endless desire for things, or there may come a day when earth will be no more.

> "That's not apocalyptic; it's not a scare tactic. That message —save the planet— is everywhere: flashing from the headlines of daily newspapers; on Glad garbage bags; UN studies; the latest reports from Washington, Paris, Tokyo, or Moscow; and blaring from evening news programs and rock concerts."

Self-directed, presonal change can be considered a model of global change. The decade of the 90's may be devoted especially to rescuing ourselves, individually and collectively. Dysfunction and disease, created by problems in our food supply, are among the most important challenges to our present and future well-being. Our medical system, relatively ignorant of food and air quality problems, labours under the delusion that diseases are static and solvable by "medical means". We even refer to diseases as "medical problems" not social, biological, environmental problems. Our medicine fosters the belief that drugs and technology can rescue us - one at a time - in expensive, high-tech hospitals. The misleading assumption is that all we need is to spend more money to pay the ever increasing medical bill for problems which need fundamental solutions at their source.

Our experience with the success of Nutritional Therapy allows us to be optimistic; many people get better, even from chronic suffering by the simple expedient of changing their food supply. Many diseases can be prevented by similar changes in diet. Our excitement about diet revision, however, does not make us giddy and irrational. We have often been discouraged reviewing popular books which advocate get-better-quick schemes on false grounds. The following giddy hyperbole is an example:

> "Yes, these Natural Healing Foods stop symptoms... break down viruses, toxins, pollutants in your body...wash away the damage done by bad habits or past sickness... actually reverse or protect against 30 common and deadly diseases..."

There are no 'healing foods" as such, and no guarantees that any given food selection will work for everyone. Nutritional Therapy is based on more intelligent premises, especially that careful and complete diet revision is necessary to restore and maintain good health. Diet Revision is hard work. The information in this book has been simplified so that any motivated reader can make sense of what is really going on. Books that over-simplify complex matters may be more readable, but risk being false and misleading.

Good diets must be custom-fitted to individual needs. The Core Program is an all-purpose diet revision method, a diet design technique that leads to healthier food selection and eating practices. The Core Program can be a therapeutic approach to the management of a wide range of food-related illnesses, a deceptively simple alternative to expensive medical care for many people with common diseases. The program is presented in this book along with explanatory essays, with the hope that more people will have access to this safe and effective solution to health problems. I also hope that professional readers will be inspired to try the Core Program themselves, help their families and share the insights which I found to be revelationary and revolutionary. As Osler suggested, the physician really understands only the disease he suffers himself. Insightful physicians do share the benefit with their patients and clients even if they must act at odds with their drug-oriented colleagues. No-one is well-educated in diet revision therapy; this is truly a pioneering effort. I have faith in the intelligence and good intentions of the general reader, and dedicate this book to better-informed, more self-sufficient, healthier citizens of a changing world.

Stephen J. Gislason M.D.
Vancouver B.C. , January 1991.

How To Use This Book

Nutritional Therapy is distinctly different from other nutrition and diet books. Several techniques are involved in nutritional methods; the emphasis is on matching a food supply to the biological properties of each person. This is not a trivial task and is seldom attempted in a logical and realistic manner. Nutritional writing usually focuses on the nutrient content of foods and readers are urged to select foods because of the presence of a desirable nutrient or the absence of an undesirable substance; drink milk for calcium and avoid butter because of cholesterol are typical recommendations. This simple-minded level of nutritional advice plagues us everyday in the popular media. There are many other important details of food-body interaction that receive little or no attention. The least desirable subject is the disease-causing, pathological properties of food.

The **pathology of food-body interactions** is complex and forces us to take a more thoughtful approach to food selection. The idea of the Core program began with the simple assumption that the food supply may be involved in causing or promoting many illness patterns which were not well-understood. What safe experiment could be carried out to reveal the contribution of the food supply? The most promising techniques were not minor modifications to existing diets but more radical changes in food intake - very limited food choices or fasting and cleansing methods which had been used for centuries in many cultures. Diets invented for food allergy management were similarly radical forms of diet revision. Oligoantigenic diets (meaning a little bit of antigen in the food) were prescribed for food allergy management. The idea was to retreat to a limited set of well-tolerated foods and once you were better, add foods back in an orderly manner. This basic strategy is incorporated in the **Core Program.**

The Core Program is **human software.** The program can and should be modified by the reader according to his or her own experience. It is a flexible program of permanent diet revision for sustained, good health; not a rigid program of temporary dieting for weight loss or brief remission of symptoms. The strategy of the Core Program reflects successful outcomes reported by many patients who carried out diet revision therapy. The recommendations are based on good observations and sound biological information; not speculation, preference, or opinion.

The Core Program is **self-directed**, even if you have professional supervision. As you reconstruct your food supply from an early hypoallergenic diet, you decide, every day, if your body-input recipe is okay or not okay. If it is not okay, you modify your food choices until you feel better and then proceed with further food introductions.

The text has been written as simply as possible without compromising the accuracy of the instructions nor the informative value of the explanatory texts. It is intended as a teaching text and the reader should expect to study the relevant instructions and explanations. The theory behind the Core Program incorporates scientific concepts, which are of personal as well as professional interest. Several references to the medical literature are provided for the reader who needs more specific details, although no attempt is made to exhaustively reference each topic. Wherever possible, direct quotations serve to illustrate the insights and perspectives that give life to the whole concept of diet revision. This collective voice becomes the "we" speaking through individual biases and interests towards a better picture of **what is really going on (WIRGO)**. The Sufi parable quoted after the table of contents reminds us that the same thing looks and feels differently to different people.

This is a book about science and it is about **doing your own science**, using your own body and mind as the laboratory. The science part requires more learning, more thought, more enquiry and some safe, effective experiments. You may need to change some of your habits, your assumptions about food, and your interpretations of symptoms. You will need to be open to changes in the way you think and behave. This is not "pure science", but applied science, since you have a vested interest and want practical results. Your goal is to feel and function better. If anyone thinks that changing diet is a simple matter with little effect on body-mind states, then do the Core Program, as written, and report back in 3 weeks!

The **professional reader** should benefit from this introduction to a successful method of diet revision therapy. The concepts and general approach to disease management by looking for and remedying the underlying causes of disease should appeal to physicians. The committed and professional reader should consult other books in this series for more information. More detailed discussions of food chemistry, nutritional concerns, and food-related illnesses have been moved from this text to *Nutritional Programming. Core Program Cooking* provides kitchen-level assistance, and the *"Core Diet for Kids"* is a parallel description of the Core Program directed at children's problems and needs. The references to the medical literaure should also be helpful and provide a gateway to further enquiry.

The book is divided into three sections; the first is an introduction to the many considerations that motivate us to do diet revision; the Core Program instruction set in section 2; and further explanatory material in section 3.

Section 1 reviews the most important reasons for diet revision. In chapter 1, we ask why so many people are sick in this modern, affluent world and why their food supply is a major factor in creating their illnesses. The importance of the food supply is defined as a biological determinant. The idea of diet revision is introduced as a major player in any **Health Care Program,** old or new. Four objectives of diet revision are considered in subsequent chapters:

> **Health Improvement**
>
> **Disease Prevention**
>
> **Problem-Solving**
>
> **Therapy**

Health Improvement is really the theme of the entire book. We think first of relatively healthy people who want to use nutritional methods to optimize the health and performance. These ideas merge naturally with the ideas of longevity, how to maximize both the quality and quantity of life. Thoughts on **longevity** then suggest we must consider disease issues, talk about the prevention of disease, and the remedies for dysfunctional patterns that make us old before our time.

In chapter 3, diet revision to **prevent cardiovascular diseases and cancer** is reviewed. In chapter 4 we begin to consider how proper diet revision is an essential strategy for **solving health problems** which seem to be overwhelming our society at great cost in terms of dollars and human suffering. We argue that **addiction** to food, alcohol and drugs are all related and further point to an important connection to the mysterious body of illnesses we will call "food allergy". The problems of eating disorders, alcoholism, overeating, gaining weight, and the difficulties of weight loss are tied into the addiction-food-allergy complex.

In chapter 5 we try to develop a context for understanding a plethora of **ill-defined illnesses**. We consider the idea that disease is a consequence of a collection of problems in the environment, especially in the food supply, and that delayed patterns of food allergy are important, neglected mechanisms of disease. In chapter 6 we continue to explore the fascinating subject of food allergy. The overview of food allergies is necessarily brief, but should alert you to health problems that are likely to respond to diet revision.

Chapter 7 further develops the heretical idea that the **food supply** is all important in causing **mental illness.** Our further heresy insists that the distinction between mental and **neurological illness** is spurious; we may have two departments at the university and in the hospital, but in the human body the departments are all integrated. Again we invoke problems in the food supply as explanations of neuropsychiatric disease. Chapter 8 displays typical **case histories** of patients who recover dramatically with diet revision therapy. These histories were chosen to illustrate how real people get sick in complicated patterns which evolve over time, not with neatly packaged, single diseases.

Section 2   The Core Program

The Core Program   **instruction set** is arranged in a self-help version with explanatory material added. These instructions should allow a well-motivated reader to undertake successful diet revision. Our preference is that physicians, nutritionists and other skilled therapist become familiar with this **methodology** and help guide their patients through the stages of transformation. The **stages of transformation** experienced by patients undertaking diet revision are reviewed in Chapter 9; this is an overview which emphasizes the experience of change, at both a physical and emotional level. Some of the reasons for Core Program **food selection** is reviewed in Chapter 10. In Chapters 11-14, the **5 Phases** of the Core Program are described in detail. Common experiences on this path are described. Self-monitoring and problem-solving methods are simply explained.

The Core Program often works uneventfully if the instructions are carefully followed. Many will succeed in health improvement, disease prevention, and solving their own health problems. Some problems are more complicated than others and difficulties may persist. There are too many possible problems to cover all contingencies in this text. The supervising physician's role is to provide help in troubleshooting, symptom interpretation, problem-solving,   behavioral   management   and   supportive   counselling.   Without knowledgeable professional supervision, you may encounter some difficulties which you cannot readily solve. If in doubt, consult your physician.

Section 3: More Information

More explanatory material is presented in this section. Chapter 16 briefly reviews nutrition. Food allergies are the most important problems, resolved by the Core Program and are given special attention in Chapter 17. Chapter 18 is a consumers guide to food test and treatments with advice about ineffectual methods.

The Elephant: A Sufi Parable

An elephant belonging to a traveling exhibition had been stabled near a town where no elephant had been seen before. Four curious citizens, hearing of the hidden wonder, went to see it. When they arrived at the stable it was very dark and they sought to identify this mysterious creature by touch. Each thought he knew something because he could feel a part. Later they told their friends about the elephant. One, touching the trunk thought it was a rough hollow pipe, awful and destructive. Another, who had graps an ear said it was large, like a rug, and flapping in the wind. The one who had felt its leg said it was mighty and firm like a pillar. The fourth who had felt the elephant flank said it was warm, rough, broad and had no boundaries.

None could form the complete picture; and of the part which each had felt, he could only refer to it in terms of things which he already knew. (Adapted From Indries Shah, "The Sufis" Anchor Press, Doubleday)

Disclaimer

The instructions, information and advice in this book are intended to help you identify and solve health problems. The instructions are based on the premise that better-informed people can make valid choices about their life-style, health consequences and seek self-directed change in illness patterns. You are responsible for the outcome of your current habits and will surely suffer if your food choices and eating behavior are not correct for the biological design of your body. While the greatest risk lies in continuing wrong habits, there is always doubt, uncertainty, and risk in making changes. Many of the problems of change are discussed in this book. You are responsible for the outcome of any changes you make in your food selection and eating habits; be sure you understand the concepts, goals, and methods of the Core Program before you embark on diet revision. The book is not intended to replace the diagnostic and treatment services of physicians. You are advised to seek proper professional advice and supervision whenever and wherever possible. If there is any doubt in your mind as to your proper course of action in resolving your health problems, you should follow the advice of your physician and other professional advisors. You should seek further information and advice until you are better informed and more confident in pursuing your own self-responsible course of action.

Nutritional Therapy Table of Contents

Section 1

Section 2 The Core Program

Section 3

SECTION 1

Introduction to Nutritional Therapy and Indications for Diet Revision

ABCD Abdominal pain, Bloating, Constipation, Diarrhea: the symptom complex typical of food allergy, found in various degrees of severity and attributed to different diseases. The old term is "Irritable Bowel Syndrome (IBS)" is discarded and replaced by ABCD.

AD Autoimmune Disease.

ADS Adaptive dysfunctional state: the concept that "normal" states often involve degrees of malfunction with symptoms at a manageable level. Adaptation to dysfunction allows many people to carry on, but with compromised quality of life and increased risk of chronic or catastrophic disease.

Allergy is immune-mediated dysfunction and disease.

Antigen is any substance which stimulates an immune response, usually proteins.

Antibody is a protein manufactured by immune cells to identifyand combine with antigen.

CFIDS Chronic Fatigue Immune Dysfunction Syndrome also **CFS**, chronic fatigue syndrome: different descriptions of the delayed patterns of food allergy.

Clearing refers to the improvement and eventual disappearance of physical symptoms and emotional-behavioral disturbances.

CD Core Diet: the personal and custom-fitted diet which each person defines by following the Core Program; a basic, safe set of foods and cooking practice.

CP Core Program: a specific path or algorithm for diet revision therapy; a copyrighted plan of diet revision.

DRT Diet Revision Therapy: the concept and methods of treating dysfunction and disease by altering the food supply of a person.

EMS Eosinophilic Myalgia Syndrome .

ENF Elemental Nutrient Formula: a mixture of pure nutrients, designed to replace food, free of extra chemicals and allergens; a hypoallergenic formula supplying complete nutrition.

Four-F 's Feeding, fighting, fleeing, and sexual interests.

Hypersensitivity: increased adverse reactions to substances in air, food and water. Hypersensitivity reactions are often immune mediated or "allergic" with four or more basic patterns of immune response.

Hypoallergenic: low risk of allergic reactions.

GIT GastroIntestinal Tract synonyms or components include digestive tract, stomach, bowel, intestine, gut, and colon.

SGRHN Surgeon General's Report on Health and Nutrition 1987: a U.S. review of the role of food and nutrition in disease and recommendations for diet revision, incorporated into the Core Program.

SLE Systemic Lupus Erythematosis, a severe immune mediated disease,

TOS Toxic Oil Syndrome

WIRGO What Is Really Going On Here?

Chapter 1

Introduction To Nutritional Therapy

This book is about getting better by changing your food supply.
It is also about the nature of food problems and modern disease.

We believe that wrong food choices and deteriorating food quality are important causes of disease in industrialized countries. To function well, the human body depends on a regular supply of well-balanced nutrients, without toxins or problems of excesses and deficiencies, or problems of additives never experienced before in the history of life on earth. The Surgeon General's Report on Nutrition and Health asserts that at least half of all deaths in the USA are related to faulty diet.

The basic strategy of Nutritional Therapy is to resolve faulty biology by diet revision. Let us assume that half of all health problems can be improved or resolved by diet revision. If we wanted to define the most promising cost-effective technology for a modern health-care program why not consider the technology of diet revision? Bad food choices, and problems in the food supply are not minor issues but should be the most important concerns of health maintainence programs now emerging to face the challenge of the next century. Diet revision can be a method of health improvement, a method of problem-solving and a therapy with enough power to reverse disease and restore health. All benefits can be made available every day, without expensive technology, without elaborate tests, without intervention from anyone else; you do not have seek anyone's permission to change your food supply.

We will develop the biological insight that food-related illnesses are now prevalent in our communities, and that changing patterns of food-related illness are causing a great deal of confusion. Food contains both old and new problems. The new food-related illnesses are a consequence of our changing, maladaptive food-production and consumption habits. We will explore the nature of this change and attempt to clarify the issues involved. The success of the Core Program depends on willingness to change, thoughtful food selection, self-awareness, and control over appetites and desires. People who are successful develop a caring and considerate attitude which addresses their own needs first; their success positively influences those around them. This process of self-conscious change rescues us, individually and collectively, from careless habits and destructive practices

Who Should Do Diet Revision Using The Core Program ?

In this section a variety of motives for doing diet revision are examined. The most important, generally acknowledged reasons for diet revision are considered in the following chapters. Experience suggests that the pursuit of lasting diet change is never just a technical exercise, involving food lists, recipes, and nutritional supplements. Significant diet revision always involves the whole person in transforming old, often destructive habits into new healthier patterns. Important insights develop as we attempt to change our food habits.

One of the myths of medical diagnosis is that disease is an orderly process, and that neatly packaged diseases are supposed to present, just as the textbook says. We perceive modern illness as a more random or chaotic process. **Disease is disorder.** The source of disorder can seldom be localized. Often, no-one thinks that food and drink have much to do with creating the chaos, but on closer examination, what is more likely to produce biological malfunctioning on a daily basis? The **Core Program** is a method of regaining control of a confusing, chaotic set of circumstances and symptoms. Careful application of the Core Program method will reveal the fundamental significance of the food supply in the production of disorder. We are talking about self-observation, self-control, self-diagnosis, self-healing, and self-determination. The Core Program is, therefore, a final common pathway for ordering chaos, for satisfying many urges toward better health.

Many people will find the plan useful simply as a guide to good eating practice. Some may seek specific improvements in their health status, better complexions or improved athletic performance. Some will want to change their food to prevent cancer. Others will need to interrupt compulsive eating or addiction to alcoholic beverages, coffee, tea, or chocolate. Others will have specific goals, such as weight loss or cholesterol management.

Others will have immediate health concerns and will seek a solution to common digestive problems or food intolerances, which are already known to them. Some people will be seeking solutions to serious food allergic disease or other major, chronic illnesses including ill-defined viral-like illnesses. Others will seek the end of migraine headaches, or mysterious muscle pains. Others will find a solution to chronic illness which they have not previously related to their diet. Yet others will realize, often for the first time, that their mental and emotional disturbances are caused by their ingestion of wrong food and drink and seek relief from their suffering by the simple expedient of diet revision.

Increasingly, well-informed people want to contribute to solving ecological problems, or want to change exploitative agricultural and food marketing practices. They understand their food choices not only as biologically relevant, but also as politically relevant.

The Surgeon General's Report on Nutrition and Health

The Surgeon General's Report on Nutrition and Health (SGRNH)[1] describes the:

> *"...convergence of similar dietary recommendations that apply to prevention of multiple chronic diseases. Five of the ten leading causes of death in the USA are clearly related to wrong food choices. Diseases of nutritional deficiencies have declined and have been replaced by diseases of dietary excesses and imbalances- problems that now lead rank among the leading causes of illness and death, touch the lives of most Americans, and generate substantial health care costs."*

The Core Program incorporates all the major recommendations in the SGRNH, and extends some of the recommendations further, for further benefit. The main difference is that the recommendations in the SGRNH are directed to policy-makers, addressing the general needs of a population of people. Core Program recommendations are directed to individual needs.

Definitions

Terms which describe our food supply are used differently in different contexts. Let us begin by defining our terms. **Food** is defined as all the materials we ingest. Our food supply includes solids foods, water, and a variety of other liquids including alcoholic beverages. We define **nutrition** as the study of food and its interaction with the body. **Pathological nutrition** is the study of the diseases caused by food. **Nutritional therapy** is the rational design of diets which prevent or correct the diseases caused by food. We define the term **diet** as the food eaten and beverages drunk. A diet can be traditional, spontaneous, or designed rationally. Spontaneous diets are often disorganized and chaotic and deserve the description **"wild diet"**. Affluent people on wild diets seem to eat whatever they want, whenever they want, from any source whatsoever, as long as its handy. People often deny the health problems caused by their wild diets and are surprised when the diagnosis of a food-related illness is made. They are surprised to realize that their suffering occurs at all levels of their being from rather obvious digestive symptoms to mental disturbances which seem remote from their food supply. Improper, wild diets characterize modern society and undermine our civilization at the fundamental level of biological functioning.

Rationally designed diets are usually only offered for weight-loss or specific illnesses such as diabetes. Medical therapy includes diets for special needs, but medical therapy has not had a standard method of diet revision for investigating and treating food-related illness. The result is that a very large population of people suffer unnecessary disease at great cost to themselves and society.

Nutritional therapy is based on removing the cause of illness, by correcting a faulty food supply. The supreme technique of nutritional therapy is, therefore, diet revision, not vitamin pills. The Core Program is an all-purpose method of diet revision; developed to fill the need for a practical medical management of food-related illnesses. We use the Core Program daily in treating patients with the wide range of diseases described in this book.

This **Core Program** began with observations that certain food-selection patterns are associated with dysfunction and disease. In one person, for example, the daily ingestion of multigrain bread, milk, cheese, bran muffins, beef, coffee, orange juice, and wine is associated with chronic fatigue, sleepiness after eating, nose congestion, flushing, headaches, generalized aching, stiffness and episodes of unexplained depression. When the food list is changed to rice, vegetables, chicken, peaches, and pears, the symptoms disappear and the person reports increased energy, and a renewed sense of well-being. Similar observations are repeated in a large sample of people of all ages. A variety of other dysfunctional patterns are found to improve with proper diet revision.

Diet revision is an experiment in the best tradition of **science**. There are five essential steps in scientific experimentation:

1. You realize you don't know	What's wrong with me?
2. You make a hypothesis	Something wrong with my food ?
3. You do an experiment	Change your food and observe.
4. You tally your results and decide	What food Selection is best.
5. Resolve uncertainty; go back to #1	Recheck doubtful results/foods.

In order to do meaningful experiments you keep the situation as simple as possible and have to decide what level of evidence we want to achieve. Wild diets are so complex, so chaotic at times, that the only way to begin a diet revision experiment is to stop everything; proceed through complete withdrawal; and wait until existing disturbances settle. Fortunately, this clearing process usually occurs within 1 to 2 weeks. The Core Program, featured in Section 2, as a safe and effective method. The program involves reasonable compromises between liveability and conclusive experimentation. **The goal of the experiment is not to pinpoint the exact problems with the existing food supply, but rather to invent an alternative food supply which is relatively free of problems.**

Problems With Modern Diets

Modern diets are biologically new and full of complications beyond the design specifications of the human body. Current eating practices are out-of-step with our biological machinery and dysfunction and disease are inevitable. The majority of modern citizens are removed from growing their own food, or buying directly from the farm or market-garden. Most food now comes in packages, bottles, and boxes through an anonymous network which manipulates the body in mysterious ways. Foods can now make people ill in progressive and subtle ways that they and theri doctors fail to understand. The living membrane on our planet's surface has been radically altered in the 20th century and we now face an unprecedented environmental crisis. Human disease patterns are evolving rapidly as human populations grow beyond the capacity for their environments to sustain them. Problems in food, air and water supplies increase drastically as planet problems multiply. We believe it is essential to view individual disease and dysfunction in a whole-system's view of Planet Earth. Our food choices will change for local personal health reasons but also in the next decade we will change collectively, some voluntarily and others because there will be no choice.

Why Are We Ill?

Food contains problems for many people. There are many ways that food interacts incorrectly with the human body causing harm. Highly esteemed whole grains, for example, may be the cause of serious digestive diseases, skin disease, chronic lung disease, arthritis, and brain disturbances for a variety of reasons, which we shall explore in some detail. Many people have been conscientious in following "good dietary advice"; eating whole grains, supplementing bran and fiber, taking supplements, and abstaining from apparently noxious nutrients like alcohol, animal fat, salt, and sugar. When this strategy fails and they grow sicker, they are confused and feel wronged when they discover the cause of their suffering is their compliance with "good dietary advice"!

The industrialized countries have collectively conducted an experiment in new food selection practices with increased our consumption of meat, dairy products, cereal grains; food additives, synthetic, and manufactured food products. Perhaps, now the negative consequences are becoming apparent. There are many adverse environmental factors. The food itself is changing as the atmosphere and soils deteriorate. It may be that the grain supply is contaminated with agent "X" which promotes illness through a variety of mechanisms. It may be that meat, dairy products, eggs and cereal grains, especially processed into composite, semi-synthetic foods in large quantities, may be improper food for many modern people. We will emphasize the role of food intolerances, especially food allergies as common, important mechanisms of disease. We will also attempt to explain why food allergy has yet to be properly recognized in the medical model as the proper explanation for prevalent illnesses.

Denial and ignorance about food-caused illness is unfortunately common among professionals who really should know better. The medical model attempts to understand the "causes of disease"; but food causes tend to be discounted. Even gastroenterologists, who aspire to understand digestive diseases, may deny food causes of common, digestive-system disorders. Biology is used selectively in medical practice, with large chunks of proper biological science missing from day-to-day medicine. Curious blind-spots have devloped in medical vision. There is a high awareness of infection caused by unseen microbes, but many physicians cannot imagine and often deny the unseen processes of biochemicals, allergens or toxins working in the bodies of their patients. They cannot imagine the flow of molecules from food through the digestive tract, through the blood and into tissues of the body. Allergic symptoms are among the common problems that physicians treat with antibiotics, because they assume that bacterial infection causes most symptoms. They seem to difficulty imaging the unseen processes of immune defense or the actions of toxins delivered in food, air and water. They need to reminded of food chemistry, food allergy and environmental problems. Physicians are also likely to misdiagnose and may sometimes deny chemical toxicity problems which increasingly occur in the workplace, homes and schools.

Ignorance is one thing, but a small minority of vocal "authorities" invest unusual time and energy denying that illnesses are related to problems in the food supply. These "authorities" often use terms, appropriate to defense attorneys, referring to "alleged food allergy", claiming at the same time to be "scientific", and scoffing at patients who believe they have health problems from food and air. We are alarmed at their indifference and question their knowledge, judgment, and motives. The worst offenders claim that suffering and dysfunction are "in the mind" of the afflicted people. The problem with these "authorities" is not just ignorance of basic biology, ecology, biochemistry, immunology, and toxicology, but also a regrettable denial of the sickness and suffering of fellow human beings. The denial is all the more unacceptable as planet-wide biological calamities become obvious. Intelligent people must not deny evidence of human, animal, and plant sickness as a result of atmospheric crises, climate changes, improper food choices and widespread pollution.

What Else Can We Think?

Denial is used to avoid recognizing the need to change our habits and methods. A proper biological method of medicine must begin by recognizing and solving problems in food air and water supplies. A steady flow of molecules from the environment enters the body of each individual, through the air breathed and the food and liquids ingested; this body-input determines not only health and disease in the long-term, but also the moment to moment functional capacity of the individual.

A person's performance can change dramatically with changes in this molecular stream. The quality and composition of air, food, and water changes continuously. The illusion of food continuity in the supermarket conceals changes in the growth, contamination, storage, spoiling, transportation, and merchandising of food products. To understand environmental reactivity, we must deal with changes, variability, and inconsistencies, and seek adaptive flexible responses to changing circumstances. The biologist sees living creatures connected to and interacting with their environment. It is normal for a biologist to think in terms of populations, food supply, seasons, weather, and social-behaviors, and to do field studies which reveal patterns of adaptation to specific environments.

> *Anyone who has worked with animals or fish in closed environments knows how critical environmental conditions and diet are in determining both the behavior and the physical status of the residents. When a fish in an aquarium displays disturbed behavior, you do not call a fish psychiatrist; you check the oxygen concentration, temperature, and pH of the water. You have to clean the tank and change the fish diet.*

Each person interacts with home and work environments, chemical soups, which determine biological fate. In industrialized countries, the micro-environment of each person is controlled by human constructions and is generally polluted by toxic substances, the extent of which is seldom measured, and the effects, poorly understood. As environmental problems multiply, new ill-defined illnesses will increase. Food and ingested liquids are selected by socioeconomic and cultural factors more than biological factors. Food selection is part of more complex behavioral patterns, often determined by the advertising and availability of junk and fast foods. Common abnormal eating behaviors include cravings, compulsions, binge-eating, and excessive food intake with obesity, food addictions, aversions, and anorexia.

Pristine Nutrition

We suffer from our ingested affluence. The great abundance and variety of food and drink available to us is a challenge to our biological identity, invented a long time ago under quite different circumstances. Our prehistoric ancestors were hunters and gatherers, eating leaves, roots, seeds, fruits, insects, meat and fish. With the advent of agriculture, increased grain and animal consumption became the norm. Eventually nonnutritious extras appeared in our diets. Spices, teas, coffee, and sugar greatly influenced European colonization of the New World, and continue to play important roles in the world economy. Fermentation became popular and introduced a new element of chaos in human affairs.Prehistoric hunters and gatherers hardly exist in the world today, but are of great interest to nutritional theorists and medical epidemiologists. S.B. Eaton and M. Konner state, in their review of prehistoric nutrition:[2]

> "Differences between the dietary patterns of our remote ancestors and the patterns now prevalent in industrialized countries appear to have important implications for health, and the specific pattern of nutritional disease is a function of the stage of civilization. Physicians and nutritionists are increasingly convinced that dietary habits adopted by Western Society over the past 100 years make an important etiologic contribution to coronary heart disease, hypertension, diabetes, and some types of cancer. These conditions have emerged as dominant health problems only in the past century and are virtually unknown among the few surviving hunter-gatherer populations whose way of life resembles those of preagriculture human beings."

Food occupies much of our time and attention, even when we insist on getting it quickly. Every North American city has been infested by fast food outlets. The resultant clutter of garish food signs and drive-ins provides a characteristic look to our suburban landscapes. Tea and coffee are the most frequently consumed beverages. Most Americans obtain their daily food energy from bread, doughnuts, cookies, cake, alcoholic beverages, milk, hamburger, processed meats, eggs, potatoes, and pop. Time magazine, in its August, 1985 cover article, "The Fun of American Food", states:[3]

> "As the restaurant becomes the new American theater, and the young, the well-off, and the restless may eat out five or six nights a week...Dining out is often less a culinary experience than a social one. Restaurants have become a form of entertainment, a place to meet friends, a chic locale to see and be seen in. Why else would hungry customers endure the noise, crowds and 90-minute waits, all for the privilege of sitting at cramped tables, and eating disappointing fare?"

Food manufacturers and vendors may be quite oblivious to our unique biological needs. Food entertains us and our habits of socializing with food and drinks usually precedes our concern for the well-being of individuals. The Time magazine article further states:

> "Since Ray Kroc opened his first McDonald's in a Chicago suburb back in 1955 (burgers: 15 cents), fast food has grown to a $45 Billion business...what they (Americans) want more than anything is to get out of the house for dinner. Nothing is more American today than avoiding a home–cooked meal..the average family spent 39.5% of its food dollar on restaurants in 1983...The typical American now eats out 3.7 times per week. From the trendy bistros of Manhattan's East Side to the ubiquitous 'franchise row' that lines the main drag on the outskirts of Anytown, U.S.A., eating out is in...McDonalds serves 6% of the American population every day."

The Time statistics remind nutritional theorists that the modern diet is different from the three well-balanced, home-cooked meals which dietetic textbooks postulate. This desire to eat together tends to be exploited by restaurants, encouraging us to consume high-fat, high-calorie foods, alcoholic beverages, coffees, and desserts. But restaurant meals have a biological cost. For some, the tab for dinner is just the initial cost of an expensive illness, lasting hours or days. The entertainment value of eating is so compelling that many people would rather risk major suffering from incorrect food choices, than give up the restaurant visit with friends. There are many opportunities to eat selectively and well, but the picky eater risks rejection by less careful, or more robust friends. Recognition that food ingestion can cause real suffering is only now emerging strongly. Often, as we treat children and young adults for food allergy, grandparents will vigorously deny that "good food" can cause illness. They are defending their old values against both the changes in the physical properties of the world, and also the changing concepts about what is healthy and proper nutrition.

An emerging, new sophistication in food presentation will recognize individual health needs and biological goals. Meals will be judged not simply on their appearance, taste, and smell, but, more importantly, on the biological consequences inside the body of the eater. A waiter or waitress who asks if you have any special dietary needs or food intolerance will get full marks for consideration and generous tips. Rules for labelling of food packages should logically apply to restaurant menus. As the scientific description and understanding of food-related illness emerges in the next decade, we can expect to develop a different social and legal awareness of the biological meaning of food. Alcoholic beverages are the first major component of the social meal to be regulated by social and legal constraints. Social progress clearly involves changes in the eating and drinking behavior of people.

Stress or Allergy?

Food-related illnesses are confusing to sufferers and interpreters alike. Many theories of symptoms and disease causation thrive in this confusion. "Stress" is one of the most common terms mentioned by our patients when they relate their medical histories. Many sick patients have been told repeatedly by physicians and many other professionals that their illness is caused by "stress". The term "stress" is losing its meaning and often explains nothing. The worst use of the term "stress" is to conceal ignorance of biological causes. The biological meaning of the word "stress" is often lost in popular usage. Emotional responses are not stressful, nor are emotions symptoms of stress. Hard work is not stressful.

The environment changes continuously and each person must **adapt** continuously. When changes are too great or too sudden, a failure of adaptation occurs, with malfunctioning of mind/body as a consequence. Any interaction between individual and environment which is maladaptive and produces symptoms can be called **stress**. Any event, agent or component of the environment which causes a maladaptive response is called a **stressor**. You may live in a perpetual state of change; travelling, eating-out, trying new foods, changing jobs, growing, learning, succeeding, failing, suffering illness and injury. Your biological success is determined by how successfully you can maintain a reliable supply of proper food, air, and water. If you replace proper food with an assortment of odd materials bought at different stores and restaurants, your chances of successful adpatation are rather slim. The most stressful events are those changes in our environment and food which control systems in your body can neither control nor predict. Events which cause unstable changes in our body function require adaptive responses. If responses work, the instability is reduced and no stress occurs. If the responses do not work, then body systems, seeking balance, become confused with maladaptive consequences.

Biological stress (unpredictably changing body input) is reduced to a minimum by regular patterns in stable environments, doing the same things every day. Food selection has the greatest impact on basic body states, and regularity in food consumption and correct food choices may be the simplest method of reducing biological stress. Biological stressors are the real, physical factors that challenge our body's adaptive mechanisms: bad air, noise, bad chemicals, wrong food, confusing information, and ill-considered drugs. If food input is neither predictable nor controllable, major body stress occurs with all its negative consequences. You can think about this as you eat in different restaurants and consume a great variety of packaged, bottled, canned foods, treats, and snacks. Wrong food ingestion is likely to be the most common, most persistent body stress that you suffer.

Hans Selye was the father of the stress concept. As a young scientist, he set out to learn more about how animals and people get sick. Intuitively, he took a whole-systems approach. The early ideas of "stress" were based on observations of physical changes in animals exposed to injury, prolonged pain, or to challenges with toxins and allergens. It is curious to review how the original idea of stress has been exaggerated in popular usage to describe all manner of relatively innocuous circumstances. Stress has become a mythical dragon, beyond any biological definition. A patient will describe "stress" when he has to work overtime, or when she has relatives visiting. All manner of emotional experiences and trivial discomforts are now called "stress".

Allergy As Stress

Selye made important observations about allergic disease. In his 1956 book "The Stress of Life",[4] he described injecting rats with egg white, the protein fraction of the egg:

> "...one group of rats was injected with egg white, just to see how much stress this foreign protein would produce. Much to my surprise, egg white did not act merely as a stressor, but produced a very specific and strange syndrome. Immediately after the injection the rats seemed to be quite all right, but soon afterward they started to sneeze and sat up on their haunches, scratching their snouts with the forepaws. A few minutes later, their noses and lips became greatly swollen and red, giving the animals a very peculiar appearance."

Selye's description of the allergic effects of a foreign protein is a good introduction to food allergy. Human patients experience similar reactions to ingested protein as do the rats to injected protein. If Selye had chosen to concentrate on the general theory of allergic response, our current vocabulary would probably use the word "allergy" instead of "stress". We are likely to discover in the next few decades that immune defenses (Allergy), operating within us, are far more potent determinants of body-mind states than any number of nonspecific events that people refer to as "stress". A healthy person copes with a remarkable range of adversity and emerges intact, whereas a sick person cannot cope with the ordinary transactions of daily life.

The original design of the-Core Program was based on the management of food allergies; a complex set of problems that are poorly understood, seldom diagnosed, and seldom managed properly. We believe that food allergy is a logical consequence of operating the human body with food and probably afflicts everyone in some degree or other.

Allergy is immune-mediated dysfunction and disease. Allergy, is a collection of the adverse effects of immune defense against the environment; food air, and water. If we use the term allergy in its broadest meaning then allergy must be the most common pattern of human reactivity. Even the symptoms of a cold or the flu could be described as "allergic", since we mostly feel the adverse effects of the immune defense against the virus, and not just the action of the virus itself. All of the body responses that Selye investigated as "stress" are implicated in allergic responses. Allergy is the whole-body response to challenges from the outside. Allergy is the stress! Symptoms are the result of allergy-stress and not the cause of it!

Food allergy often co-exists with digestive and absorption disturbances, and metabolic or biochemical problems, and is never a simple problem to understand, nor solve. Even some "experts" in food allergy deny that immune mechanisms play a role in the wide range or disorders that we will discuss; some seem to prefer dealing with uncertainty by denial; others lack curiosity or a broad clinical experience which would alert them to the many problems which can be explained as food allergy.

Politics and Health Care

The arguments in favor of diet revision are reviewed in this book. When you add up all the diseases and all the suffering that can be related to problems in the food supply, you have to ask: why are techniques of diet revision not used as primary therapy in medicine? When you look more closely at the **medical model** you see expensive techniques deployed to rescue individuals from calamities which, in the most part, were avoidable. You will also see evidence that the participants in medical systems are unhappy with what is going on. You find out that it is too expensive and that somehow it must change. You find government people euphemistically referring to the "health-care system", and when you look closer you find they are talking about a high-cost **medical intervention system**, which is directed at treating the end-stage disease, but not preventing disease. This system is interested only in people who have lost their health.

Look even more closely at the medical intervention system, and you will not find a cause-oriented program but an effect-oriented system. Medical attention is focused on ever more expensive machines which take better pictures, surgical suites to repair the damage done by usually preventable misadventure, and more drugs. Thus, patients complain that they are x-rayed and given drugs to relieve their symptoms but no-one is interested in the origin of their suffering and no-one helps them correct the underlying causes. If their disease is not well-enough developed, they are admonished for complaining and sent away ... come back when you have really got something to show for your troubles.

The importance of altering the course of a disease process by changing diet has somehow been pushed aside by the more glamorous, instant-gratification methods of modern medicine. The problem of the concealed cause, and the uncorrected bad habit requires the **co-dependency** of patient and physician. Both must conspire to maintain the status quo; and both must agree neither will threaten each other if their co-dependency has negative consequences. Human relationships can be factored into three-way transactions. Often two people are visibly interacting and a third is hidden in the background. Triangulations overlap in complex patterns. The **physician triangulates** the relationship with the patient by making implicit contracts with drug companies, hospitals, and laboratories; all profit from the patient's misadventures. The physician is often selling a drug to the patient, justifying its cost and assuming some liability for its adverse effects. The **patient triangulates** by contracting with food suppliers, alcoholic beverage vendors, tobacco promoters, advertisers, and restaurants, where all appetites are profitable. **Governments triangulate** relationships with all parties concerned in a complex of no-win situations. Taxes on the "bad stuff" are profitable; the cost of adverse health conditions is listed somewhere else, and can be easily blamed on the doctors. **Universities triangulate** relations, trading prestige for money, connecting faculty with drug companies, funding agencies, with patients, with benefactors, with hospital boards; everyone but the patient profits from illness. Laboratory research is especially tidy and profitable - it keeps the real world at a safe distance. Only unpopular radicals shout "the emperor has no clothes!" and proceed with the attempt to remedy the conditions which cause diseases.

We are proposing a standard method of **diet revision** as a practical, **universal therapy** for a wide variety of diseases. Diet revision therapy (**DRT**) fits into the medical model as a first-stage combined diagnostic and treatment procedure. Diet revision is **safe and inexpensive.** Diet revision can be used as a triage procedure to quickly identify patients who have food-related illness and to send this group into well-supervised but cost-effective programs of lasting diet revision. The nonresponders would proceed through further diagnostic and treatment procedures.

But DRT is not an easy process. DRT challenges traditions and co-dependency relationships. DRT challenges cherished beliefs about "good food" and the concept of the "four food groups", a nutritional dogma still taught at universities. DRT challenges vested interests whose profits are threatened by changes in market preferences. Physicians often believe that major changes in personal habits are impossible to achieve, and interfere with the patients enjoyment of life. Physicians who are unprepared to deal with nutritional concerns may claim that DRT may be "dangerous".

Is anyone left who will support diet revision therapy? The truth is that diet revision therapy is desperately unpopular despite its promise as a vital concept for reforming the "health-care" system. Patients will support DRT, once they realize they don't have to be sick. Some physicians have a natural inclination to biology and enjoy the detective work involved in solving the health problems of patients; they support DRT. Many health professionals have food-related illness and begin to question their own assumptions. If they become ill or a family member suffers from food allergy, they become the strongest advocates of DRT. Patients who make diet revision work for them save money, restore well-being, and regain autonomy. Expensive patients become inexpensive patients. We see disabled patients go back to work. Government agencies may eventually see the light and support DRT to save money, if they can ever get their priorities straight. Even the food industry will support diet revision, as soon as they realize that they too can profit from new food products and realize at the same time that their old products are safe, however bad they may be. Most people will not change their eating habits.

Planet Ecology, Politics and Food Choices

The Core Program includes primary foods, popular all over the world and, at the same time, excludes other foods that are staples in current North American diets but often are not well-tolerated. The Core Program is not based on the popular meal-planning concepts of the "four food groups", but is based instead on a set of more advanced nutritional concepts. The health-seeking goal is to return to a diet of simple, carefully selected, natural foods. Fresh or frozen vegetables, fruit, poultry, and fish are the basic food choices. Rice is chosen as the staple grain. These are primary foods that allow you to reconstruct daily menus, with confidence of good nutrition, and stable life-long eating habits. Under ideal circumstances you could eat only organically grown vegetables and fruits from your own gardens or neighborhood market-gardens. But probably, the garden is a distant retirement dream and organic vegetables are scarce and expensive. You must do your best with the food that is available. Your intention is to simulate eating from the garden by buying and preparing fresh or frozen vegetables, fruit, poultry and fish, according to your own preferences and tolerances.

Food choices influence agricultural practices, government policies, packaging industries, incinerators and garbage dumps. You can support local farmers who grow organic vegetables and fruit[5] and support stores that reduce packaging waste and encourage recycling of bottles, plastic bags and containers. You can compost organic waste and return nutrients to the soil. Many have argued that vegetarian eating practices would have enormous benefits for global ecology. Efforts to save animals and environments require thoughtful, selective food choices. Meat consumption is wasteful, in biological terms. Land devoted to raising feed for cattle could produce human food directly. Forests disappear in developing countries to make room for grazing cattle. Clearing new land for cattle grazing in Brazil, for example, destroys the Amazon rain forest, a precious and irreplaceable global resource. The cleared land is soon barren and abandoned by poor settlers, who are ignorant of the drastic consequences of their ill-fated quest for economic independence. Other industrialized countries have a long lead in ill-considered exploitation of forests and other natural resources.

By reducing our intake of meat and other animal products, we improve our health, reduce the suffering of animals, and reduce the heavy burden on planet resources that meat-production entails. Francis Lappe made the point in her 1971 book, "Diet for a Small Planet", that eating vegetable foods was biologically more efficient than eating animals. An organic, vegetarian diet saves the planet and saves us at the same time. John Robbins in his startling book, "A Diet for New America"[6], makes a strong case for a new level of consumer awareness and vegetarian diets. He is appalled by cruelty to animals, waste, and inefficiency in our food production system. Robbins states:

> "We live in a crazy time when people who make food choices that are healthy and compassionate are often considered weird, while people are considered normal whose eating habits promote disease and are dependent on enormous suffering."

While we find nutritional value in recommending increased fish consumption, we are concerned by destructive fishing practices, especially drift-net fishing and purse-seine fishing for tuna which kill about 100,000 dolphins per year. Whales and dolphins are close relatives, intelligent mammals, and should receive the same protection afforded human beings under law. In April 1990, three U.S. tuna canners, StarKist, Bumble Bee, and Chicken of the Sea announced they would not purchase any tuna caught in association with dolphins. StarKist also announced that they would refuse to buy fish caught anywhere with gill or drift nets, destructive fishing methods. Japanese, Taiwanese, Korean and Russian fishing vessels have been the most consistently implicated in destructive fishing practices which threaten, not only the fishing resource they exploit, but also ocean ecology as a whole. Other problems with fish caught close to polluted shorelines include contamination with heavy metals and dioxins; these are particular problems with bottom-feeding fish, crustaceans, and shellfish. Fish-farming, properly managed, may be a viable option to unsustainable ocean-fishing practices. Important changes in fish procurement and quality are necessary for this food to remain a desirable component of our long-term diet.

An immediate ban on pesticide use would be desirable for human health and planet ecology, but is probably not feasible in the short term. The use of these pesticides should be phased-out over the next two decades. Buy organically grown produce whenever possible; but realize in the short term that safe food will be in short supply and expensive. In the interim let us insist on better food monitoring with regular publication of levels of agricultural chemicals in foods displayed in stores. Every consumer should ask their local supermarket to supply with food quality information and to give them the choice among produce-suppliers. Dr. David Suzuki, the well-known Canadian geneticist and defender of planet earth argues that pesticide use is folly. Suzuki states:[7]

> "Spraying powerful poisons that kill all exposed insects is no more management of pests than killing everyone in New York city would be managing urban crime. Once embarked on the use of chemical pesticides, we become dependent on them because of the enormous ecological upset that results."

Suzuki goes on to describe the biomagnification of pesticide toxicity, because small, regular-ingested amounts of these poisons can be concentrated in our tissues and in secretions such as cows' and human mothers' milk!

As the decade unfolds changes in food supply and selection will be increasingly rapid and profound. Global warming will threaten major agricultural areas of North America and grain production will decrease in a timely manner as we realize that wheat disease is an endemic illness. Beef, dairy and other animal product consumption will drop dramatically as grain resources diminish, improving health and also reducing waste of global land and water resources. Increased vegetable and fruit consumption will encourage the renewal of local family farms in the immediate vicinity of city markets. Each urban area will wake up to its own survival needs and begin to restore productive agricultural land within its boundaries and in its immediate vicinity. Subsidized family produce gardens will return as a welcome feature of the suburban landscape. Regional agricultural planning hopefully will include hydroponic greenhouses, intensively-cultivated, organic, garden and fish farms; these will assure year-round, local food supply. Chemical pesticides and fertilizers will be phased out as sustainable biological methods take over. Long-distance shipping of food will decrease as fossil fuel becomes more expensive and strict controls over carbon dioxide emission become mandatory. Equally important changes must occur in our attitude toward nature, the spirit food, and our relationship with planet earth. As we learn to take better care of ourselves, we renew an awareness for the sacred dimension of mother earth; food is the gift and eating is a sacrament, connecting us spiritually with mother earth. You cannot receive this sacrament at McDonald's nor even at an expensive French restaurant.

As Gary Snyder suggests in his wonderful book *Practice of the Wild:* [8]:

> "Deep Ecology thinkers insist that the natural world has a value in its own right, that the health of natural systems should be our first concern, and that this best serves the interests of humans as well...Environmental concerns and politics have spread worldwide. In some countries the focus is almost entirely on human health and welfare issues. It is proper that the range of the movement should run from wildlife to urban health. But there can be no health for humans and cities that bypasses the rest of nature."

> "A sophisticated postindustrial 'future primitive' agriculture will be asking: is there any way we can go with rather against nature's tendency?"

During the next decade, we hope those involved in designing the Core Program will be able to increase efforts to investigate food origins, in terms of ecological integrity, nutrient quality, and levels of contamination, and recommend only those foods which pass increasingly stringent standards as safe and desirable. We anticipate increasing use of the elemental nutrient formula concept (ENFoods), in the treatment of increasingly common, food-related illnesses until remedial environmental measures take effect in the next century. Without a solution to food problems, more and more people, who can afford it, will be retreating to the safety of space-aged ENFoods.

---

[1]Surgeon General's Report on Nutrition and Health 1988 U.S. Department of Health and Human Services DHHS(PHS) Publ No. 88-50210; U.S. Govt. Printing Office Wash DC.

[2] Eaton SB, Konner M. NEJM 1985;312:283-289

[3]Fast food speeds up the pace. Time August 26, 1985;44-45.

[4]Selye H. The stress of life. New York: McGraw-Hill, 1956

[5]Alternative Farming Systems Information Center, National Agricultural Library, Room 111, Beltsville, MD 20705, (301) 344-3724.

[6]Robbins J. Diet for a new America. Stillpoint Publishing, Box 640, Walpole, NH 03608 USA ;1987.

[7] Suzuki D. The folly of chemical pest control. Globe and Mail; April 9 1988

[8]Snyder G. The Practice of the Wild. North Point Press; Berkely Calif; 90; 1990.

Chapter 2

Diet Revision for Health Improvement

Energy and Athletic Performance

With increased interest in improving health and athletic performance, nutritional ideas have been tested to increase energy dynamics in muscle, and to improve endurance. Physical fitness is dependent on many metabolic adaptations. Fitness begins with increased ability of the circulatory system and the lungs to deliver enough oxygen to rapidly metabolizing cells, especially muscle cells. The word "aerobic" now part of the fitness vocabulary, points to this oxygen-dependent metabolism. Just as important is the ability of the circulation to carry increased amounts of metabolic waste products away from active tissues to processing organs like the liver. The heart may triple its resting rate during exertion, and must receive adequate circulation, balanced electrolytes, and other metabolic considerations to sustain this dramatically increased work-load.

The idea of physical fitness centers on increasing tolerance for bursts and sustained physical exertion. Short bursts of intense activity have different energy requirements than sustained muscular work. Short exertions may be fueled by glucose alone. Sustained exertions require the metabolic machinery to use fatty acids and the branch-chain amino acids as fuel. Extra oxygen is stored by muscle in myoglobin, a hemoglobin-like molecule. Myoglobin supplies the extra oxygen required by peak demand fuel consumption, which exceeds the ability of circulating hemoglobin to rapidly deliver increased amounts of oxygen. The glucose supply is exhausted when exercise is prolonged; lactic acid accumulates with the consequences of muscle fatigue and pain. With sustained athletic conditioning, muscle cells become more efficient in switching to fatty acid consumption as a primary fuel; more prolonged exertion is then possible.

Weight loss is dependent on exercise and appetite regulation works better in those who enjoy daily exertions. Depression is improved by daily recreational exercise. Sexual interest is increased by exercise. There is a small risk of heart attack and sudden death with vigorous exercise, estimated to be 0.3-2.7 events per 10,000 exercise hours in men.

Peak-demand energetics

Peak-Demand Energetics are very different from normal-activity energetics. Every endurance athlete knows about "hitting the wall". The failure of muscles and their support systems to sustain continued work is inevitable at some level of exertion, and usually occurs abruptly. Muscle metabolic work increases 50-fold at maximum capacity, and there are obvious limits in sustaining peak performance. The limited ability to sustain aerobic fuel burning is the principal constraint on sustained exertion. As metabolism shifts from aerobic to anaerobic fuel consumption, toxic metabolites accumulate in active tissues, decreasing their efficiency. During sustained exertion, water is lost through the lungs and sweat, and is probably the most important nutrient to be replaced.

Sugar has received undue attention as a fuel in endurance athletics. Its popularity is undeserved. It has been demonstrated [1]that prolonged exercise to exhaustion regularly produces low blood sugar. This exercise-induced hypoglycemia is defined as blood levels less than 45 mg/dl. The surprising observation is that hypoglycemic athletes can continue to exercise for 15 to 70 minutes with blood sugar levels of 25-48 mg/dl. According to the popular hypoglycemic theorists, who worry about blood sugars of 50-80 mg/dl, these low levels should be a complete disaster. This hypoglycemia fails to affect the endurance of the athletes, and taking sugar does not help them feel better. The secret of the hypoglycemic athletes seems to be the ability to use fatty acids as their primary fuel.

A grueling regimen of a low carbohydrate (CHO) diet and intense workouts for four days have been used by some athletes to deplete muscle stores of glycogen, the storage polymer of glucose. The depletion seems to encourage muscle cells to store more glycogen when CHO is next available. With CHO refeeding, the athlete is then prepared for endurance exertion (one hour or longer). Another version of the glycogen manipulation idea is the depletion-taper regimen. A week before the big event, the athlete works out to exhaustion, then begins an increasing carbohydrate intake and lighter exertion prior to the competitive event. Maximum CHO intake may be 600-800 gm/day. CHO-loading may not be a very good idea. A more sustained body intake of essential nutrients with careful consideration of problem exclusion should give better results than efforts to trick the metabolism to perform unusual feats.

Athletic training programs require slow, graded increments in workouts and performance demand. The athlete's diet must supply a balanced source of energy nutrients. There are many pet theories on best diets for athletes. The pre-game steak and beer meal is definitely a poor idea. Athletes perform better on an empty stomach. Nutrients supplied as an Elemental Nutrient Formula (ENFood) may become the optimal pre-performance food. A custom formulated ENF, with adjustable amino acid and fatty acid concentrations and altered micronutrient ratios, promises to become as useful strategy in performance nutrition. Choices about specific fuels for muscle work can be better made at the biochemical level of an ENF more precisely than at the level of regulating food intake. Protein powders and other dietary supplements now sold for athletes are not ENF's and may create problems more than benefits for unwary athletes.

The Core Program recommends the best foods for athletes: vegetables, fruit, rice, and carefully selected meat, poultry, and fish. Vegetables supply complex carbohydrates, which act as sustained-release energy sources. The intake of complex carbohydrates should account for more than 60% of the total caloric intake. Fat should be less than 25%, and proteins 12-20%. The modest amounts of fatty acids as vegetable oil are often sufficient to maintain proper blood and tissue levels of these important fuel molecules. Free sugar is avoided since it induces hectic metabolic shifts involving insulin, glucagon, and bursts of sympathetic regulation, all undesirable features when good muscle metabolism is desired.

The consumption of excess protein is a common mistake athletes make. There is no need for large amounts of protein. Most athletes have vigorous appetites and consume diets with an excess of 3000 kcal per day. Protein intake should remain at 12 % of the total caloric intake, unless exercise is designed to produce muscle hypertrophy, requiring up to 15 % protein. Excess protein consumption is likely to degrade athletic performance. Since proteins are among the most reactive molecules in food allergic disease, any symptomatic athlete should carefully review his or her intake for reactive foods; these usually are the staple foods like milk, eggs, wheat, and meat. Protein powders sold as "body-building" supplements are also a source of trouble. Athletes on high protein diets often present with migraine headaches, asthma, digestive disturbances, and major brain dysfunction with incoordination, falling, and confusion. They are disabled by their high-protein foods! Athletes may also have food-induced asthma and exertional anaphylaxis. Occasionally foods will sensitize an athlete who, during or after exertion, develops a threatening allergic response with shortness of breath, choking, and collapse (anaphylaxis). If the athlete's diet is changed appropriately, the exertion reaction does not occur or is significantly reduced. We routinely recommend that patients with allergic disease avoid sudden unusual exertion. We recommend to athletes that they identify sensitizing foods and avoid them carefully for many days prior to demand-events.

Amino acid supplements to a high performance diet are interesting alternatives to eating high protein food. **Leucine** in particular seems to promote muscle growth, acting in concert with insulin. The other two branch-chain amino acids, **isoleucine and valine,** may also supply muscle fuel if impairment of glucose utilization occurs. Other amino acids, particularly, tyrosine and phenylalanine, will influence neurotransmitter function and may be used to improve performance. The technique of amino acid proportioning has not been worked out, and is a frontier for performance nutritional programming. It is probably unwise for individual athletes to experiment on themselves, especially by taking high disproportionate doses of any amino acids.

Longevity

Many articles are written about the promises of good nutrition in extending life. Aging seems to be orchestrated from a genetic lifespan program, read out sequentially from DNA as our life unfolds. The genetic program establishes a lifespan range of about 100 years. Our eating habits and environment decide how well each of us will do within the range of the lifespan program. The average lifespan in industrialized countries ranges from lows of 69.7 in Hungary and 69. 9 in Romania to a high of 79.1 years in Japan. The food selection of a native Japanese diet resembles the Core Program, with rice as a staple and higher vegetable, poultry, and seafood content; traditional Japanese cuisine does not involve wheat, milk products, and red meat as staple foods.

Eastern European countries have some of the worst habits of industrial pollution, and indifferent diets; their citizens have the highest death-rates and lowest life expectancy. Among affluent, successful countries, Switzerland, Iceland, and Sweden compete for second place with life expectancies of 77.1 -77.6 years. Canada ranks fifth with Spain at 76.5 years and the USA trails significantly at 75.0 years, below the United Kingdom at 75.3 years.

We can assume that optimal diets, good air and water will permit the longest, healthiest life. The only measure which reliably extends the lifespan of experimental animals is food restriction; less food means longer life! Food inevitably contains problems and food processing in the body has a cost or penalty. Less food usually means better health. Ironically, fear of nutritional deficiencies dominate popular diet theories in countries suffering from food surpluses and overindulgence.

Osteoporosis or bone-thinning is also an aging problem in affluent societies, afflicting women more than men. This is a problem of disuse atrophy and loss of anabolic hormones. Postmenopausal women, who lose the anabolic hormone effects of estrogen and progesterone, and who do little or no physical work, lose bone mass and strength progressively until their spine collapses and their bones break from minor trauma. This problem has been attributed to lack of calcium. Calcium supplements alone may not prevent or reverse bone loss. Combined therapy involves diet revision, calcium and other mineral supplements, exercise, and optional hormone replacement. Milk is promoted as "good for bones" but we have no evidence to support this claim. Indeed, the evidence points to the opposite conclusion: that milk-drinking women with high protein intake get osteoporosis.

Patients with **food allergies** have provided us with interesting insights into the aging process. Many patients with chronic food allergy look tired, feel tired, stiff and older than their chronological age. They complain of feeling old. Fatigue, aching, stiffness, weakness, loss of pleasure and failing interest in work and play are typical symptoms of aging and food allergy. One of the principle mechanisms of chronic disease is inflammation and food allergy is capable of sustaining long-lasting inflammation in any tissue of the body. Chronic inflammation is a smoldering fire that gradually destroys healthy tissues, leaving scarring, calcification and gradual loss of function in its wake.

Mental changes are also important clues to the relationship of food allergy to premature aging; difficulty concentrating on tasks, balance problems, memory loss, and sometimes, confusion are symptoms of senility and food allergy alike. Food allergy patients will express concern that their mental decline suggests Alzheimer's disease, which indeed it does, but fortunately, memory impairment usually clears with diet revision. Conversely, people recovering on the Core Program report rejuvenation; increased energy, activity, improved memory, sharpened mental acuity and increased enjoyment of daily activities.

---

[1]Felig P et al. Hypoglycemia during prolonged exercise in normal men. NEJM 306(15):895-900.

Chapter 3

Diet Revision to Prevent Major Diseases

Heart Disease and Stroke

Diseases of blood vessels are a major cause of premature disability and death in our society. Heart attacks and strokes are the most obvious consequence of damaged arteries and increased clotting of blood. People with coronary artery disease have a higher risk of developing Alzheimer's disease. These problems are strongly linked to the high fat, high protein diets popular in Europe and North America, and seldom occur among vegetable-eating populations who seldom eat dairy products, meat, and other high-fat foods. Other well-known risk factors are high blood pressure, smoking, excess body fat, and inactivity.

Food allergy may contribute to these problems in important, but unrecognized ways. Food allergic reactions may occur within blood vessels, damaging bloods cells, vessel walls and triggering the clotting mechanisms. The design of proper diets for disease prevention must take multiple factors into account. A "low cholesterol diet", for example may remain a problem for people who are allergic to skim milk, egg whites, and cereal grains. A "high fibre diet" may be a problems with people allergic to cereal grains. High fibre intake is achieved on a Core Diet by increasing the intake of vegetables and fruit.

High Blood Pressure is treatable in the same manner. According to the Canadian Coalition for High Blood Pressure Prevention and Control, nondrug strategies should be the priority for hypertension control in the 90's. Smoking cessation, low fat diet, weight loss, exercise, reduced alcoholic beverage consumption, increased potassium intake with decreased sodium are the important steps to avoid the problem of high blood pressure.

The Core Program is designed to reduce cholesterol, total fat, saturated fats, increase vegetable fibre, and reduce food allergy, all desirable measures in the effort to prevent blood vessel diseases, heart attacks and strokes. Potassium and calcium supplements are advocated with reduction of sodium salt intake. The Program can be enthusiastically recommended, along with exercise and relaxation, as the most important defenses against cardiovascular disease.

The only modification to the Core Program needed for people with no evidence of digestive problems or food allergic symptoms is to include 1 or 2 portions a day from the cereal grain group (whole wheat bread, breakfast cereals and pasta).

Atherosclerosis

Atherosclerosis is often referred to as "hardening of the arteries". This is actually a complex disease of the arterial wall which sets the stage for most heart attacks and strokes. The process of atherosclerosis involves high-cholesterol fat accumulating in the walls of arteries in plaques, which grow to obstruct blood flow through the artery. As the plaques age and grow, they become scarred, and often calcified. Restricted blood flow to any organ reduces its ability to function and obstruction leads to death of tissue. Sudden obstruction of a narrowed blood vessel is often caused by a clot forming in a narrowed region of the vessel (thrombosis). If the tissue is vital, such as heart or brain, arterial obstruction may be lethal or, at best, disabling.

Serum cholesterol

Serum cholesterol is a predictor of coronary heart disease, and current recommendations set target goals of less than 200 mg% for blood levels. So-called "normal levels" range from 180-300 mg%, depending on age and sex. Strict vegetarians may have serum cholesterol levels of less than 100 mg%, considerably less than their lactocarnivorous peer group. A 10 year collaborative study on serum cholesterol levels and heart disease showed that a decrease in serum cholesterol progressively decreased the risk of heart attacks. A 1% drop in serum cholesterol levels yielded a 2% drop in risk of heart attack. A 25% reduction in serum cholesterol, therefore, reduced the incidence of heart attacks by 50%. Some of the cholesterol in food is partly digested, or not absorbed, and does not appear in the overall body cholesterol equation.

Most body cholesterol is synthesized in the liver, at the rate of 1000 mg/day. A similar amount of cholesterol per day is secreted in bile by liver cells and circulates through the gastrointestinal tract (GIT). A portion of GIT bile cholesterol is lost through the feces. One way to decrease total body cholesterol is to increase GIT loss. The use of binding resins or fiber, like plant fiber, or the semisynthetic resin, cholestyramine, to trap bile salts and cholesterol can lower serum cholesterol levels. Cholesterol is incorporated with protein into transport packages, travelling in the blood. These are often referred to as lipoproteins. In the blood, **low density lipoprotein (LDL)** is "bad cholesterol" since it seems to accumulate in blood vessel walls, plugging them. This fatty tumor growth in arterial walls is known as atherosclerosis. Half of all deaths in the U.S. are caused by atherosclerosis, and half of all Canadians and Americans have high fat diets, associated with elevated blood LDL. **High density lipoprotein (HDL)** is another form of transport cholesterol. HDL is "good cholesterol". The ratio of HDL to LDL should be as high as possible. You can bet that a vegetarian, non-smoking, non-drinking athlete will have the lowest cholesterol, highest HDL/LDL ratio, and the least risk of coronary artery disease and stroke.

Surgery or Diet Revision?

Dramatic and expensive operations have rescued many patients from the consequences of bad eating practice, and failed to help others. Coronary artery by-pass operations cost $11 billion per year in the USA; at $30,000-40,000 plus disability costs per patient (not to forget pain and suffering and risk of operative death); 330,000 operations are performed per year in the USA. Another 190,000 angioplasty procedures are performed at a cost of $7,000 each. Surgical procedures which attempt to restore blood-flow to the brain are also popular. Surgery to remove fat blockage from the carotid arteries, supplying blood to the front half of the brain, is commonly attempted, without convincing evidence of benefit, and considerable risk. This operation, carotid endarterectomy, has never been properly evaluated. Another operation to bring blood flow from outside to inside the head was carefully studied before it was applied as a standard surgical procedure. Scientifically appropriate studies of extracranial to intracranial bypass surgery, coordinated at the University of Western Ontario, have shown the disappointing results of no substantial long-term benefits. This more technically demanding, delicate, surgery to bypass plugged arteries inside the head, was theoretically promising, but failed to deliver the hoped-for benefits.

The Metabolic Solution of Atherosclerosis

A metabolic solution to the fatty artery problem is more desirable, cheaper, and safer than attempted surgical rescue. Brown and Goldstein, in an article on LDL receptors and atherosclerosis, state:[1]

> "If the LDL-receptor hypothesis is correct, the human receptor system is designed to function in the presence of an exceedingly low LDL level. The kind of diet necessary to maintain such a level would be markedly different from the customary diet in Western Industrialized countries (and much more stringent than moderate low cholesterol diets of the kind recommended by the American Heart Ass'n). It would call for the total elimination of dairy products as well as eggs, and for a severely limited intake of meat and other sources of saturated fats.

> "We believe the change is not warranted for the entire population. There are several reasons. First, such a radical change in diet would have severe economic and social consequences. Second, it may well expose the population to, other diseases now prevented by a moderate intake of fats. Third, experience shows most Americans will not adhere voluntarily to an extreme low-fat diet. Fourth...people vary genetically. Among those who consume the current high-fat diet High-fat diet of Western Industrialized societies, only 50 % will die of atherosclerosis; the other 50 % are resistant to disease....people who have a strong family history of heart attacks or strokes and who may therefore be more susceptible to the damaging   effects of LDL, might well be encouraged to follow a diet extremely low in cholesterol and saturated fats – even if their LDL level is near the mean normal level."

A solution to major endemic disease problems should be aggressively sought by diet revision. The cost of neglecting bad dietary habits is too great for a society to afford. "Low Cholesterol" diets, popular for the past 25 years, do not address all the problems of arterial disease and may mislead some people at risk; the advice may be too moderate and too general. In his best-selling book "The Pritikin Promise", Nathan Pritikin advocated a more stringent low fat diet to combat cardiovascular disease. His opinions are interesting and relevant. He, like many nutritional theorists, chose one food demon, fat-cholesterol, to attack, but he also recommended limiting protein foods like poultry, lean meat, and fish to 3.5 ounces per day. Pritikin advocates high vegetable intake, and even a partial vegetarian diet. He discourages the ingesting of vegetables oils. The observation that olive oil is a protective component in an otherwise high fat diet, reducing cholesterol and increasing

HDL softens Pritikin's notion that all fat is bad. Similarly, inclusion of fish in the diet seems to be protective; fish fat contains the fatty acid, **EPA**, which may be the protective component. The general design of the Pritikin program is worthwhile, and may serve as a good starting point for diet revision in asymptomatic people with increased risk of cardiovascular disease.

Dr. Dean Ornish of the University of California treated patients with a very low fat diet, similar to strict versions of the Core Program, and the Pritikin diet. He demonstrated marked improvement in the conditions of patients with established coronary artery disease. Ornish's patients combined strict diet control with exercise, yoga and meditation. Fat intake was less than 10% and oils were banned. Increasingly, we are encouraged to think that corrective diet and life-style changes will reverse established blood vessel disease, reduce risk of disability or death, and dramatically improve the quality of life. The 40 million Americans who have heart disease, and the insuring agencies who pay their medical bills, should carefully consider the benefits of complete diet revision therapy! To improve the health of modern citizens and at the same time reduce the sky-rocketing costs of health-care, we need to strengthen the concept of self-responsibility for disease-prevention. Each person will have to alter disease-causing habits, change poor eating habits, and stop smoking and drinking or be accountable for the health problems they choose to retain.

Theories of vascular disease may be too simple. Other food-related problems, especially food allergy are important contributors. Cardiovascular and cerebrovascular events are thought of, simplistically, as just one disease. In our whole-system's interactive model, all factors which influence body function are considered. No single dietary factor, such as an elevated cholesterol level, will be solely responsible for the calamatous events which physicians are used to treating. The total impact of the food supply must be considered before a comprehensive model of diet-disease relationships will develop.

What about the protein content of foods? The Pritikin diet and other low fat diets may not work because of the high content of of allergenic proteins in cereal grains, skim milk, and egg white. Skim milk is as allergenic as whole milk. Egg white is the allergenic protein which is avoided on hypoallergenic diets, but may be permitted on low cholesterol diets. Protein antigens, arriving in the blood through GIT, may trigger an immune response which inflames and damages the arterial wall. Many people with food allergy develop migraine, angina, heart rhythm abnormalities and may be more likely to develop blood clots and inflammation of blood vessel walls, all features of the life-threatening complex of vascular disease. Dr. William Hollanderof Boston University suggested that atherosclerosis was an autoimmune disorder with immune complexes injuring blood vessel walls. Immune complexes could contain food antigens. There is no data on record which limits this possible association; everyone needs to pay attention to symptoms which suggest this type of reactivity in their body. If there is any possibility that attacks of migraine, heart-symptoms, or brain dysfunction is linked to food ingestion would it not be prudent to investigate, using diet revision? We have no difficulty in recommending aggressive diet revision, sufficient to remedy an existing problem, and vigorous enough to prevent vascular disasters. We tell people to imagine that they live in a little cottage by the sea, think quiet thoughts, walk everywhere, tend their organic vegetable garden, cultivate their fruit trees (never sprayed), and go fishing once or twice per week. Now you have a perfect setting and a perfect diet (a Core Diet) for enduring good health.

Current recommendations for fat intake are shrinking progressively from 35% of total calories to 20%. Typical American diets contain as much as 42% fat, an extravagant surplus. Our needs are supplied by 15-25 grams of fat per day. Bare minimum requirements are 1-2% of total calories for adults and 3% for infants. If you have normal cholesterol levels, your Core Diet level of fat intake should be less than 20% of daily calories with 70% fat as vegetable oil; our **target is 14% fat intake.** If you have elevated cholesterol and/or triglyceride levels, your total fat intake should be less than 10% of total daily calories. **Safflower or sunflower oil** are chosen as the principal oils because of a high content of **linoleic acid.** Olive oil is an alternate oil, a mono-unsaturate with increasing credentials as an antidote to coronary artery disease and with anti-inflammatory properties. The inclusion of oily fish in the diet increases the intake of beneficial fatty acids (EPA and DHA). If fish intake is low, these fatty acids can be taken as a supplement. A customized Core Program oil mix contains 2 parts safflower one part olive, and optionally, one part flax oil. Supplemental EPA and GLA are considered optional fatty acids. The average daily intake is 3-4 teaspoons of oil.

Cancer Prevention

Increased cancer incidence in the USA and Europe point to problems in food, air and water. Cancer tends to occur increasingly as we age, and alarming increases in brain tumors, breast cancer, kidney cancer, lymphomas, myeloma, and melanomas have been observed in the past two decades in people older than 55. An equally alarming 32% increase in cancers of children less than 15 years of age point to environmental carcinogens. Lymphomas increase with pesticide exposures. There are many different kinds of cancer with marked regional variation in incidence of any given type. Clearly local environmental factors play a determining role in deciding who gets cancer. In affluent countries, research tends to remain in the laboratory, focused on the cancer itself, rather than going out into the community and solving cancer problems at its source.

The story of solving the problem of esophageal cancer in the Lin Xian county of China illustrates how basic, down-to-earth research can resolve a local cancer problem. Researchers there traced a high incidence of esophageal cancer to nitrosamines and fungal carcinogens in favorite foods of the populace; at the same time, they discovered that molybdenum deficiencies in the local soil increased the nitrite content and reduced the vitamin C content of their produce, depriving them of a protective factor. Changes in the food supply to reduce nitrosamines and fungal contamination; and adding molydenum to the soil were rational changes designed to reduce this unusually prevalent form of cancer.

Carcinogens

Some cancers are caused by specific chemicals. There are at least **350 certified carcinogens** producing 8 different tumors in animals and man. Human cancer is known to be produced by at least 130 different chemicals.[2] Radioactive isotopes have already been identified as carcinogenic. Industrial carcinogens include asbestos, benzene, cadmium oxide, chromium, nickel, vinyl chloride, soots, and tars. Several medicinal drugs are carcinogenic. Dioxins from pesticides and municipal incinerators are now a great concern. The most potent carcinogenic drugs are those used to treat cancer! Many cancer patients trade remission of today's cancer for the induction of a subsequent cancer in years to come. **Food additives** have been closely scrutinized as potential carcinogens, and several, like saccharin, cyclamate, Ponceau 3R, and Red No. 2 (amaranth), have been banned by the FDA because of concern about possible cancer causation. Natural foodborne carcinogens, the aflatoxins are produced by aspergillus fungi which grow in or on peanuts, wild soy sauce, and grains. It is ironic that foods advocated by some "health food" fans are most likely to be contaminated with aflatoxins. Many other substances are suspected. The surface of the gastrointestinal tract is most intensely exposed to ingested carcinogens. Fortunately, stomach cancer has been declining in the US for many years. Some have suggested that increased vitamin C is responsible, reducing in the formation of nitrosamines. Cancer of the colon, on the other hand, is not declining, and suggests that the late stages of food-processing in the GIT produce a carcinogen. The incidence of colon cancer is positively correlated with the intake of animal food and fat, and negatively correlated with the intake of vegetable foods. Increased vegetable consumption, with inclusion of the Brassica group (cauliflower, cabbage, broccoli, brussels sprouts) is now recommended.

Generally applicable dietary themes emerge from the results of many studies in industrialized countries: The risk for breast and colon cancer is correlated with total fat consumption, for example. Increased breast, colon and colon cancer is observed in animals fed a high-fat diet. Poylunsaturated fats (vegetable oils) promote animal breast cancer, while omega 3 fatty acids (flax and fish oils) tend to protect. Increased fibre consumption tends to protect against colon cancer, but the best type of fibre has not yet been determined. Vitamin A is protective against some cancer and this effect may be more linked to high intake of carotenoid vegetables (dark yellow, orange and green) than intake of the oil-form of vitamin A (fish liver oils). Vitamin C probably is protective against nitrosamine-induced cancers, especially esophagus and stomach and lung. Vitamin E may enhance this protection. Dr. Garland and associates at the University of Southern California suggested[3] that sunlight and vitamin D reduced the risk of colon cancer; the risk of colon cancer is highest in populations exposed to the least amount of sunlight. Other evidence also suggested a protective role of vitamin D in breast cancer. High oral intake of vitamin D in fish-eating Japanese populations also correlates with low incidence of colon and breast cancer. Generally, American and Canadian diets are low in vitamin D and supplements are required. Cancer prevention involves modifying your food supply. Core Program diet revision includes features recommended in the SGRHN for cancer prevention. The paths of risk-factor modification for many illnesses converge toward similar lists of things to do and not to do.

Steps to Reduce Risk of Cancer

* Do Core Program diet revision
* Maintain a normal body weight
* Eat from the garden
* Vegetables supply 60% of daily calories
* More than 20 grams of fiber content per day
* Eat vegetables of the Brassica family
* Low animal-fat, low cholesterol diet
* Reduce red meat consumption
* Limit milk intake and dairy products,
* Avoid smoked, barbecued foods
* Eat only a few eggs per week (3-4)
* Avoid nitrates, nitrites
* Avoid other harmful food additives
* Take vitamin-mineral supplements

---

[1] Brown MS, Goldstein JL How LDL Receptors Influence Cholesterol and Atherosclerosis. 1984. Nov. Sc. American 58-65

[2] Soderman JV. Identified carcinogens and noncarcinogens: carcinogenicity-mutagenicity database. CRC Press, Chemical Class File, 1981:1, Target Organ File 1981:2 Cat #3200BF.

[3] Garland C et al Int Jour. Epidemiology, 1980;9:227-231

Chapter 4 Diet Revision

Food, Addiction, Weight Control

Excessive Eating with many adverse health consequences is the most prevalent eating disorder in our society. Food choices play an important role in disorderly eating patterns. Craving and compulsive eating are features of food allergy, and diet revision with the Core Program is an effective way of unraveling this complex problem. Patients and their families experience many problems when they attempt diet revision. We first encounter withdrawal symptoms, similar to drug and alcohol withdrawal. Next, we encounter cravings for specific foods, especially sweet things, and a mini-grieving process which suggests that loss of habitual foods is a major emotional event. Finally, we encounter the phenomenon of specific foods triggering intense cravings and compulsive or binge-eating. Eating these trigger foods often interrupts or ends the attempt to do diet revision. We recognize an **underlying "addictive" cycle** to these abnormal eating behaviors, observed in many people, both adults and children. The individual substances which trigger the addictive cycle are not well known, but the problem cannot be blamed on sugar alone. Thousands of other molecular species in the food supply are also implicated, including "Agent X", unknown environmental contaminants.

The Addictive Loop

How can we explain the curious and biologically perverse phenomena of craving and compulsive eating of injurious foods and drinks? Cravings may be interpreted as urges to find missing nutrients, but the foods found in compulsive searches are not biologically correct. Instead, food cravings are a symptom of an addictive loop. The term **addictive food allergy** was suggested to describe the connection between compulsive eating and illness. The puzzle of cravings and compulsions may be solvable by biological thinking. We can look for molecular information in food which triggers **recursive loops** and keeps people locked into self-destructive cycles. The compulsive eater is seldom spared symptoms and real suffering as a consequence of eating the "addictive" food. The term "addictive food allergy" may be too glib, but does describe the common experience of craving, and then, compulsively eating foods which produce illness. Among our patients, there is a consensus that eating-control is difficult to achieve, even when wrong food choices involve serious illness. The consensus is also that some foods trigger compulsive eating, uncontrollable by ordinary acts of consciousness.

The basic pattern of using and abusing addictive substances is a recursive loop; strong cravings (and other symptoms) lead to ingestion (or injection); followed by a brief period of stimulation and satisfaction; followed by depression and renewed cravings. Often the first, brief response is increased energy and increased activity. The loop recurs with specific timing, presumably because of the duration of effect of specific drug-like substances; the nicotine loop in smokers can be as short as 20 minutes; the food loop tends to be 1-2 hours long. **Normal eating** is controlled by a similar loop with cycles of hunger and satiety. Normal hunger builds slowly and rhythmically, but can be over-ridden by normal activities. If food is not eaten, normal hunger builds in pulses of increasing intensity, but the normal person can carry on with activities and does not develop distressing symptoms. The abnormal addictive loop is more intense, exclusive, and leads to the wrong results. Cravings build quickly, and interrupt other activities. In the abnormal state, missing the next "fix" leads to withdrawal symptoms which can be severe, even within a 4 hour period. **Often the addictive food and drink is not satisfying** at all and the most dysfunctional people keep eating and drinking with only the briefest interruptions, never satisfied.

The attempt to change eating behaviors often reveals the addictive process in a typical sequence of **withdrawal, clearing, cravings, falling-off-the-wagon, binging, retreating and clearing,** often in a repeating sequence over months and years. We recognize the same patterns with foods, alcoholic beverages, and drugs. Our concept of "clearing" refers to the disappearance of both physical symptoms and cravings. A clearing period on an elemental nutrient formula (ENFood) and water is the most dramatic recovery experience that an addicted person can have. Often, people with food allergy or other food-related illness are abnormal eaters. Most people report **sugar cravings** and/or binging. "Sugar" means a wide range of candies, cookies, desserts, baked goods, pop, ice cream, and junk food. Sugar is only one component among many that may cause trouble. But these foods definitely trigger strong cravings and compulsive or binge eating. Cravings for milk, bread, cheese, peanuts, fruit, or potato chips are as common as cravings for sweets. Even people with obvious milk allergy, with a protective aversion to drinking milk, will compulsively eat cheese or ice cream, maintaining their milk-allergic illness.

Many follow the Core Program with little difficulty and get better uneventfully. They respond well to the explanation and reassurance of withdrawal effects and cope well until their symptoms clear. Evidence of withdrawal symptoms and attendant frustration disappears by day 4-10. The "clearing" effect is the beginning of a whole new mode of existing. Clearing tends to open your appetite to new foods, and, with a little patience, Core

Program foods start looking attractive. Minor relapses seem to increase determination to stick with safe foods and diet revision proceeds to a successful conclusion.

Others have more difficulty, continue to eat reactive foods and follow a roller-coaster path of physical and mental disturbance. The people in trouble tend to have the behavioral profile of addiction. They go through obvious **withdrawal** in the first week on the Core Diet, often with angry or tearful protests, and refuse to eat Core Program foods. The worst-afflicted will relapse quickly with anger and denial; they will go to any length to maintain their old food habits. The more successful of the addictive people will do well for awhile and then relapse, often in a recurring pattern. Complete abstinence from foods that trigger compulsive eating is the only way to avoid recurrence of the addictive cycle.

If you follow the Core Program food list, without exceptions, food cravings tend to go away. If food exceptions are made every 3 or 4 days, the incoming problem may be sufficient to sustain cravings, and spoil the clearing effect. If people close to you also have problems managing their food cravings and compulsions, your attempt at diet revision may fail. They will sabotage your efforts to maintain control, often unintentionally. It is essential to seek the support and cooperation of people who share your meals.

Alcoholic Beverages and Addiction

Alcoholic beverages are foods with great potential for abuse. These foods trigger cravings and compulsive eating-drinking just as other foods do, but the health and social consequences are more drastic. **Alcoholic Beverages (ABs) can be devastating** to individuals and their society. The direct material and medical cost of **Alcoholic Beverage Abuse (AB Abuse)** in the U.S.A. alone is estimated to be over 20 billion dollars per year. Absenteeism in the U.S. government due to AB abuse is estimated to be in excess of half a billion dollars per year. The inestimable social cost is expressed in the suffering, despair, and behavioral aberrations of alcohol-abusers, their families, and their community. Dr. Sidney Cohen, a drug abuse expert, has described alcohol as "the **most dangerous drug** on earth".[1] We do, however, consider it a major error to attribute all the problems caused by alcoholic beverages to alcohol alone. We will, therefore, use the acronym, "AB "and refer to **AB abuse** rather than "alcohol abuse". In nutritional programming language, AB abusers become ABABs, pronounced A-BAB.

ABs must be considered "food". The ingestion of ABs is so closely linked to food selection, eating behaviors, and socialization that no consideration of diet and food-related illness is realistic without knowledge of ABs. The regular abuse of ABs (AB abuse) is called "alcoholism". A practical definition of **alcoholism** is: regular ingestion of ABS, sufficient to produce dysfunction or damage, at a physical and/or a socio-economic level. The label "alcoholic" is resisted by most alcohol abusers. The stigma attached to the identification of AB abuse remains curious and obstructive to any intelligent perspective of this common problem. The best guess estimate is that 10% of our population is disabled by AB abuse and another 30-40% have seriously compromised their well-being by regular AB ingestion. Among our patients, who carefully control their food intake, the ingestion of ABs falls to a minimum; either no AB ingestion, or only occasional glasses of white wine, or mild ABs like apple or pear cider. Very few of the successful patients drink beer, ale, whiskey, or liqueurs, since these chemical brews are often toxic.

Alcoholic Beverages Are Foods.

The Recursive Loops involved in AB abuse must be driven by addictive molecules in the beverages. Alcohol or ethanol is one addictive molecule, but are there others? **Hand-to-mouth loops** can contain any molecular message. When hand-to-mouth loops contain AB, the consequences of not interrupting the loop escalate rapidly. If coffee or chocolate are in the loop, there are negative consequences, but usually less severe compared with ABs. The cost of compulsive eating and drinking is measured within the body (endogenous) of the ingestor and without (exogenous), in the environment, influenced by the altered behavior of the AB abuse. Any brain chemical in an HML tends to produce a **microscopic endogenous cost** (invisibly altered brain information processing) and a macroscopic, **amplified exogenous response** (shouting, fighting, shooting, knifing, car accidents, and so on). Both the nervous system and the immune system have the impressive ability to amplify a tiny body event on the molecular level into a large physical world event.

The AB Abuser or Alcoholic is a person who cannot moderate AB ingestion. Not all AB abusers are "drunks". But all drunks are AB abusers. The compulsive aspect of drinking is experienced by all AB consumers. The moderate drinker, however, learns to avoid toxic AB doses, and is happy to abstain from AB for days or weeks without effort. Some AB abuses follow a binging pattern with periods of heavy drinking leading to total disability, followed by withdrawal, and then substantial periods of sobriety. The phenomena of AB abuse is not limited to the effects of alcohol, but involves the **entire chemistry** of the different fermented foods, yeasts, additives and contaminants.

What are ABs? They all are **yeast fermentation products** of staple foods. ABs are grape-yeast, grain-yeast, potato-yeast brews. The basic process of manufacturing an AB is mashing carbohydrate-rich fruit, grain, and vegetable material, and fermenting the mash in a container for a regulated period of time. The fermented mash tends to be toxic, and good

AB makers know how to reduce the toxicity of their products so that people are less likely to get immediately and unmistakably ill after drinking the brew. Amateur wine and beer makers often make themselves and their friends conspicuously ill, because they lack the professional's finesse for disguising the toxicity of the ferment. The sediments of wine, beer, and any alcoholic base for distillation contain the yeast corpses, and substrate residues. Sediments must be removed to improve the taste and clarity of the brew, and to reduce its toxicity. Wine clarification removes the rest of the particulate matter before consumption. Red wines are made from the whole grape mash and tend to be more chemically complex and toxic than good white wines. The best white wines are supposed to be made from the juice of gently squeezed grapes and should be free of chemicals and contaminants associated with grape skins.

Distillation of raw alcoholic brews concentrates the alcohol and leaves behind many chemicals that are not volatile at distillation temperatures. Whiskeys, therefore, are concentrates of ethanol and other volatile aromatic chemicals, which are chemical stressors. The chemical stressor value of whiskeys is increased by aging in devices such as charred oak caskets which give Scotch whiskeys their color and flavor. AB manufacturers spend a lot of money advertising their own charming version of the whiskey-aging process. These ads are supposed to appeal to the sophistication of the whiskey-connoisseur, but, rather, should alarm the reader as to the stressor and toxic properties added to the already harmful brew. Wine connoisseurs use the chemical sensors in their nose to select from among various aromatic chemicals present in the wines. The pretense of wine sampling in restaurants should allow you to screen for corks contaminated by obvious mold growths or wines which have turned to vinegar. Obviously wines containing sediments have not been carefully bottled and are rejected.

Ales and beers are raw filtered products of fermented grain mashes with hops, often chemically treated to manipulate color, foaming characteristics, and stability. These food liquors are somewhat nourishing, but they are also diuretic and toxic. Many male beer-drinkers get characteristic belly fat, breasts, and skinny limbs. It is hard to imagine how their deteriorating body shapes and soggy brains could be associated with manliness. Beer vendors tend to spend a lot of money advertising their imaginary link between beer-drinking and healthy, athletic, fun-loving adults. There is no credible link between beer drinking and healthy athletes, or beer drinking and happy young adults.

Beer is intrinsically toxic and could be expected to degrade athletic performance as much as any other skilled, energetic activity. More realistic scenarios of beer-drinking, and all other AB ingestion would show the consequences of drinking too much, too often: noxious, smoked-filled rooms, demented discussions, arguments, illness, smashed cars, beaten wives, abused children, and wrecked careers. Our attention should focus on AB-caused illness; to the diarrhea, dermatitis, and dementia of the alcoholic pellagran; or the staggering, and absurd mutterings of the brain-damaged alcoholic with Wernicke's psychosis.

Appetite, Body Size, And Shape

People come in different shapes and sizes. Any traveller knows about regional differences in the "look" of people. Some nations specialize in fat, others in lean. Family groups develop characteristic shapes and sizes, but there are always exceptions. The shape and size of each person is an expression of their food supply and their work, interacting with their genetic blueprint. An Eskimo needs to be fat to stay warm just as a a marathon runner or New Guinea tribesman has to be lean to stay cool and agile. We can think of the regular food supply of an individual or group as having qualities that determine body shape and overall appearance. The food supply of any person will influence the "look". As a person in our society gains excess weight, they tend to develop other symptoms and signs of a dysfunctional eating pattern. Their face may flush for example, and allergic shiners develop with "bags under the eyes". Water retention may make hands, ankles and feet puffy. Distension of the abdomen may increase the obese look. Inactivity and loss of muscle tissue means loss of body contours, sagging, and drooping postures. These changes are physical signs of food allergy. Social acceptance is partly determined by the "look" of a person and weight gain, especially with other signs of food allergy, spoils anyone's good looks. The "ugly" appearance of fat rippling the skin, known as "**cellulite**", is most apparent on the buttocks and thighs. Cellulite can be changed only by reducing the amount of fat stored under the skin. The rippling is caused by connective tissue partitions in the fatty tissue which attach the skin to the underlying fascia, a firm membrane which packages muscle. Buttock and thigh fat wants to fall down as you stand, and the fibrous tissue anchors it against gravity, producing the rippling effect on the skin. No surface cream, special exercise, vibrator, or electric current will alter the basic tissue architecture or the skin appearance.

Fat as Body Shape

Patterns of fat storage are expressed as different body shapes. This tells us that genetically-determined control-factors, such as hormones, interacting with the food supply, determine the distribution of fat. There are likely many **body shape factors (BSF)**. Female shapes are produced by female hormones. This means that fat cells have receptors on their surface that make them responsive to control signals. Breast and buttock fat cells receive special signals to encourage them to grow into those wonderful shapes that make women attractive to men. Men too will develop similar fat deposits if they ingest too much estrogen in their food supply or manufacture abnormal amounts in their body. Male hormones are anabolic steroids which promote muscle and bone growth with less fat, the athletic male look. Changes in food choices are the most available means of altering body size and shape. It is difficult to find people with 25 pounds of stored lettuce, broccoli, or carrot surplus.

High vegetable diets tend to be weight-reducing, even with high carbohydrate content. The calories work differently. Rice, as a staple food, supplies good food energy, but it is difficult to gain weight with rice. Most of our patients with food allergic diseases cannot eat milk products or grains, and rely on rice and vegetables. Their fat intake drops and they loose weight. The most common experience on the Core Program is initial weight loss during clearing and in early **Phase 2**. Continued weight loss depends on staying with the Core Program and increasing physical activity.

Women who spend a lot of time, energy, and money in a futile effort to alter body shape through expensive creams, and machinery would be grateful for an effective BSF, which blocked the fat uptake receptors on buttock and thigh fat cells. For now the best approach to body size and shape is to choose the right food and exercise regularly.

Eating Behavior

Human relationships are built around shared pleasurable experiences. Eating together is the principal bond among people Some people get fat because they share an eating relationship with friends and spouses. Often spouses start getting fat after marriage, as an expression of mutual caring through a **pleasure bond**. Others get fat because they are lonely and idle at night. Others get fat because food pleasures are the easiest, most available form of self-gratification. Compulsive eating often emerges in early childhood as a dysfunctional pattern. If cravings and compuslisive eating are associated with physical symptoms, mood, and behavioral disorders, the diagnosis of food allergy must be considered. Dysfunctional eating patterns tend to persist into adult life with obesity as one of the many consequences.

The expression "diets don't work" refers to a basic truth of weight reduction diets. Most fail because the dysfunctional behavior patterns are only temporarily suspended and return in full force when the diet program is over. Many compulsive eaters try weight reduction diets, succeed for a few weeks, and then fail; the net result is frustration, guilt and low self-esteem. Some have been told that their sense of deprivation, guilt, and the failure complex keep them from losing weight and are encouraged to keep their kitchens stocked with all the foods they like; ice cream, cakes, cookies, bread, potato chips, pop are all fair game.

This upside-down approach is intriguing in a world of puzzles, paradoxes, and mirrors but does temptation really work?   None of the patients we have worked with succeed with kitchens stocked with tempting, fattening foods. The idea of indulging yourself does not work. There are many important reasons why abstinence from "forbidden foods", both in the short and long-term, is required for health restoration and weight loss. Food addiction is similar to alcohol and drug addiction. We do not advise the alcoholic to keep his home stocked with bourbon and scotch whiskey. We advise no alcoholic beverages at home; stock up soda and carbonated water, and fruit juices. We advise compulsive eaters to follow all the rules that an alcoholic follows. Avoid temptation!

The Core Program emerges from a tradition of careful, deliberate choices based on intelligent understanding of the biological issues. We are not interested in guilt or failure and take a level-headed, common-sense, problem-solving approach to diet reconstruction and behavior modification. A clear and simple instruction of the Core Program is to clear your kitchen of unwanted foods and avoid all tempting social events, especially during clearing and early Phase 2 food reintroductions. People stuck in addictive loops have to abandon their old habits and seek a completely new pattern of eating, working, and exercise. They may have to avoid familiar binging triggers for years before they have enough self-control to cope with temptation.

Appetite Regulation

Computer-like centers in our brain, especially the **hypothalamus,** regulate eating behaviors. These neural computers gather chemical data from the blood and receive messages from various regulatory tissues in the body including insulin, sex hormones, and peptides secreted by GIT as it processes food. The appetite computers must integrate information about body weight, temperature, activity level, season, and reproductive cycle (in women) to decide how much food is needed today. The appetite computer establishes a weight and temperature "set-point" and tries to maintain these values even when the food supply varies a great deal.

There are numerous opportunities for this regulatory system to fail. Often appetite and weight regulation is unstable for short periods of weeks but produces dramatic, lasting changes in size and shape. The human appetite system works at about the same level it did in reptiles millions of years ago. The strategy of the reptilian brain is to establish the most efficient path to reliably available food, then to lock in the behavior and repeat it without further modification. Our appetite system tends to run automatically at this primitive level and defies conscious attempts to alter any well-programmed behavior.

Food factors determine the intensity of repeating appetitive behaviors. Some food factors establish strong repeating behaviors and are called **addictive triggers**. Food vendors know that salt and sugar assure repeat business. Salt and sugar are the two principle markers of food in an animal's environment. At the reptilian brain level, therefore, the taste of salt and sugar signal the successful discovery of food. The repeated discovery of salt and sugar sensations at specific locations in the environment lock-in food-seeking behavior toward those locations. Our experience strongly suggests that milk and wheat proteins also lock-in intense repeating behaviors. This is probably a property of milk and wheat proteins (specifically peptide digestive products of these proteins). Successful food manufacturers offer foods made with wheat flour, milk, sugar, and salt. These ingredients can be turned into doughnuts, pizzas, pancakes, waffles, pies, cakes, cookies, ice cream, milk shakes, and a host of other "fast foods" with an assured market.

Three properties of reptilian behavior are worth noting:

Perseveration is the tendency for a fixed behavior to repeat or persist, even when the path is blocked or the real benefit of a behavior disappears. Eating behaviors are highly automated and resist change.

Frustration Whenever seeking-behaviors are blocked, anger or rage is the response. The least degree of drive-blocked discomfort is frustration which. occurs when you want a McDonald's hamburger and your friend, or spouse refuses to cooperate, making disparaging remarks about the plastic nature of the food. An argument may follow, reducing your valuation of the other person, as well as your appetite.

Displacement, occurs when there is no further supply of the gratification for the appetite or drive; seeking behaviors shift laterally to find an alternative. The most obvious displacement occurs when no McDonald's outlet is found, and seeking displaces toward Burger King or Dairy Queen. If there are no fast food outlets, displacement may shift laterally toward another convenient salt-sugar-wheat-milk food, like pizza or doughnuts. Displacement rules say that you can substitute another kind of behavior for eating if there is no food available; you may spend money and consume goods, for example. The most destructive displacements turn hunger for authentic nourishing food into ingestion of destructive substances such as alcoholic beverages. A more desirable disposition of appetitive drives requires that you "jump" out of the cycle of ingesting things for immediate gratification and incorporate the world through eyes, ears, and skin, rather than through the mouth. The learning path involves specific techniques: sport, yogas, meditations, as well as lifestyles promoting skilled, thoughtful, well-integrated activities.

Eating Disorders

Specific patterns of compulsive eating have been recognized. Most literature treats "eating disorders" as personal and social problems, not related to food choices. We are most interested in the biological causes of abnormal eating patterns and the similarities between food, alcohol, and drug addiction patterns. **Bulimia, or "Ox-Hunger,"** is an eating or appetite disorder which afflicts women more than men. The essential features of bulimia are binge-eating, interrupted by deliberate efforts to avoid the consequences of over-eating by vigorous exercise, fasting, self-induced vomiting, and purging with laxatives. The bulimic pattern is associated with guilt feelings, secrecy, and overt depression.

The incidence of bulimia appears to be increasing. Indeed, bulimia has all the appearances of one of the common diet-related endemic diseases. There are many theories of causation and a variety of treatment strategies. Too few therapists postulate a biological cause; an infectious agent, an environmental agent, food allergy, or other problems in the food supply. If a similar endemic involved more explicit physical symptoms, an epidemiological approach would search for a physical or infectious agent as the cause of the malady. A good theory would postulate **"Agent X"** in the food supply, which disorders appetite regulation in a predictable manner. Agent X need not be a single substance, but may be a collection of operators in the food supply, affecting susceptible individuals.

Self-induced vomiting in the bulimic patient is a rather complex behavior that involves both a rational component - avoiding the consequences of eating the wrong food- and an irrational, compulsive component The idea of a recursive feeding loop, running amok, helps us to locate the irrational behavior at a primitive, addictive level. The rational concern is not just avoiding weight gain, but also avoiding the awful feelings and the depression which follows binging. Many bulimics with food allergy, initially vomited spontaneously after eating offending foods, only to feel much relieved; and then learned self-induced vomiting as a method of avoiding food-symptoms. Many bulimics have a split personality; one part of their personality knows that they crave and compulsively eat foods that make them ill, but they will still seem suprised that food allergy is involved and resist advice that favorite foods such as bread and cheese may be a problems. They are involved in typical addictive denial. Their denial that food makes them ill is often reinforced by treatment programs that fail to recognize food allergy symptoms and discourage efforts to change food choices.

Often **depression** is associated with binge-eating and binges increase along with depression during the late fall and winter in northern climates. Patients with seasonal depression (seasonal affective disorder or SAD) tend to binge like animals preparing for hibernation, gaining weight through the winter unless vomiting and purging efforts rid their body of excess calories. Excess calories tend to be carbohydrates, often dariy and wheat-based foods with high sugar content.

Psychogenic explanations of binge-eating focus on the personalities of the women involved. The personality profile suggests that women who are high-achievers, perfectionistic, lonely, dissatisfied, and frustrated are at high risk. A phobic fear of being too fat is usually mentioned as the cause of fasting, purging, and vomiting. The psychological or psychogenic explanations take the easy route. That is, they simply restate a description of the problem as its cause. If the patient says: "I am intense, frustrated, and concerned about my body weight..."; the psychological rendering just turns this around: "Women become bulimic because they are intense, frustrated, and are concerned about their body weight." This is no explanation at all! Many smart people with eating disorders, wisely and appropriately, do not accept these "psychological" nonexplanations. Our patients often describe., "... something inside is not working properly; there is something chemically wrong with me". One patient stated it succinctly:

> *"I think there is a little gizmo in my brain gone crazy...if you can only get in there and fix it, I`ll be OK again."*

Weight Gain, Loss and Obesity

A major concern in our society is weight gain. **Obesity** means that the pattern of food selection and amount eaten is out of synch with biological needs. All obesity is mute testimonial to over-eating. Excess fat accumulation is an artifact of disordered eating behaviors with food energy intake exceeding energy expenditure. Even if compulsive eating stops, fat stubbornly persists, even with heroic efforts to lose weight by food restriction. Stored fat is stored energy. The only way to lose weight is to exercise; use the stored energy by hard, physical work!

Obesity may be defined as body weight greater than 20% of an average body weight (determined from statistical tables). In terms of individual perception, obesity is defined as looking and/or feeling too fat. For most of us, the esthetic judgment is more important than a statistical reference. The amount of fat stored in us may be compared to our **lean body weight,** a measure of structural and functional tissues. If the fat proportion exceeds 30% in women and 25% in men, then obesity exists. Some women feel too fat if their fat proportion exceeds 25% and would seek dietary and exercise remedies. Lean body mass includes muscle tissue which tends to use up food energy.

In our society, aging is associated with reduced activity, increased weight; reduced muscle mass, and increased fat. As the muscle mass progressively declines, energy needs decline, and food excesses are stored as fat in a progressive manner; a vicious cycle. Body fat is energy storage which acts like a savings account. Food surplus tends to be saved with interest and stored as fat. People who remain fat have a frugal metabolism and it is difficult to withdraw and spend the savings. One pound of fat is worth at least one day's hard physical labor. Reduced food energy intake tends to induce energy conservation, and body weight is maintained until severe food shortage results in weight loss.

Weight loss requires spending energy, stored as fat, with hard
physical work. Fat does not evaporate!

The extra food may be ingested slowly and gradually, although most people gain weight in spurts, as a consequence of binge-eating or periodic indulgences in extra foods, alcoholic beverages, desserts, and snacks. Rapid weight gain may be associated with hormonal changes, as in pregnancy or low thyroid states, or whenever life-style changes, injury, or illness reduce physical activity. Without a balanced reduction in food intake or change in food selection, reduced physical activity produces weight gain. Bursts of weight gain represent maladaptive responses to a variety of stressors.

Many warnings associated with weight gain say, "Watch out if you get too fat - later on, in the distant future, you will have diabetes, coronary artery disease, etc...". The truth is you do not have to wait to feel ill. Within minutes or hours of eating too much of the wrong food, you already are tired, confused, and irritable. You may have gastrointestinal symptoms, a headache, a congested nose, a rash, and so on. It is not possible to overeat, or even to eat as you please, without risking discomfort, dysfunction, and disease. A **"less is best" rule** suggests:

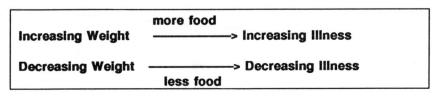

A mistaken assumption is that we should be able to enjoy ourselves by eating and drinking whatever and whenever. Obesity is often the result of compulsive eating or binge-eating, combined with wrong food choices, and lack of exercise.

Every year, new weight-loss books appear on the bookstalls, and magazines run endless articles on the subject. Millions of people have proven that it is easier to gain weight than to lose it and dieters have also proven that weight-loss attempts by calorie restriction, following a temporary "weight-loss diet", may succeed for a short time, but ultimately fail. Any therapist who has worked with obese patients has many stories of spectacular initial successes, with equally spectacular relapses, weeks or months later. Obviously, there are unsolved problems in the obesity business. Newsweek has valued the weight loss industry in the U.S.A. as a $33 billion per year industry and suggests that Americans spend an estimated $1 billion per year on a variety of liquid diet formulas; some over-the-counter, and some dispensed in commercial weight loss programs like Optifast. Another $370 million per year is spent on over the counter weight-loss pills and potions which have no value.

Commercial weight loss programs offer a variety of services and products which may be helpful, but may prove to be too expensive or otherwise inappropriate. The best programs offer supervision, education, and a rational behavioral management plan with prolonged follow-up. Without a sustained exercise program, and permanent change in eating habits, no weight loss program should be considered. Medical supervision of weight loss programs is often advocated but may prove to be an impractical, cost-prohibitive approach.   Each person should be aware enough to assess the risk of weight loss against the established risks of continuing bad habits.

Medical supervision may not be available, affordable, or effective in weight loss programs. Further, without special expertise, physicians are often cast in an supervisory and advisory role which they cannot fulfill. Many tests, including routine blood tests and cardiograms, will fail to predict calamities. It would not be practical or affordable for every person undergoing diet revision and exercise programs to have blood tests and exercise stress tests. The physician's function is often to absorb the liability, for some other party, if things go wrong. Many people will get sick, develop cancer, have heart attacks and be otherwise high-risk persons while they pursue changes in the diet, body size or fitness levels, regardless of medical supervision. Years of neglected health are responsible for most calamities, more than the attempt to do better. It is backward to think that reasonable diet revision is risky, when the real danger is the dysfunction and disease caused by years on the original diet.

> *Advice, which creates fear of change, works against individual prerogatives and argues against self-responsibility. There are safe methods of weight loss, such as the Core Program, which can be undertaken by self-responsible people*

Dangers of Rapid Weight Loss

Having placed limits on the feasibility of medical supervision of weight loss programs, and the onus on ourselves for self-responsible changes, let us quickly examine some of the hazards of rapid weight loss with surgery, very-low calories and high protein diets. The most drastic weight-loss measure are surgical attempts to modify eating behaviors and to interfere with the digestion of food. Stomach stapling operations reduce the amount eaten, and intestinal bypass operations spoil digestion, reducing the absorption of nutrients. Rapid weight loss often follows these operations. One hazard is the development of **gallstones;** up to 54% of obese patients undergoing stomach bypass operations developed gallstones postoperatively. Relapses are also common after dramatic weight loss from intestinal by-pass surgery, and are complicated by worsening health from chronic diarrhea, malabsorption, and untreated food allergy.

Gallstones also follow rapid weight loss on very-low calorie diets (500-600 Kcal/day). An incidence of 19% gallstones in men and 9% in women have been reported. High blood fat levels (triglycerides) and higher blood calcium levels seem to predispose to stones. One suggested solution would be for patients undergoing rapid weight loss to take ursodeoxycholic acid, a bile salt, which can dissolve stones before they have a chance to develop. A better alternative is to plan slower weight-loss with diet revision and exercise, maintaining daily caloric intake at least 1000 Kcal. Other problems occur when patients lose weight rapidly on high protein diets or high protein liquid formulas. These problems are obvious if the mechanisms of weight loss are better understood. Caloric deprivation with consumption of proteins leads to excess ammonia production; the ammonia is processed by the liver and excreted by the kidneys as urea. This nitrogen (ammonia) may accumulate and becomes toxic, especially to the nervous system. The use of proteins as fuel is, therefore, not desirable.

The brain is essentially in charge of organizing adaptation to food restriction or fasting. Body arousal, temperature, and metabolic rate are all adjusted by the autonomic nervous system and a hormonal control system. The **sympathetic nervous system** arouses us to "fight or flight" responses. We feel sympathetic nervous system activity as excitement, tension, restlessness, anxiety, or fear. Fasting suppresses the sympathetic nervous system. Overfeeding stimulates it. The metabolic effects of increased sympathetic activity are to stimulate the withdrawal of fat from fat storage cells, the breakdown of liver glycogen to supply extra blood glucose, and the new synthesis of glucose from other nutrients like amino acids. The pancreas is discouraged from secreting insulin and encouraged to release glucagon, measures which tend to increase blood sugar. The typical response to a rapidly falling blood sugar (**hypoglycemia**) is a sympathetic surge; sweating, tremor and anxiety are typical symptoms as adrenalin raises the blood sugar. True hypoglycemia is recognized by the symptoms of this emergency response. Prolonged caloric deprivation generally is not associated with low blood sugar, since metabolic adjustments prevent this occurrence and sympathetic activity is suppressed.

One danger of fasting, followed by abrupt refeeding, is the sudden release of sympathetic activity. This surge of catecholamines may provoke heart rhythm abnormalities and may cause fatal cardiac arrest. This danger has be noted in women on severely restricted weight-reduction diets, particularly when artificial **protein powders** were used as the only source of food. [2] Although the direct toxicity of protein was not considered in the analysis of these tragic deaths, the allergenic properties of protein powders are a major concern and may also trigger heart rhythm abnormalities. High-protein diets do not have the benefits their advocates have claimed; they are associated with sodium loss, decreased sympathetic activity, increased ketosis, and no improvement in body protein conservation. [3] Protein foods should be eaten as structural foods close to the level of their actual need, about 12 % of total daily calories.

Secrets of Weight Loss

Once fat is stored, it requires little energy to maintain. The fat person tends to be more efficient than the thin person, and holds tenaciously to the stored fat. In order to use up the stored fat, you must operate with an energy input deficit for a long period of time. This requirement makes intentional weight-loss difficult to achieve. A state of major imbalance must be maintained to lose weight progressively. Fat cells seem to send out control signals, demanding more and more calories as they enlarge.

An appetite regulating protein, **adipsin,** has been described in mice which inhibits eating behaviors. Adipsin seems similar to, or identical with, complement D, one of the circulating proteins that participates in immune defense. One theory of obesity is a failure of feedback regulation of appetite, perhaps as a result of deficiency of adipsin or similar regulatory hormone. Adipsin deficiency may be genetically determined or induced by unknown materials in the food supply. Perhaps enlarging fat cells progressively lose the capacity to produce adipsin. Excessive weight gain is common in the food allergy complex and may represent interference with feedback regulation of appetite controllers by complement consumption or some other complicated event. Another regulatory protein, **cachectin,** has been described as causing progressive weight loss. People with chronic diseases, such as cancer, lose weight inexorably, even with forced nutrient intake. Cachectin is a hormone-like substance which apparently is made by macrophages, immune cells, in the course of their work as defenders against infections and malignant cells. Cachectin increases the withdrawal of stored fat, and inhibits further fat deposition. It is fascinating to realize that cachectin also destroys cancer cells. In its anti-cancer mode, it has been called the "Tumor Necrosis Factor" (TNF). The wasting of cancer patients may be a manifestation of vigorous immune defense against the cancer. Cachectin-TNF will soon be available in therapeutic quantity for trials in human disease. It is a member of a potent new pharmacopoeia of Biological Response Regulators (BRR), which are now emerging.

The rate of fat withdrawal from stores is also hormone regulated and dependent on enzymes called **lipases.** If your fat withdrawal system functions less well than your deposit system, you get fat even on a modest diet. Currently, there is no simple way to activate lipases through drugs or hormones. Attempts to administer thyroid hormone are unsuccessful in increasing fat withdrawal. Undisclosed food characteristics may influence the balance between fat deposit and withdrawal. The best way to activate lipase is do physical work. If your lifestyle does not include significant physical labor, you require active daily exercise at the level of tennis, badminton, running, bicycling, swimming, or other aerobic exercises; a minimum of 20 minutes of aerobic exercise per day is required to make any significant change in the metabolism of fat. Sustained exercise is better for fat consumption than bursts of more intense exercise. Frequent outings involving long walks, hiking, skiing, or cycling, are also desirable.

Insulin is the hormone which most promotes fat deposition. Sugars increase insulin secretion and provide the substrate for fat synthesis. Early-onset diabetes, a disease of insulin deficiency, is diagnosed by weight loss, fatigue, and increased urine volume. The deficiency of insulin does not allow fat deposition and weight gain. Late-onset diabetics have a different problem since their sugar intolerance appears when they are overweight. The excess fatty tissue probably interferes with the other functions of insulin, but obese diabetics have enough insulin to gain weight readily.

Most weight loss dieters experience the increased-efficiency effect as calories are restricted. In healthy experimental subjects, a daily deficit of 1500 Kcal produced a maximum weight loss of 25% at 24 weeks, when a new equilibrium was established. No significant weight loss may be seen in a sedentary obese person until energy intake has dropped below 800 Kcalories. The quality of food choice at this restricted level of intake is crucial. Fat, sugar, and high protein are definitely avoided. Sugar in excess is converted directly to fat. High sugar foods are addictive and maintain cravings for more sugar. Fruit and fruit juices, high in sugar, lead to recursive-looping, and are not desirable on weight reduction diets.

There are only **two allies** when you want to lose weight: **hunger and work.** Weight loss is directly equated to physical work; not food deprivation. The jogger or swimmer is losing weight. Even the walker is losing weight, although more slowly. Hunger must be restored as a normal, welcome feeling. There is nothing wrong with hunger! In order to establish new healthy eating patterns it is essential to practice being comfortably hungry for periods as long as 4-6 hours before eating. A normal rhythm might be 4 hours between meals. The less you move, the longer you have to be hungry; another way of looking at weight loss.

The Core Program and Weight Loss

A change in food selection habits, permanently, is required to sustain weight loss. Most diets do not address this problem, and are eventually futile. Success in long-term weight reduction is strategic, and not a matter of willpower. The Core Program emphasizes correct food selection and does not require food restriction, nor calorie counting. With caloric restriction alone, cold, fatigue, and sluggishness are experienced as physical activity and energy expenditure decreases. If we only consider the balance sheet, relating energy intake to output, we should prefer increased energy expenditure as the better means of controlling weight. The choice of food by its quality and impact on eating behaviors is initially more important than the choice by quantity or caloric content. Diets, which emphasize changes in the proportions of protein, fat carbohydrate, fiber, and so on, do not have special properties for weight control. The proportions recommended on the Core Program tend to work very well, but only if the food choices are correct. Vegetables foods have the most to offer a weight loss program since they have low nutrient density (you can eat a lot more) and seldom trigger cravings and compulsive eating. The timing of meals is relevant to regulating eating behavior. More food should be eaten earlier in the day. Compulsive eating is most difficult to control at night. It is often necessary to restructure evening activities; start new and physical activities instead of sitting all evening. Avoid alcoholic beverages. They are destructive to weight loss and long-term health goals. Even moderate amounts of ABs may trigger compulsive eating. The social context of drinking ABs is seldom conducive to selective eating and impulse control.

Liquid Diets

Properly formulated liquid diets can be a very useful adjunct to weight loss programs. We advocate the development of an entire technology of chemically-defined formulas to support the treatment of food-related illnesses, obesity included. Unfortunately, many formulas on the market may fail to serve your best interests, and may pose some risks. Low calorie liquid diet formulas may have inferior ingredients and some formulas with many "natural" ingredients and allergic materials are undesirable. High protein liquid diets pose the greatest risk of allergic reactions, and metabolic abnormalities and should be avoided. The choice of ingredients in the mix is vitally important. Currently, there is no effective regulation of formula contents. Liquid weight-loss diets are often made from cheap raw materials, especially skim milk powder, egg white, soya or hydrolysed vegetable proteins; all present major food allergy problems. Food cravings and other symptoms may continue with the ingestion of allergenic proteins and lead the user back to compulsive eating. Flavoring, emulsifiers and other additives also make a big difference. Some formulas are made to fortify skim milk and are, in our opinion, not desirable options for weight loss.

Avoid:
1. Very Low calorie liquid diets
2. High Protein liquid diets
3. Herbal protein mixes

Elemental Nutrient Formulas (ENFood)

Elemental Nutrient Formulas (ENF) are discussed as clearing options in Chapter 11 ENF's are important Core Program options to replace food with a hypoallergenic "chemically defined" nutrient formulas. There are essential differences between liquid diets, sold for weight loss purposes, and elemental nutrient formulas (ENF). ENF's are not low calorie, contain no proteins, and provide balanced, safe, nutrient intake without food allergy effects. The chief advantage of an ENF is that superior, more purified ingredients are used in an effort to avoid all the problems of food allergy, and the weird biochemical mixes of a wild food supply. One key to understanding the difference an ENF and other formulas is knowing that proteins are the main food allergy problem and are not allowed in an ENF. The nutrients, derived from proteins, are amino acids and these are provided in their free form in an ENF. The proportions of nutrients in ENF provide balanced nutrition with the sense of satiety; the satisfied feeling when you have had enough to eat. While ENF's are not designed specifically for weight-loss purposes, they may serve well in this application.

---

[1]Cohen S. The substance abuse problems.New York: Haworth Press, 1981.

[2]Landsbergic L, Young J. 1978. NEJM: 298; 1295-1301

[3]DeHaven JH et al. Nitrogen and Sodium Balance and Sympathetic Nervous System Activity in Obese Subjects with a Low-Calorie Protein or Mixed Diet. 1980 New Engl Jour Med:302:9;477-482

Chapter 5   Diet Revision

The Solution of Modern Diseases

In the previous chapters we discussed the general reasons for diet revision. In this chapter we will introduce the idea of food allergy as a powerful explanation of many contemporary diseases and outline the problem of ill-defined illnesses. We can be specific about some problems which we know, from experience, improve with diet revision. Many ill-defined illnesses, problems called by different names, and explained by different theories, will turn out to be variations of the prolific delayed-patterns of food allergy.

No simple explanation would cover the range of disturbances that food ingestion causes. Our basic understanding of modern illness bears repeating: it is a myth of medical diagnosis that illness is an orderly process; illness is a more random or chaotic process. Disease is disorder. We seldom see patients with only one problem. The concept that we are dealing with single diseases, and not multiple processes, misleads the unwary to construct wrong theories, and to ignore the evidence that suggests food causes. Food interacts complexly with our bodies and disease causation is, therefore, a complex affair. We can assume that chemical, metabolic, and allergic processes interact to produce unwanted events - symptoms and malfunction of our organs. We can assume that our behavior is influenced by our food and that food selection is determined by our behavior in rather complex, looping relationships. Health problems tend to cluster in groups and evolve over time. Many factors contribute over time to the final end-stage disease, listed as diagnoses in medical records.

Food allergy is often their best explanation of the many health problems we discuss in this chapter. There are disease progressions over time that can only be explained as persisting immune-mediated dysfunction. Increasingly, our major unsolved diseases are attributed to immune-mediated mechanisms. Evidence points to the food supply when we need to explain the mystery of persisting immune-mediated disease.

Dr. William Knicker, a prominent American Allergist and Immunologist has stated:[1]

> "The estimated group of 40 million citizens with classical allergies is possibly the most
> underserved of all diseases in the U.S; medical marketing surveys suggest that many
> atopic individuals are not yet diagnosed or are poorly treated. In addition, there are
> countless millions of other individuals who have unrecognized adverse reactions to
> various antigens, foods, chemicals, and environmental or occupational triggers."

Medical Diagnosis

Each of us develops patterns of dysfunction. Symptoms are unpleasant experiences, markers of dysfunction, which tend to occur in specific patterns and sequences, intermittently, in every person. From a physician's point of view, the dysfunctional experiences of the patient are interpreted as symptoms or indicators of disease. Physicians are taught to elicit patients' reports of specific symptoms in a certain order. The practice of diagnosis is deliberately designed to ignore a great deal of the information a patient provides. Physicians are used to dismissing certain patterns of dysfunction which they know from experience resolve spontaneously, or at least, are not immediately life-threatening. This diagnostic screening strategy serves us well in emergency situations where triage is needed. A physician tries to organize a patient's symptom account into diagnostic descriptions similar to:

> *...Crampy, periumbilical abdominal pain, associated with vomiting,
> but not diarrhea, which becomes steady and moves to the right lower
> quadrant in eight to twelve hours...*

This description is diagnostic of acute appendicitis. The medical diagnosis is completed by finding tenderness in the lower right abdomen over the appendix area, and finding an elevated temperature and white blood cell count in the laboratory. Other disorders may approximate this pattern and are considered as "differential diagnoses". Appendicitis may also present in an atypical fashion, leaving much to the physician's discretion.

Diagnostic categories always oversimplify a complex situation, and inexperienced physicians tend to take the definition of disease too seriously. Most patients outside teaching hospitals often fail to meet rigid diagnostic criteria; their suffering has to be managed in a different way. Many disease processes evolve slowly over many years and early symptoms fall through the triage screen and patients continue to suffer until their disease is sufficiently advanced that it shows up on tests. New patterns of illness also are missed when the established criteria for well-known diseases are not met. Since the food supply of an individual is an important biological determinant, diet revision should be an early diagnostic and treatment strategy in medicine, especially when the precise nature of the disease is unclear. We propose a process interpretation of dysfunction over a category definition; in other words we are more inclined to ask what is the source of the problem and how does the problem develop in the body than what is the problems called?

Diagnosis as Entities

Diagnostic classifications tend to be descriptive. A collection of symptoms is given a pattern and a syndrome name, and, thereafter, it becomes an entity. The word "depression" has been elevated from the status of vague description to a proper medical diagnosis. The term "arthritis" simply describes joint inflammation. As we further categorize arthritis, we develop descriptive criteria for many different types of arthritis. The diagnosis "rheumatoid arthritis" requires a definite collection of symptoms, especially symmetrical joint swelling and pain. Objective measurements give some diagnoses even more credibility. We may require the presence of a specific circulating antibody before the diagnosis of Rheumatoid Arthritis is made, even when most other features of the disease are present.

The recognition and approval of diagnostic entities involves a complex, quasi-political process within the medical world. The admission of new syndromes to the entity-description-system is generally resisted, unless groups of well-established investigators, publishing in major medical journals, endorse the new entity. As new illnesses emerge, especially the multi-symptom, multi-factorial problems of food and environmental illnesses, their victims pass through a limbo of ignorance and misunderstanding, often lasting years. They are denied the rights of sufferers of "legitimate" disease and may be mistreated by arrogant physicians, ignorant bureaucrats, and self-serving insurance companies. Their complaints are dismissed, rather than investigated. Their needs are ignored rather than met with compassionate concern.

We believe that the patterns of food allergy, described in this book, are common, prevalent health problems that are seldom diagnosed and treated properly. The range of food-related illnesses also extends well beyond food allergy and accounts for even more common diseases. And yet, most textbooks in medicine and the majority of post-graduate teaching articles in free, drug-company sponsored journals never mention food allergy or food-related illness! A sick patient who does not fit into a standard diagnostic category, tends to be ignored or dismissed. When a patient falls into this diagnostic limbo, curious things begin to happen. We have catalogued a number of "diagnostic default" explanations are often offered by physicians, instead of proper diagnoses. Stress, tension, colds, flu, viruses, or references to psychosomatic illness are the favored defaults. In the worst cases, patients are blamed for inventing symptoms or failing to respond to drug therapies. Patients are confused and feel diminished when they do not fit a disease category - "...I have a lot of pain and can barely walk on many days, but the rheumatologist says the blood tests and X-rays are OK and I don't have real arthritis...".

One physician, who served on a British committee to investigate food allergy, exemplified a dogmatic and patronizing attitude towards her patients; she was quoted:

> "You can't just dismiss them as aging hippies or Yuppies. They are entitled to the full attention of physicians because their lives are engulfed by a whole series of wide-ranging, if minor miseries...After a simple social and psychiatric history I give them a thorough physical examination. Then, if necessary, I have to say the condition is not organic and stand by my reputation."

Many patients report encounters with physicians who have similar attitudes, and are left with the bitter frustration that they were hopelessly misunderstood. They have received no benefit, and conclude that the physician really doesn't know what is going on. There is always doubt and uncertainty about the nature and origins of our problems, and no single person can ever have all the answers. Dogmatic physicians (they really do not know what is going on) are losing their credibility. Any patient, encountering psychosomatic explanations and dogmatic dismissals, should seek help from another, more insightful physician, with an interest in solving biological problems and not dispensing self-righteous opinions.

The Avalanche Effect

Although, we are often presented with a major illness, apparently of limited duration, close scrutiny of the medical histories of many patients reveals an evolution of symptoms over several years. Patients often discount or fail to report long-term, chronic or recurrent symptoms. They are encouraged to report only major events and are discouraged from linking their symptoms together as a complex which evolves over time. Many years may be spent in the **adapted dysfunctional state (ADS)** with stable symptoms or smooth adaptation to slowly decreasing level of funtion and/or slowly increasing disability. Symptoms of a mild ADS are often intermittent and ambiguous. A new factor such as a change in eating habits, a viral infection, an injury, childbirth, or a drug reaction may precipitate a sudden decompensation with collapse into a more severe, disabling illness.

For example, a 34 year old woman presents with an illness of 10 months duration. A consultant's medical history states that she was well until 10 months ago when she developed a flu-like illness with lymph node swelling, fatigue, aching, and sore throat; when she did not recover as expected extensive investigations for infections and other problems were inconclusive.

She described a 10 month debilitating illness with chronic congestion, sore throat, generalized aching, stiffness, digestive problems especially bloating, and extreme fatigue associated; she had quit work 4 months ago and spent most of her days in bed. The medical reports went on to describe many test results that were not helpful in making the diagnosis nor directing treatment. The impression of the illness, on casual review was that it was a new event, but on closer examination of her history, a different story emerged. She revealed that she had had chronic "sinus problems" for 15 years (nose congestion, mucus in her throat, cheek and forehead pain from sinus congestion); muscle pains, tension and stiffness had been occuring for over 10 years but were limited to her shoulders and upper back and she used to actively treat this discomfort with exercise; massage and ASA, keeping it under control; as a child she had episodes of mysterious illness with fevers, middle ear infections, nose congestion, and eczema. She described increasing work "stress" for a year prior to her collapse; the "stress" translated into a series of relevant behavioral and diet changes - she worked longer hours, she stopped exercise classes, increased her cigarette consumption from 10 to over 20 per day; increased her coffee consumptions from 2-3 to 8-10 cups per day; took more ASA for headaches and muscle pain; increased her intake of fast foods, muffins, crackers, cheese, and yogurt; indeed about 70% of her daily calories were supplied by milk products, wheat, and eggs; the 10% vegetable fraction was mostly potato.

What really happened was not a sudden new illness in an otherwise healthy, professional woman, but an **avalanche effect** from a cascading series of negative events over many months to years. Her history suggested that she had had delayed pattern food allergy since childhood in a mild and intermittent form; she existed in an adaptive dysfunctional state and perceived herslf to be "well" even during the hectic year which shifted her food intake, smoking, and other habits into a maladptive range. This perception " I am OK" during the progressively symptomatic stage of ADS is typical of highly-motivated, goal-oriented people. Some admit they are "workaholics".

The addictive nature of the work, eating, drinking patterns is obvious; complete with denial of the growing evidence of dysfunction. The medical model permits and even encourages this sort of self-deception. When the Doctor reassures an ADS patient, who presents with symptoms too early, that everything is OK because the tests are normal, he/she is really encouraging the patient to go back to working on the illness until it is a fully-expressed, finished product. When you go too far out of range, you can expect a sudden, dramatic collapse, the avalanche; but you never know when it will occur.

If we amplify the details of her childhood history, we would reveal more convincing evidence that she had chronic symptoms from food allergy, perhaps even beginning in early infancy. A similar illness is often seen in children. For example, a nine year old girl presented with an illness, apparently of 4 months duration which left her bed-ridden, unable to attend school from 3 months. She had nose congestion, sore throats, lymph node swelling, coughs, muscle aching, extreme fatigue; she felt tearful, despondent, and could not concentrate on her school assignments, nor remember what she had learned the day before. She had been carefully studied with many tests, and mother had been told that the cause was " a virus, there is nothing to do but wait." Her mother described an unusual eating pattern; she craved milk and yogurt and consumed these foods with toast, often with the exlusion of all other foods, especially on her worst days. On careful review of her history, it was obvious that she had had symptoms since infancy, and mother knew that she was allergic to milk during the first year when she had relentless colic, bloating, continuous colds, and severe diaper rash while on a milk formula, and complete remission of symptoms on a soya formula. Her symptoms seemed to clear after 2 years and her physician advised resuming dairy intake, telling mother that "infants outgrow their milk allergy". The child went on to display chronic respiratory symptoms, and had odd "mysterious" illnesses with fevers, aching, headaches, and somtimes abdominal pains for the past 5 years; although none of the prior illnesses were as severe as her present illness, the pattern was well-established before the avalanche effect occured. The myth that "children outgrow their food allergy" has been prepetuated by pediatricians who do not notice how the food allergy pattern shifts and evolves over time and who do not study adults who display the slow, logical progession of food allergy over decades.

The 9 year old girl and the 34 year old woman are on a continuum of a disease-making process that continues through life. The undercurrent is a set of problems in the food supply and the surface expressions are the result of many factors combining at any given time. Both these examples have food allergy or "milk-wheat disease", one of the most prevelant forms of food allergy. Both improve dramatically with complete diet revision; both do better if they continue to live without milk or wheat in their diet. The 34 year old woman must stop smoking before she is well again; as she recovers with initial diet revision, she finds that each cigarette she smokes makes her dopey and sick; the cigarettes alone will inflame her throat, enlarge her lymph nodes, and rob her of mental and physical energy. When she is completely clear, she finds that she can no longer stand the company of smokers.

Per Bak and Kan Chen, writing about castrophe theory,[2] state that:

> "Large interactive systems perpetually organize themselves to a critical state in which
> a minor event starts a chain reaction that can lead to a catastrophe."

They describe their theory of "self-organized criticality" to explain how complex systems (such as a person interacting with his/her environment) may suddenly collapse. Castrophe may strike because of ordinary events, often repeated; no new, dramatic ingredient is required. An avalanche or earthquake waits to happen, sometimes for long periods, quietly accumulating probability until finally the system shifts or collapses. The concepts of human illness tend to emphasize a less sophisticated concept of "one illness, one cause", supporting our bad habits and false-beliefs that everything is OK.

As the world changes, so do our illness patterns. Our medical model, with its rigid diagnostic categories and overly simplistic views of human biology, has trouble keeping up with changes. We may have to change the way we teach and practice medicine. No medical specialty has assumed the clinical responsibility of applying knowledge of environmental principles, ecology, or toxicology. Public heath physicians have been the only professionals with a community perspective in medicine, but tend to get bogged down, inspecting restaurants for cleanliness and tracking infectious illnesses; massive violations of good environmental practice have eluded public health scrutiny and control for too many years. Milk and wheat disease, although well-documented in many specific instances has never been investigated systematically as an endemic problem in North America. Allergists often express an interest in understanding environment problems, but often limit their knowledge and practice to a few selected environmental problems, like allergy to dust and pollens which results in hay fever or asthma.

Chronic Fatigue Syndrome

Most patients we see have a combination of health problems, extending over a long time period; often complaining of disturbances in many parts of their body. Often the symptom list is long and perplexing. They have a multisystem, polysymptomatic disorder, and often do not respond to therapies offered them. They often have little tolerance for drugs and experience major side effects with many drugs. In terms of our well-established diagnostic entities, these complex disorders may not be well understood, and may be called Ill-Defined-Illness (IDI). We believe that IDI is often food-related and can often be solved by diet revision therapy.

The problem of non-recognition and denial of emergent, complex illnesses is exemplified by the plight of patients who suffer from a non-specific but chronic, often disabling illness with fatigue, weakness, muscle pains and other symptoms, suggestive of immune dsyfunction. This complex has been referred to as CFS, the "Chronic Fatigue Syndrome" or CFIDS, "Chronic Fatigue Immune Dysfunction Syndrome".

Unconcerned journalists have called CFS "Yuppie Flu". Another description of a similar symptoms-complex refers to "myalgia" or muscle pain and "encephalitis" or inflammation of the brain. The myalgic encephalitis (ME) description points to prevalent symptoms in patients with delayed-pattern food allergy; aching, fatigue, reduced exercise tolerance and cognitive dysfunction (especially difficulty concentrating and   remembering). The "candida theory" has also become a popular explanation of IDI with fatigue. Many of the articles in a journal for chronic fatigue suffers[3] address the problems of dsicrimination and even abuse of these patients. A coalition of CFS advocate call themselves CACTUS to "bring the reality of chronic fatigue immune dysfunction syndrome top national attention." A significant section in this journal reviews the ignorance and denial that long-suffering patients face from some professionals and some media. Government agencies have not been particularly supportive. No-one writing in this journal seems to know that CFS is often food-related illness and no-one has made it clear that therapy should begin (and often ends successfully) with adequate diet revision. The favored theories are the most simpistic; viruses are the most popular.

The symptom complex described as CFS or CFIDS includes:

Fatigue	Sore throat
Lymph node swelling	Muscle pain
Muscle weakness	Headaches
Depression	Sleep disturbance
Fever	Memory loss

The two patients described above fit the CFIDS description, but we already know (in their case) this is delayed pattern food allergy or milk-wheat disease; and we know these patients get better with Core Program diet revision! We are again reminded of the Sufi parable quoted at the beginning of this book. The observers are relative blind to WIRGO and come up with a variety of descriptions and a variety of names for the polypmorphous events that different patients manifest.

Fatigue and pain are two of the most common human symptoms and often dominate IDI patterns. Multiple causes can be suggested for fatigue. The simplest medical investigation looks for anemia, thyroid problems, and evidence of liver or kidney disease. Food supply and metabolic problems are usually not considered. Toxicity from industrial and domestic sources is rarely considered. Similar syndromes have been described in the Medical literature over many years. Neurasthenia is old term that suggests the same illness pattern has been recognized for many years. Dr. A.J. Rowe[4], Dr. T.G. Randolph[5], and Dr. Fredrick Speer were among the first American allergists to associate CFS with food and inhalant allergies. Dr.Speer referred to the "allergic-tension-fatigue" syndrome, [6] [7] and described "motor fatigue":

> *" People...complain of weakness, fatigability, and achiness... many find it difficult to carry on sustained activity of any kind and require more than normal amounts of physical and mental rest"*

Dr. Speer stated that "no patient should be classified as having a neurosis until allergy has been considered." His good advice is still being ignored. Stephen Strauss and associates and the National Institutes of Health noted a high prevalence of allergy (of the immediate hypersensitivity, IgE variety) in patients with CFS.[8] While this correlation is interesting it may mislead both patients and physicians into reliance on skin testing to define "allergy". The authors of this paper failed to differentiate food from airborne allergy and failed to mention the delayed patterns of immune activity to food antigens. These references to a limited definition of allergy need to be clarified in a sophisticated model of disease before Dr. Speer' advice becomes fully operational. The majority of patients we see with CFS do not have skin test positive food allergy but they do have symptoms of food allergy and they do get better with diet revision.

Allergy, Toxicity

Air and food-borne chemical toxicity has been identified as the cause of many illness patterns. Patients with "environmental hypersensitivity" have been identified, especially by a group of American physicians who call themselves "clinical ecologists. They often acknowledged patients' illnesses when other physicians dismissed their suffering as psychosomatic. Unfortunately, the clinical ecology movement remained outside the power structures in American medicine and failed to convince skeptical colleagues that environmental issues were important. Their concern about chemical pollution of the environment was politically unpopular and threatened many powerful lobbies who attempted to discredit both suffering patients and their sympathetic physicians.

Drs. Rae, Laseter and their associates at the environmental Health center in Dallas, Texas, have published studies on the role of pesticides in producing human illness.[9] They report finding pesticides in the blood of 200 sick patients who suffer environmental sensitivity. DDT was found in 62%, hexacholobenzene in 57.5%, Heptachlor epoxide in 54%, Beta-BHC in 34%, Endosulfan in 34%, Dieldrin in 24%, and Chlordane in 20%. Other pesticides were also found. Only 1% of the patients tested were free of pesticides! They treated patients in a specially designed, pesticide-free and chemically reduced environment within a hospital and carefully managed their food intake. Dr. Rae suggested that brain dysfunction, expressed by depression, irritability, altered sensation, movement disorders, attention and memory deficits, could be blamed on pesticides. Dr. Rae states:[10]

> "Airborne chlorinated pesticides are ubiquitous, resulting in a broad public exposure to potentially hazardous material.... By 1980, over 400 synthetic chemicals have been identified in human tissues...At low levels of exposure, the effects may differ in different individuals ... Behavioral changes could promote interpersonal difficulties because of the affected individual's depression , irritability, level of activity..."

Alan Anderson, writing in Psychology Today,[11] reviewed the importance of nervous system toxins from the environment in causing psychological malfunction. He stated:

> "Of the 100,000 or so chemicals now in use by American industry, 575 are deemed dangerous in large doses by the Federal Government, and many of these are known to be associated with catastrophic illness, from cancer to respiratory disease. Perhaps no class of chemicals is more subtle and treacherous in its effects, however, than neurotoxins, which can damage the nervous system even in modest doses and cause a variety of behavioral and emotional symptoms – among them, hallucinations, loss of memory, confusion, depression and psychosis."

Among the neurotoxins cited; lead, mercury compounds, pesticides, herbicides, fungicides, aluminum, styrene, tetrachlorobiphenyl, and dioxins may contaminate our food supply. The Environmental Protection Agency in the USA reported that the magnitude of chemical contamination of the USA in 1987 was 9.7 billion pounds of chemicals into streams and 2.7 billion pounds into the air. We have a hard time even imagining what a billion pounds looks or feels like; remember that a billion is 1,000,000,000. The allowance of toxic chemicals for each citizen is about 50 pounds.

Ironically, if a sick person approaches your average physician saying "I am being poisoned", he is sent to a psychiatrist. The patient must reply "Just because I'm paranoid, doesn't mean they aren't trying to poison me!".

Individual sensitivity to contaminant chemicals varies, and is interactive with other chemical stressors. The biological effects of agricultural chemicals in the human body at any level are not so well-known that any authority can assure you all is well. Chronic exposure to low doses of chemicals is likely to lead to biological chaos, chronic illness, and sooner or later, avalanche into catastrophic illness. People who use pesticides on a regular basis obviously risk toxicity and should reconsider this use. The effect of agricultural chemical contamination of the food supply is not clearly known; changes in immune function, brain disturbances and cancer are the first concerns. Pesticides are generally distributed in the environment and need not be sprayed directly on crops to contaminate them. Even DDT which is banned in North America still shows up here carried on air currents from distant countries who continue to use it.

PCB's and Dioxins are groups of highly toxic chlorinated hydrocarbons, originating in agricultural and industrial chemicals and persisting in the environment for many years. PCB's (polychlorinated biphenyls) are the best known source of dioxins. PCB's have been used extensively in industry since the 1930's. Swedish scientists first noted PCB's in birds in 1966. Since then, many studies have documented the existence of PCB's in animals, plants, and fresh water supplies. Recent spills of PCB's from transformers in electrical systems; criminal efforts to sell PCB-contaminated fuels; and orphan containers of PCB wastes looking for disposal sites have been newsworthy reminders of dioxin hazards. Industrialized society is not prepared to cope with its own poisons.

The herbicide-defoliant Agent Orange gained notoriety after it was sprayed over 6 million acres of Vietnam to kill foliage. Agent orange was a mixture of 2 common herbicides; 2,4,5-T, banned in 1985, and 2,4-D, which remains the most used herbicide in the USA at about 65 million pounds per year. Cancer is the main consequence of 2,4-D exposure with high incidence of lymphatic cancers in Canadian and American farmers who sprayed the herbicide on their fields over many years; and concern has been voiced about brain tumors seen in test mice exposed to 2,4-D. Cancer causation is most likely linked to dioxins; there are 75 related poisons in the dioxin group; 2,4-D's most toxic component is TCDD (tetrachlorodibenzo-para-dioxin). TCDD is also produced by combustion of wastes in municipal incinerators, and by chemical industries, and pulp mills. Schecter [12] reported finding alarmingly high levels of TCDD in the breast milk of American and Canadian mothers. Evidently, dioxins are widely distributed in our food supply, and are stored in the fat of our bodies, once ingested. Elevated dioxin levels have been found in poultry, pork, beef, milk, eggs, and fish. Dioxins have appeared in beached-paper containers of food products, including milk and fruit juice cartons. Dr. Shecter was quoted:

> "Breast-fed infants represent a population with daily exposure to dioxins and related chemicals and I am very concerned about the potential health effects at the levels we found."

The mechanism of dioxin toxicity has been studied; it binds to a special receptor inside cells and then binds to DNA[13], altering the reading of the DNA code that runs the cell. A small alteration in the interpretation of DNA has profound effects on the life of a cell and its progeny. The idea now is that dioxins work much like regulatory hormones with a malevolent purpose. With a half life of 5 years this compound could conceivably cause profound and delayed-onset disease in low concentrations.

Writing in the Annals of Allergy, Selner and Staudenmayer encouraged "allergists to expand their environmental intolerance to include chemicals found in everyday practice."[14] They point out that chemicals can produce the same symptoms as IgE-mediated allergy, and can mimic flu-like illnesses. Evaluation of chemical toxicity is not, however, a medical office task. Nor is it a laboratory task in the local hospital or university laboratory; nor can government agencies routinely test individuals for chemical contamination; the measuring technology is simply not available. Doctors who propose to test patients in their office by offering chemical tests - injected, dropped under the tongue, inhaled, even ingested are playing childish games with very complex and serious problems. Worse hocus-pocus occurs with muscle testing and vega meters; nonsensical techniques which are nevertheless popular.

The effects of chemicals are multiple, additive, and stretch-out over time. Reluctantly, we have to accept that there is no convenient technology to assess the role of chemical toxicity in any individual. Obviously, whenever modern citizens are ill, there are multiple causes to consider and chemical toxicity should not be easily dismissed. Physicians must assume that patients symptoms are legitimate. Patients must assume that the physician does not know what is really going-on. You need a very sophisticated research lab to detect intracellular dioxin-receptor complexes. The physician must assume that you are suffering changes in intracellular function that cause symptoms and realize that these intracellular changes cannot be measured in the clinical laboratory!

The best position re: diagnosis and treatment of chemical toxicity may be summarized:

The differential diagnosis of mysterious illness should now include allergy, environmental toxicity, other food problems and viruses as the top four potential causes. Our theories should not state that single agents act alone to produce illness, but that multiple factors combine to produce the unwanted results.

At times we wonder if food is becoming too unsafe for people to eat; certainly it seems so with some sick, hypersensitive individuals. Various detoxification regimes have been promoted to "detoxify the body". Some employ fasting, vitamin and mineral supplements, chelating agents and even sweating in saunas or hot tubs. We doubt these methods have any value but we do not have all the answers. Serious research into chemical contamination and decontamination is urgently needed. The Core Program is designed to reduce intake of food additives and contaminants. The most austere clearing program employs an elemental nutrient formula, composed of nutrients in their pure form with no other food intake. The advantage of an ENF is to allow a sick person to return to a baseline of normal functioning, without the intake of the numerous adverse substances that may have been present in their food supply. Over time, the body has a tendency to excrete toxic materials; however, the potential for long-term toxicity of dioxins and other poisons means that only avoidance will protect us from their ravages. On the Core Program, clearing of symptoms may take weeks to months to years; we encourage patients to continue careful eating for several months before giving up hope that they will get better, even when initial results are disappointing.

Viruses and Allergy

Mysterious illness is often blamed on viruses. Since viruses are just bits of genetic code, are universally available, and have a proclivity to subvert the normal functioning of all living organisms; it is probably appropriate that we think of viral problems at all times. The Epstein-Barr (EB) virus has been blamed for the CFS. EB virus causes infectious mononucleosis, which presents with symptoms of the CFS which usually resolve within 6 weeks. Mono symptoms are also the symptoms of chronic delayed pattern food allergy; the major difference is that food materials, not the virus maintain the pathological immune activity for months or years. Too frequently the EB virus explanation is accepted uncritically. Now the EB virus antibody titre is measured in the blood and, if it is high, people are told they have "chronic EB virus infection"; go home and wait for it to go away.

Myalgia and encephalitic symptoms have also been blamed on viruses; the symptoms often resemble a mild polio attack. Resident brain viruses, herpes simplex and zoster, are among the suspects.

Dr. DeFreitas of the Wistar Institute in Philadelphia reported finding bits of retrovirus proteins in the cells of patients with CFS. The retrovirus family includes HIV, the virus of AIDS and HTLV-II, a virus associated with hairy-cell leukemia. HTLV viruses attack lymphocytes which are the infantry of the immune system. The HIV virus eventually destroys T4 lymphocytes, leaving victims vulnerable to infections by organisms that rarely bother immune-competent individuals. The early symptoms associated with HIV positive patients has been called the "AIDS Related Complex" are similar to the symptoms of delayed pattern food allergy in patients with no HIV. We can speculate that HIV triggers an allergic hypersensitivity in the early stages of infection, and early symptoms of the illness can be controlled by regulating the food supply, air and water. If the HIV eventually destroys enough T4 lymphocytes to damage the defence against infection, food control loses efficacy. Our concept of ADS and avalanche allows us to view HIV infection in a hopeful manner. The presence of HIV alone will not decide that you get AIDS; other factors will decide; if you could control those other factors, you can remain well. Diet revision looks very attractive.

Even if viruses such as the Epstein Barr Virus, Herpes, HIV play a role in IDI, they are not the only cause of chronic illness patterns. Host factors, not the mere presence of the virus, determine what the illness is and what the illness does. For example, viruses may act as non-specific immune-system activators and increase allergic hypersensitivity to food and airborne antigens. We often record the history of a viral illness, which runs its course in a matter of weeks, but leaves the patient in an altered state, hypersensitive to foods, drugs, and chemicals encountered in the environment. Often, it seems like the "flu" or a "mono" infection, but the patient will state that "it never goes away".

If the symptom complex fits the description of illness patterns, outlined in the next three chapters, we set about to do vigorous diet revision, even if the patient does not think that their problem has anything to do with their food. Because of variable and delayed symptoms after eating food, most of the patients we see have not identified food causes of their illness. We find that diet revision improves the majority of these patients and, in the best case, restores normal functioning. Patients with known food allergy will think they have recurring "Flu or Colds" because their recurrent symptoms from food allergens are the same symptoms experienced with a viral infection. Active food allergy may reduce the effectiveness of immune surveillance against viruses, making our story even more complex; often we see patients with recurrent herpes outbreaks, increased incidence of warts, and crops of molluscum contagiosum, all viral infections. Immune hyperactivity is associated with selective immune suppression! We wonder if food allergy is one of the mechanisms which turns HIV positive individuals into AIDS patients? A variety of immune cell and immunoglobulin abnormalities show up in the food allergy complex, but none to date have proven consistent markers of the disease. Since their are several kinds of food allergy we would not expect to find simple patterns. Food allergy research provides a wealth of interesting measurements of "immune dysfunction" and should be considered by anyone interested in CFIDS or ARC. (See the following chapters and section 3 for further explanation).

Other Examples of Food-Related Illness

A new syndrome, the Eosinophilic Myalgia Syndrome (EMS), first reported in the USA in '89, involved severe muscle aching with itching, rashes, and breathing problems. EMS was linked to the ingestion of capsules containing the amino acid, l-trytophan. L-tryptophan is a perfectly normal, essential amino acid which present in all food; high levels are found in milk. Subsequent investigation showed that the problem-causing l-tryptophan was manufactured by one Japanese company, Showa Denko and contained a specific impurity (DTAA) which activated immune cells. The company had used recombinant DNA technology to modify the bacteria used to synthesize tryptophan and evidence suggests that the modified bacteria began to synthesisize trace amounts of DTAA, which, as bad luck would have it, acted as a hypersensitivity-inducing agent. The attempted changes in the bacterial production of DNA are the result of interesting and very important early research on the gene regulation of cellular metabolism. The first discovery that nutrients regulated gene expression involved trytophan in bacteria; when the concentration of tryptophan decreased, the gene, coding the synthesis of the amino acid, would be turned-on and when trytophan increased the gene is turned off. The exact mechanisms of gene control have been intensively studied and the regulatory parts of DNA well-identified. The application of this knowledge in modifying bacteria to produce trytophan more efficiently would have been irresistable.

EMS is similar to the presentation of muscle pain, asthma, and other inflammatory activities in a general population of patients with food allergy and a related group of patients with auto-immune diseases. EMS perhaps provides another clue to immune-mediated disorders and should be viewed as an example of endemic food-related illnesses; not as a unique, separate disorder. The Showa Denko impurities may be representative of a class of substances found in the food supply that induce hypersensitivity. Patients with EMS should give diet revision a try; they may just have delayed pattern food allergy. An troubling side-issue of EMS is the U.S. FDA's move to remove all products containing tryptophan; an obvious case of over-reaction. Trytophan from many different sources continues to be safe with many potential benefits. In Canada, tryptophan was placed on a prescription list, and continues to be available as an alternative to sleeping pills or an aid to the treatment of depression. As an essential nutrient, trytophan is a necessary ingredient of elemental nutrients formulas which we highly recommend for the treatment of allergic disease, inflammatory bowel disease and a host of other applications. Tryptophan is also essential in therapeutic formulas for infants and children with inborn errors of metabolism. The National Council for Improved Health[15] "is actively opposing HR3688, a federal bill to ban the sale of L-tryptophan, a supplement millions of Americans have taken for years." Members of this council believe that the U.S. FDA discriminates against the nutritional industry in favor of drug company monopolies.

EMS has been compared to the Toxic Oil Syndrome (TOS) which appeared in Spain in 1981. The TOS was blamed on a cooking oil sold in unmarked 5 liter bottles, which was contaminated with aniline. Fatty acid anilides were thought to be the agents of this disease, although studies of this localized food-related illness were never carried to a satisfactory conclusion. TOS often presented as severe muscle aches and progressed to diffuse inflammatory disease which resulted in about 800 documented deaths.While TOS was investigated and EMS is now being investigated intensively as a curious, separate disorder, millions of people are suffering TOS and EMS-like syndrome from food everyday with no benefit of research, diagnosis or treatment.

In this review, the collection of ill-defined inflammatory disorders is placed under the title "Food Allergy". The two things we know are 1) that immune activity is likely involved in these diseases and 2) that changing the food supply of the victims, improves their condition. For years, has shown major health risks from milk and wheat, but little is ever said about these problems and no major public health investigation has ever been undertaken. If we were really interested in the truth of disease, milk, wheat, and other foods should be under intensive investigation as causes of common diseases.

Other patterns of illness give us further clues about allergic hypersensitivity as a common mechanism of illness. For years, a variety of auto-immune diseases (AD) have be recognized. Systemic Lupus Erythematosis (SLE) is an immune-mediated disease which contains all the symptoms of CFS, ME, EMS, TOS and serves as a model of allergic hypersensitivity. Many of our food allergy patients have lupus-like symptoms and signs for years, but only a small subgroup crosses over or decompensates into the more severe illness, SLE. The diagnosis of SLE depends on finding specific auto-antibodies in the blood, and demonstrating target organ damage from immune-mediated inflammation. SLE is probably bad food allergy plus an added self-destructive component. We think SLE patients should be on strict diet control along with immune-suppression therapy whenever their disease flares. (More on SLE in the next chapter).

The experiences of people with mysterious, prolonged illness is cause for great concern. They present the leading edge of endemic food-related and environmental illnesses. We should assume that these emergent illness patterns are problems in our air, food, and water until proven otherwise. Our list of causes does not include "psychogenic, psychological, or psychiatric" causes. These terms only serve to perpetuate psychosomatic myths and ignorance of biological causes, especially problems in the food supply and environment, which make whole populations of people mysteriously ill.

> *The CFIDS is delayed pattern food allergy until proven otherwise. Everyone with any version of IDI should try diet revision, using the Core Program, carefully and thoroughly, before accepting other explanations or treatment of their disease!*

Some patients we have treated with Chronic Fatigue Syndrome have a complex illness which takes months or years to resolve. They seem to have lost all tolerance to foods and only feel well if they live on a minimal diet, usually with **Phase 1 foods**, supplemented with an elemental nutrient formula for several months. They are hypersensitive to chemicals in their environment, and often need special protection. They often need medication to modify or suppress their immune response. Some are threatened by tissue damage from allergic reactions to food antigens and need protection with prednisone, ketotifen and/or sodium cromoglycate. Their experience is especially distressing, since it points to our ignorance about the original causes of food problems. We need a satellite picture of human illness which reveals the changing patterns of common illnesses. It is not popular to suggest that people are being systemically poisoned by toxins, delivered in the air, water and food, but it is probably true. It is not popular to suggest that staple foods cause our endemic and new epidemic illnesses, but again, it is probably true.

---

[1]Knicker WT. Deciding the Future for the Practice of Allergy and Immunology Annals of Allergy 198;55:106–113

[2]Bak P., Kan C., Self-Organized Criticality. Sc American Jan '91;46–53.

[3]CFIDS Chronicle 1990. CFIDS Ass'n Inc. Box 220398 Charlotte, NC 28222-0398 USA

[4]Rowe, A.J. Allergic toxemia and migraine due to food allergy. Calif West Med, 33:785,1930,

[5]Randolph T.G. Allergy as a Causative factor in fatigue, irritability, and behavior problems in children. J. Pediat, 31:560,1947

[6]Speer, F. The allergic-tension-fatigue syndrome. Pediat Clin N. Amer, 1:1019,1954

[7]The allergic-tension-fatigue syndrome: Allergy of the Nervous System. Charles C. Thomas Pub. 1970:14-27

[8]Strauss S.E., Dale J.K., Wright RN, Metcalfe D.; Allergy and the chronic fatigue syndrome. J. Allergy Clin Immunol;81:5,1; 791-795;1988

[9]Laseter, J.L., Ildefonso De Leon, Rae, W.J., Butler,J Chlorinated hydrocarbon pesticides in environmentally senstitive patients. Clin, Ecology II; 1;1983 3-12

[10]Rea W.J. et al Pesticides & brain-function changes in a controlled environment. Clin Ecology II,3:1984 145-150.

[11]Anderson A. Neurotoxic Follies. Psychology Today July 1982 30-42

[12]McGuire R. Dioxin shock hits home. Medical Post November 1986;22(39):1,12.

[13]Holloway,M. A Great Poison; Dioxin helps elucidate the function of genes . Sc. Am. Nov.1990;16-20.

[14]Selner C., Staudenmayer H. The practical approach to the evaluation of suspected environmental exposures: chemical intolerance. Annals of Allergy; 55 (1985) 665-673

[15]National Council for Improved Health: 28165B Front Street #196; Temecula CA 92390 USA. 1-714-699-8622.

Chapter 6

Diet Revision for Food Allergy

In this chapter, and in chapter 11 we will develop the fascinating story of food allergy. In the next chapter, case histories illustrate how symptom patterns combine differently in different individuals, but can be recognized as variations of a few basic disease-producing mechanisms, with food allergy as a common contributing cause.

There are different patterns of allergic disease. Food allergy is not one entity or pattern. Food allergy is a name used to describe **a host of immune responses to food materials** in GIT, blood, and tissue spaces. There is, however, no aggreement about the prevalence and importance of food allergy as a general disease mechanism. Outside the community of allergists there is general ignorance and neglect of these disease possibilities, so that it is impossible to estimate the prevalence of food allergy by using medical diagnoses. The presence of food allergy is concealed in a variety of other diagnoses. Most food allergists would agree that the expressions of food allergic disease are diverse, profound, and not completely discovered or described. [1] The lists of diseases, associated with food allergy, in this chapter began with a list developed by Drs. Buscinco, Benincori, and Cantani, published in the Annals of Allergy, December 1984, supplement on food allergy,[2] representing a conservative view of food allergic disease. They were addressing food allergy in children primarily. We find similar patterns in adults, with increasingly severe disease in patients as they get older. As a medical reference text, we suggest Brostroff and Challacombe's "Food Allergy and Intolerance". [3]

Food Allergy Symptoms

Food allergy would not be so mysterious if diagnosis of **immune-mediator patterns** were easy to make. Unfortunately, only well-equipped research labs can identify immune mediators, and even then, with difficulty. You can have a dramatic fireworks display of immune activity going on in your body without showing up on routine blood tests. Victims of these internal attacks of immune activity often describe genuine despair, and are convinced of imminent disaster, as a reaction unfolds. For example, a feeling of panic, shortness of breath, increased heart rate, often with skipped beats and a pounding sensation in the chest suggests a "heart attack" as immune mediators act on the lungs, the heart muscle and conduction system. Flushing, sweating, fevers with food allergy feel like inection or the "flu". The brain is involved in immune responses and disturbances to brain function vary from mild effects such as sleepiness, fogginess and confusion to major catastrophes, on the level of strokes, multiple sclerosis, and schizophrenia.

The biological design of immune responses includes increased arousal; an emergency mode of **"fight or flight"** to face the threat of the unseen invaders. This is a primitive and powerful response system which overtakes conscious control. The associated feeling state involves at least anxiety; and fear or panic, if the reaction is intense. These attacks are amplified reactions or hypersensitivity, exaggerated alarm responses to unrecognized physical stimuli. **Hypersensitivity** is determined at a cellular level and cannot be turned on or off by will-power or good intentions. These symptoms are not the inventions of the person's psyche, although too many patients are misunderstood; their panic is interpreted as something they invented, rather than an expression of a biological defense procedure, built into their body.

A reacting patient may overbreathe and develop additional symptoms (numbness, tingling, muscle cramps) from hyperventilation. The unwary physician may blame the entire experience on hyperventilation, ignoring the original trigger of the sympathetic arousal. Some patients display more fight than flight and become unusually aggressive verbally and /or physically. We think that food allergic reactions may be the underlying cause of un- necessary violence through activation of this sympathetic arousal.

Careful observers keep a daily log of their body intake, symptoms, and environment. The major obstacles to getting at the truth of events are preconceptions and interpretations. We need to observe first and interpret later. In other words, record the observation; "I ate chop suey, egg rolls, and pork with a sweet and sour sauce at a Chinese restaurant, and, within 20 minutes of starting the meal, experienced sharp shooting pains in my left temple, lasting over an hour", rather than recording the preconceived interpretation; "I got a headache 20 minutes after eating MSG." While MSG may have been a cause of the headache, there are thousands of other molecular species in the food ingested that could also trigger the headaches. We might find, for example, on subsequent eating experiences, that eating pork, prepared in many different styles, often triggers headache.

Specific symptoms suggest allergic mechanism very strongly; nose congestion, mucus production, flushing, lymph node swelling, tissue swelling, fever, chills, pain or itching are all suggestive of immune system involvement. Much of our suffering is the result of inflammation, a universal cause of pain in all our tissues. Medical students are taught the four signs of inflammation: **redness, swelling, heat, and pain.**

An oversimplified, but convenient, description of allergic patterns separates **immediate** hypersensitivity allergy from the less obvious and more complex "**delayed**" patterns of illness. Immediate food reactions such as lip and mouth swelling are obviously connected to food intake. The connection between food ingestion and delayed symptoms is less obvious. Most people do not notice the connection between food eaten and their body pains, fatigue, or mood disturbances. The patterns of immediate hypersensitivity are distinct from the delayed responses to food ingestion, but interactions seems to exist. We hasten to add (once again) that food interacts with the body complexly and immunological reposnses combine with other adverse effects to produce the disturbances that we feel. A variety of other terms are used by other authors to refer to distinctions that are either obscure or false; we have rejected terms such as "food sensitivity, food intolerance, false food allergy, pseudo food allergy". The pseudo-distinctions which refer to "pseudo-allergy" are particulary offensive .

Food allergic disturbances can be surprising in intensity and variety. **Symptom patterns** can be sorted into body systems, expressing the greatest disturbance, or we can sort problems in other ways, according to the underlying food chemistry, metabolic mistake, or immune mechanism involved. Symptoms tend to occur in pattern clusters and in sequences which tell us something about the defensive sensing and reacting mechanisms in our body. We often suffer gas, distension, and abdominal pain, for example, from problems in the digestive tract. The more serious food allergic diseases arise from mistakes made by the digestive tract in processing and absorbing food materials.

A common presentation of **delayed pattern food allergy** involves many symptoms in many parts of the body, changing over time. **Fatigue** and chronic **nose congestion** and/or increased **mucus** flow in the throat are perhaps the most common symptoms. **Flushing** of face, ears, and neck is another common reactive symptom, often occurring during or shortly after eating. Dark semi-circles with puffiness under the eyes are known as "**allergic shiners**" and are associated with edema or "bags" under the eyes, which conspicuously mark people with chronic food allergy. An astute observer can make the diagnosis of food allergy from across the room (congestion, flushing, shiners). Often tonsils, adenoids, and the neck **lymph nodes are enlarged**. These immune-system organs contain the sensing, reacting cells, which are stimulated by food allergens ingested every day, and enlarge to defend the body against the perceived "enemies" in food.

We refer to a complex of ear, nose, and throat food allergy symptoms as **Chronic Upper Respiratory Syndrome (CURS)**. Often, respiratory symptoms are associated with headaches, digestive symptoms, abdominal pain, muscle and joint pains, itches, rashes, hives, eczema, irritability, sleep disturbances, and nightmares. Restless or irritable behavior may be linked to difficulty concentrating, mental fogginess, memory loss, angry outbursts, moodiness, crying, and low self-esteem.

Food allergy is best diagnosed from the **characteristic history of illness**. The best clue is the presence of many symptoms, in many different parts of the body, over months to years. Skin tests do not reveal food allergy. Even if some skin tests are positive, these tests do not accurately predict the responses to foods eaten. Some food allergy is obvious. Immediate reactions include itching, flushing, hives, swelling, and attacks of asthma or life-threatening anaphylaxis. Patients who experience acute reactions repeatedly must follow a carefully chosen low-allergen diet and may not be safe eating-out, and eating packaged or processed foods. **The Core Program approach is a reasonable and convenient way to reconstruct a safe food supply.**

Anaphylaxis

The most **dangerous food allergy is anaphylaxis**, which can be a life-threatening emergency. After taking a drug or eating seafood, nuts, or some other allergenic food, a person may suddenly itch, flush, swell, have trouble breathing, panic, and collapse. Anaphylaxis can be triggered by foods, drugs, injections, insect stings, and vigorous exertion. The foods most commonly associated with anaphylaxis include milk, eggs, shrimp, fish, and peanuts. The drugs most commonly associated include pencillin, aspirin and anti-arthritic drugs, morphine, radiocontrast dyes, and anesthetics. A Woman in her late 20's took the antibiotic mixture, Bactrim, and described the following anaphylactic reaction:

> "My teeth started tingling and the inside of my throat was itchy...my palms got red and swollen. I felt light-headed and agitated. My heart started to race... by the time I got to the emergency my entire body had broken out in a rash and my feet were so swollen my boots wouldn't come off. But things got worse as soon as I walked in... I couldn't breathe and I began to panic. I felt I was going to die. The Doctor in charge was very short with me. He told me to get a hold of myself, that I was just making things worse, but I was out of control. I was terrified and wanted to pass out but couldn't."

Many by-standers do not appreciate the gravity of the allergic crisis. **Immediate treatment with injected adrenalin** and life support will rescue the anaphylaxis victim. We routinely administer prednisone in the dose range of 30-60 mg along with adrenalin to reduce the second, **late phase of anaphylaxis** which can develop into a prolonged illness, if left untreated. The initial immune response recruits other, more delayed immune responses. The late onset symptoms of drug and food allergy can only be blocked with steroid drugs, like cortisone, prednisone, and betamethasone. Anaphylaxis is usually unpredictable. Anyone at risk of this type of reaction should carry an **emergency kit** containing injectable adrenalin, antihistamine, and oral prednisone; and self-administer these drugs as soon as a major reaction begins. New labelling regulations may be helpful to some people to avoid dangerous food ingredients.

Anaphylaxis can be triggered by **exertion** after eating certain foods and may be responsible for sudden deaths in athletes, asthmatics, and other people with food allergy who exercise with unaccustomed vigor. Allergy patients are cautioned to exercise in gradually graded increments, watch food intake before athletic events, and avoid sudden, unaccustomed exertion. Anaphylaxis can occur at a lower intensity and recur at frequent intervals; frightening, but not life-threatening. Many people report a recurrent symptom-complex after eating reactive foods with itching, flushing, chest pain and tightness, shortness of breath, sometimes acute abdominal pain or intense headache, often with anxiety or fear. Often, alarmingly fast heart action, and irregular heart rhythms are associated. **Moderate anaphylaxis may be mis-diagnosed as "panic attacks".** Psychiatrists may prescribe tranquilizers without enquiring about allergenic triggers, usually foods or drugs. Many food allergic patients end up in the wrong department of the hospital, investigated for heart problems, neurological problems, or get trapped in a psychiatric ward under sedation and suspicion.

Circulating blood cells, basophils, and similar cells, mast cells, distributed through our tissues, are responsible for these acute defense procedures. The mechanism of the reactions probably varies. The result is always alarming and often dangerous.

Food Allergy as Chronic Illness

We use the diagnostic term **"delayed pattern food allergy"** to refer to a collection of disturbances which involve symptoms, typical of immune responses to food materials. A technical discussion would have to distinguish among many different patterns of immune-mediated disease and would appear too complex for this discussion. To make our descriptive task simpler, the general term "food allergy" will refer to a **whole set of food-body interactions** that generations of future scientists will eventually sort out. The practical point in all the following discussions is that, even if we don't know the exact mechanisms of these problems, if you treat your disturbance as if it were food allergy, you will likely succeed in making yourself better. Remember that when you consult a physician, the doctor may have a completely different agenda from you. You just want to get better; the doctor may want to argue about definitions, invoke controversies within medical politics and may want assert his or her authority. If your symptom descriptions are not familiar to your physician, his or her agenda may be to dismiss your evidence and reassure you that "nothing is wrong," no matter how much you suffer!

The most common presentation of food allergy is a **chronic, slowly progressive illness** with many symptoms in many parts of the body. The illness may be mild and include nose congestion, headache, indigestion, flatulence, aching, stiffness and chronic fatigue. The illness may be severe and present as intractable asthma, chronic diarrhea, depression, skin disease, and/or arthritis. Since food allergy is a **whole-body disease,** a lottery selection of disturbances may evolve over many years. In many patients, we can trace the illness pattern back to infancy with slow, intermittent emergence of symptoms over many years. In other patients the illness begins abruptly with few prior symptoms and progresses rapidly. Food allergy is often confused with infections, bacterial and viral. The diagnosis may be "colds", "flu", Epstein Barr Virus, "Candida", chronic fatigue, fibromyalgia, myalgic encephalitis, or just "a virus". The food-allergy sufferer may be frequently ill with non-specific symptoms. **Flushing and sweating** are common symptoms, often with night sweats and low-grade fevers. Antibiotics, pain medications, cough or decongestant syrups, antacids, sleeping pills, tranquilizers, and antidepressants are often prescribed to no avail.

> *This multi-system and poly-symptomatic pattern of illness means food allergy until proven otherwise. A trial of the Core Program will often produce remission of symptoms, even when both patient and physician doubt that food has anything to do with causing the illness.*

The most common symptoms of chronic food allergy are:

Nose congestion	Sore throat	Cough
Headache	Aching and stiffness	Joint Pain
Nausea ,	Abdominal bloating	Abdominal pain
Indigestion	Constipation	Diarrhea
Fatigue	Depression	Irritability
Anger, excessive	Memory loss	Sleep Disturbances

The most common physical signs of food allergy are:

Allergic shiners	*Flushing*	*Throat inflammation*
Skin rashes	*Hives*	*Fever, sweating*
Enlarged lymph nodes	*Nose congestion*	*Edema*
Distension, abdomen	*Lung congestion*	*Abdominal tenderness*
Muscle tenderness	*Joint swelling*	*Fast heart rate*

Allergy expresses itself as inflammation in body tissues, targeted by immune cells and activated by food allergens. In medical descriptions, the suffix "itis" means inflammation. Thus, "rhinitis" means nose inflammation; "arthritis" means joint inflammation, and so on. A simple rule of thumb is that any disease whose description ends in "itis" could be caused by food allergy. Chapter 7 provides case histories of illness patterns in actual patients who improved on the Core Program.

Food Allergy as Ear, Nose, Throat and Respiratory Problems

DIAGNOSIS	MAIN SYMPTOMS
Rhinitis	nose congestion and inflammation
Sinusitis	sinus congestion and inflammation
Pharyngitis	throat inflammation, swelling, mucus
URI	colds, coughs, congestion
Bronchitis	coughs, shortness of breath
Asthma	coughs, wheezing, shortness of breath
Pneumonia	coughs, fever, inflammation of the lung
Hearing loss	muffled hearing, loss of hearing
Tinnitus	ringing in the ear
Otitis media	middle ear fluid, infection

Eye, Ear, Nose and Throat

The eye, ear, nose, and throat are common target organs for food allergens. **Food allergy** is suggested by: **nasal stuffiness**, increased **mucus** flow in nose and throat, **sore throats**, swelling of the neck **lymph nodes** ("glands"), chronic or recurrent **cough**, episodes of **chest pain**, "tightness", and **wheezing** with shortness of breath. Often **ear and hearing symptoms** recur; ear-plugging with muffled hearing and ringing in the ears, are common symptoms; the diagnosis of recurrent middle ear "infection" may be made with frequent antibiotic prescriptions. Patients often report **dizziness** and balance problems, suggesting allergic involvement of the inner ear. Occasionally, severe attacks of **vertigo** (dizziness, turning sensations and imbalance) sometimes with vomiting will occur with food allergy. Three related symptoms; vertigo, ringing in the ears (tinnitus), and hearing loss occur together in **Meniere's Disease.** Food allergy is one of several mechanisms that should be considered when Meniere's disease strikes. Milk, wheat and egg allergy are the most common causes of respiratory symptoms, but other foods can do this. Ingested food additives, food dyes, sulphites, and salicylates are also implicated.

Allergy to airborne materials is often confused with food allergy. Symptom patterns may be similar, but the mechanisms are different. **Inflammation** of the nose (rhinitis), sinuses (sinusitis), and throat (pharyngitis) may be due to airborne irritants and allergens and/or food allergy. Sneezing, nose congestion, and eye irritation may come from both airborne and food allergens at the same time, or at different times during the year. It is better to think of food allergy as a separate problem which might co-exist with, for example, hayfever. Often patients are given medication or shots against airborne allergens, and food problems are neglected. We have found it better to solve the food problems first, since reactivity to airborne allergens changes with diet revision and may improve.

Eye symptoms are also common in food allergy. Red, itchy eyes are the most common complaints. Blurring of vision is reported frequently and may be associated with migraine headaches. Small changes in the cornea with surface inflammation may be reported as changes in focusing ability or blurring. Migraine auras often involve dramatic visual changes with geometric figures appearing in the visual field, flashing lights, and sometimes abrupt loss of vision. Pain around and behind the eye is common in migraine. In cluster headaches, a migraine variant, eye pain, reddening and profuse tearing occur. More serious threats to vision occur with the more serious forms of food allergy; and especially as food allergy turns into autoimmune disease. The major concern is inflammation in the small blood vessels of the retina and in the retina itself; permanent visual loss can occur, prompt treatment of mysterious **retinal inflammation** with an **ENF** (no food problems allowed in!) and prednisone may save vision.

Asthma and Lung Disease

Asthma, chronic bronchitis, and "pneumonia" are all possible consequences of **food allergy**. Asthma is increasing world-wide and increasing deaths from asthma in affluent countries worries authorities. The Center for Disease Control in Canada reported a threefold increase of asthmatic deaths over 20 years, mostly in teenagers and young adults. Air pollution is one obvious concern, but other problems must be considered. Often, asthma is treated only as an airborne allergy problem or as a problem unrelated to allergic processes and the possible role of food allergy is neglected! Dr. Wraith stated in FA&I:[4]

> "Food allergy is a very important cause of asthma but is often overlooked. It is important because it may cause severe symptoms and asthma still has a high mortality despite improvements in drug therapy. It is overlooked because the usual skin tests are often negative and the history is often not helpful as symptoms appear gradually hours or days after ingestion of the food."

Drs. Pelikan and Pelikan-Filipek demonstrated lung responses top food challenges[5] and suggested:

> "The role of food allergy in patients with bronchial complaints is still underestimated by clinicians because (1) of the dearth of information in this area. (2) The involvement of foods in patients with allergic disorders is very complex and has various forms...(3) The diagnostic procedures and confirmation of the involvement of adverse reactions to foods ...is a difficult problem."

Chronic coughs may mean **allergic bronchitis** with or without asthma. Food allergy patients are often given antibiotics repeatedly since allergic symptoms and infection symptoms are similar. Antibiotics may offer no benefits and may increase the risk of further allergic reactions. Many patients report long-term deterioration after repeated or prolonged antibiotic use. This apparent adverse effect of antibiotics has been blamed on yeast overgrowth, but the real reason is probably more complex.

The mechanism of **food allergic lung disease** may involve the entry of food allergens from the digestive tract which then travel to the lungs. Food materials interact with immune defenses and arrive in the lungs via the blood stream or lymphatics. Food allergens may be found in the blood stream in circulating immune complexes which trigger the release of immune mediators in the bloodstream; these chemicals typically cause a variety of symptoms including constriction of the smooth muscle in the lungs; this brochoconstriction is the first event of an asthmatic attack. Later, the small tubes in the lung swell and plug with increased mucus secretion; this inflammatory phase is the most important mechanism of chronic asthmatic bronchitis. Patients with delayed pattern food allergy have the most severe and persistent inflammatory form of chronic asthma. The good news is that complete diet revision may allowremission of chronic symptoms.

Asthma that seems to originate inside the body (intrinsic asthma) should be treated as food allergy until proven otherwise. This assumption should lead to careful diet revision, using the Core Program. Our patients usually have asthma with associated symptoms that suggest a whole-body food allergy problem. Asthma is one of the 4 principle features of atopic allergy; associated with eczema, hay fever, and hives. Often these patients have positive skin tests to inhalant allergens, but may not show skin reactions to foods which prove to be a major problem. If all the attention is directed toward the more obvious, skin-positive inhalant allergies, an opportunity to benefit from diet revision is lost.

A **comprehensive management plan** will include solving the food allergy problem, solving airborne allergy and toxicity, and providing the right medication, at the right doses, and the right time when preventive efforts fail. The most serious airborne problems ar home are cigarette smoke, dust, molds, and house dust mites.

Drug treatment strategies have shifted away from drugs which relax smooth muscle and dilate the branching tubes in the lung to drugs which block allergic reactions and reduce inflammation. Thus **cromoglycate (intal, fivent)or nedocromil (Tilade)** by inhalation or more recently **ketotifen** orally have been favored to block allergic reactions as a preventative measure; and inhaled **steroids** (beclovent) have become "first line of defence" in treating chronic asthma. The **bronchodilators** (ventolin, bricanyl, berotec) are used to treat the acute wheezing attacks, along with steroids which lock the delayed inflammatory swelling effects. Prednisone orally is prescribed if the asthma eludes control by inhaled steroids. Patients on the Core program experience a reduction or clearing of asthma symptoms, but are vulnerable to acute attacks if they eat the wrong food. The attacks occur in a typical sequence, beginning with an immediate episode of congestion, coughing and/or wheezing, followed several hours later by a delayed, more serious episode of breathing difficulty. The initial reaction should be treated with a bronchodilator (ventolin) and a generous dose of steroid (beclovent) which attenuates the delayed response. We also recommend retreating to phase 1 foods or an **ENF** for a few days if the attack is severe.

An occasional patient will react catastrophically to food allergens with a life-threatening breathing problem as an immediate anaphylactic reaction or a more delayed **"pneumonia"** (inflammatory swelling and edema of the lungs) and will require hospital treatment with adrenalin, nebulizers, oxygen, and steroids. A milk-triggered pneumonia in infants was reported by Heiner and Sears[6]. A complex of symptoms associated with pneumonia became the **Heiner Syndrome**, not a separate, discrete disease, but a collection of problems typical of food allergy; these infants have ear, nose and throat symptom, vomiting, colic and anemia form blood loss and iron malabsorption. Removing cow's milk from the diet cures this milk-disease! We see similar collections of problems in adults to milk and other food allergens.

Food Allergy as Abdominal, Digestive Disorders

The logical source of problems in our digestive tract is the food passing through it! The best way to deal with digestive problems is to change your food supply. Remove the problem using Diet Revision Therapy! The following list summarizes the common diagnostic entities which involve food problems, and food allergy in particular:

DIAGNOSIS	SYMPTOMS
Edema, angioedema	swelling of lips, tongue, throat
Bloating	increased gas with distention
Stomatitis	sore mouth, tongue burning
Gastritis	stomach pain, nausea, vomiting
Vomiting	getting sick and bringing-up food
Diarrhea	loose to watery bowel movements
Abdominal pain	pain can be crampy of prolonged
Ileitis	inflammation of the ileum
Colitis	inflammation of the colon
Ulcerative colitis	inflammation, bleeding of colon
Crohn's Disease	inflammation, usually ileitis
Proctitis	rectal pain, burning, l swelling
Malabsorption	failure to absorb nutrients
Intestinal bleeding	blood on stools, or black stools
Constipation	infrequent, difficult bowel movements

Introduction to GIT

Digestion is achieved by, our abdominal food processor, the "Gastro-Intestinal Tract". We refer to this system affectionately as "GIT". Other names for GIT include "digestive tract, stomach, small and large intestines, bowel, colon, and gut". Inflammation of various parts of GIT is described by terms using the suffix "itis" attached to the name of the GIT part; thus we have descriptive diagnostic names such as gastritis, colitis, ileitis, enterocolitis, hepatitis, cholecystitis".

The function of GIT is to process food. Each person's food supply must be matched to the capacity of their GIT to process food. Dysfunction and disease arises when there is a mismatch. GIT is not a passive processor of food, but, rather, it actively manages and responds to food with a peculiar kind of behavior. When all is well, we ignore the presence of GIT; our awareness is limited to full or empty sensations. When there is trouble in GIT, our attention is directed to our abdomen by a variety of discomforts, pain, noise, distension, and abnormal bowel movements. Food allergy and other forms of food intolerance such as lactose (milk sugar) intolerance are capable of producing a wide range of digestive problems.[7]

GIT's surface is sensitive, knowledgeable, and reactive. The sensing, deciding, acting functions of GIT are achieved by a complex system of nerves and cells of the immune-defense network, which extends along the surface. The velvety surface of GIT is described as mucosa. A continuous sensing apparatus in the mucosa is nicknamed **MALT,** short for its formal title, **Mucosa Associated Lymphatic Tissue.** Immune sensors in MALT trigger immune responses, and local food allergy symptoms in GIT are often the result. MALT sensors in our lips, tongue and mouth trigger symptoms like tingling, itching, burning, pain and swelling.

In a similar way, **MALT sensors** along the entire length of GIT can trigger symptoms, including itching, burning, pain and swelling at the anal exit. GIT knows when the wrong stuff has entered its space, and reacts defensively to get rid of it. Vomiting and diarrhea interrupt normal living in a distressing display of GIT's reactivity. Often the food input to GIT is neglected as a source of dysfunction or disease in GIT; an oversight that the Core Program is designed to correct.

GIT's job is to take apart complex food molecules and to absorb simpler, safer molecules. Nutrients are absorbed into the blood stream, both directly and indirectly via lymphatic circulation thru GIT. The GIT **lymphatic system** is a fluid transport system that allows cells and fat molecules to flow through lymphatic filters (lymph nodes) scattered around GIT. Eventually lymph fluid returns to the blood via the large vein (superior vena cava) which returns to the heart. All food molecules are absorbed by GIT, mostly from the small intestine (duodenum, jejunum, ileum).

Digestion of food is accomplished by secretions from GIT's surface and accessory glands. The liver and pancreas are the major secretory organs which contribute digestive factors. After food molecules are absorbed, they are carried in the venous blood (portal veins) from GIT to the liver.

The **liver** is a complex chemical factory, whose function is to control the food supply for the rest of the body. The liver's main task is to take in newly absorbed food molecules for further chemical processing, storage, and slow release. Food molecules leaving the liver are distributed throughout the body in the bloodstream. The liver also acts as immune-filter, removing some of the "wrong-stuff" admitted by mistake through the GIT wall. If the efficiency of the liver filter is reduced, food allergy symptoms are increased.

Our basic strategy to solve any complex food-related or GIT problem is to stop all food input into GIT and await spontaneous clearing of the problem. The use of pure, crystalline nutrients in an elemental nutrient formula (ENFood) bypasses all the digestive processes of GIT and reduces the input of wrong stuff to a minimal level.

Oral Effects of Food Reactions

Food allergy is first detected in the mouth. Our mouths are full of immune monitoring information. If we are willing to tune in sensations originating from oral sensors, sensitive, subtle signs of food reactions may be picked up in the mouth before more major trouble begins further along GIT, or internally in body space.

Swelling reactions of the lips, tongue, and throat express the most dramatic and sometimes serious allergic responses created by **MALT**. As offending, allergenic molecules pass through the mouth, surface antibodies, attached to mast cells, react with the food antigens, triggering swelling and inflammation of the lips, mouth surfaces, and throat. The reaction may be minute, limited to swelling of a small area on the tongue, or may cause a life-threatening **swelling** of the whole tongue and throat. Small ulcers (**aphthous ulcers**) are common consequences of a localized allergic reaction. Painful sensations are common, as nerve endings of the tongue, mouth, and throat are stimulated by inflammatory mediators. Taste sensations are often reported, including a generalized blunting of taste. The tongue feels coated, or tastes abnormally, often detecting a metallic taste, which may persist long after the offending substances are ingested.

Continuous allergic inflammation in the mouth and nose may obliterate pleasant eating sensations and is associated with disordered food selection. The complete sensation of taste is dependent on proper smell, obliterated by a stuffy, swollen nose. People with blunted taste often prefer heavy doses of the primary tastes, bitter, salt and sugar. The taste-impaired lose interest in more healthy foods with subtle flavors (especially vegetables), since they cannot perceive the natural flavors. This blunting of flavor sensation is one of the routes to faulty food selection.

Gastritis, Ulcer, Hiatus Hernia

Swallowed food descends through the chest in the esophagus, into the stomach. The surface continues to be sensitive to foods making contact and reactions do occur. Pain in the central chest may come from an inflammed espophagus; this is often burning in quality, but may be a severe ache, suggesting heart attack. "**Heartburn**" is the typical burning sensation from espophageal irritation, felt as pain ascending from the upper abdomen into the chest. A **hiatus hernia** may show up on the X-ray, but treatment with diet revision will help, regardless. Further down, in the stomach a surface reaction results in upper-middle abdominal pain, nausea and sometimes vomiting is triggered; a defensive reflex which gets rid of the offending food, usually relieving the pain. Some patients induce vomiting to avoid discomforts after eating. Recurrent irritation in the upper GIT is food-caused until proven otherwise. Obviously smoking, drinking alcoholic beverages, coffee and teas are the first problems to eliminate, but surface allergy to common foods may also be responsible. A trial of Core Program diet revision can provide prompt relief. If the clearing diet is un-successful, further investigation is always required.

Ulcers in the stomach or duodenum are usually attributed to excess stomach acid and treated with antihistamines which reduce acid secretion and antacids. In the past milk was recommended; but may be contra-indicated; **milk allergy** may be an original cause of gastritis which leads to ulceration. Recent evidence has implicated a surface **infection** by the bacteria, helicobacter pylori, in chronic gastritis and ulcer disease. If adequate diet revision does not prevent recurrent gastritis or ulcers, treatment of the infection is recommended, although this is not a simple matter; triple therapy with colloidal bismuth subcitrate, metronidazole, and tetracycline is recommended- get expert help.

Irritable Bowel Syndrome

A common GIT disturbance, characterized by abdominal pain, gas, and diarrhea, often alternating with constipation, has, in the past, been diagnosed as the "Irritable Bowel Syndrome" (IBS). IBS is an inadequate description of real, usually prolonged, suffering, incorrectly attributed to "psychogenic causes". We recognize that the label "psychogenic causes" describes a lack of biological understanding more than it describes the patient's problem. The old term "Irritable Bowel Syndrome (IBS)" is discarded and replaced by reference to the **ABCD (Abdominal pain, Bloating, Constipation, Diarrhea)** complex. The treatment of IBS, usually suggested includes bulk laxatives, tranquilizers, and drugs used to modify the behavior of GIT. After failure of these treatments, not infrequently, a trip to the psychiatrist is suggested. The success rate with these methods in one study[8] was only 12%! It is surprising that proper food studies have seldom undertaken in the assessment of patients with IBS. Patients are often told that they have GIT dysfunction because of "stress, tension, or anxiety". The truth is that patients have stress, tension, and anxiety because of bowel dysfunction! Food selection, emotional experiences, and eating behaviors interact complexly. Anger, frustration, and fear will influence food selection, appetite, digestion, and metabolism; while food selection, digestion, and metabolism will help determine emotional reactivity. There is a continuous loop of causal relationships, not a one-way vector.

Dietary advice commonly given includes bland diets usually with milk, or "high-fiber" diets with increased intake of cereal grains; both food groups are contraindicated. Studies, which allegedly rule out food intolerance, have been poorly conducted, often basing negative results on limited, ineffectual diet revision. Better studies have shown different aspects of foods interacting with GIT to produce the ABCD complex. In a study by V. Alum Jones et al, food intolerance was shown to be a major factor in causing the irritable bowel syndrome in 25 patients. The GIT disturbance was related to increased levels of Prostaglandin E2 (PGE2), synthesized and secreted by GIT itself. Prostaglandin production is inhibited by ASA, and symptoms may be blocked by ASA taken before meals. Another British study[9] implicated dairy products and grains in IBS; of 200 patients treated with diet revision, almost half improved. An Italian study[10] showed similar improvement on a restricted diet and increased GIT permeability was demonstrated in 3 patients. **Complete diet revision**, using the Core Program should help most ABCD suffers and careful food reintroduction should sustain remission. If careful diet revision is not successful in reducing symptoms, a careful investigation for other causes of GIT dysfunction should be carried out.

A common symptom of gastrointestinal food allergy is **rectal itching** and/or burning, and a perianal dermatitis.The irritation may also cause burning on urination. Yeast (candida) overgrowth occurs on the skin around the anus, groin, vulva, and vagina. These common symptoms may be related to food intake. Anti-fungal creams will clear the skin irritation in infants, children, and adults if proper diet revision also clears the original cause of allergic inflammation.

Wheat Disease

Whole grains have become popular foods. The idea of "wheat disease" is therefore unwelcome and widely discounted. Unfortunately, we must rank wheat disease, second only to milk disease when we review the experience of our patients. The four cereal grains, wheat, rye, oats and barley contain similar proteins, capable of exciting a variety of allergic responses and participate in a variety of diseases. Other problems in the grain supply remain to be defined; these include contamination with pesticides, ethylene bromide, and molds, especially egot and aspergillus. The Core Program excludes all cereal grains in phases 1 to 4, because of the high incidence of observed problems with cereal grain ingestion. In the past decade especially, a renewed enthusiasm for "whole grains" and increased dietary fiber has led to increased consumption of these cereal grains, and increased incidence of problems associated with these foods. We are now encouraged to eat whole grains, in unrefined form, often in combinations of whole grains.

The diseases which every textbook acknowledge are related to intolerance of cereal grains are **Celiac Disease,** and the skin disorder, **"Dermatitis Herpetiformis"**. These disturbances are caused by wheat proteins, collectively called **"Gluten"**. Gluten is a mixture of individual proteins, classified in two groups, the Prolamines and the Glutelins. Celiac disease presents as chronic diarrhea, with abdominal bloating, sometimes pain, and evidence of malabsorption certain nutrients. Often, an assortment of related whole-body problems accompanies celiac disease. We think the related problems are typical of delayed pattern food allergy. Celiac patients have increased gastrointestinal permeability[11] and demonstrate the whole-body effects of food allergy, including brain dysfunction, arthritis, and inflammatory lung disease. The celiac patient should seriously consider complete diet revision, not just gluten exclusion in an effort to avoid problems downstream from their GIT. A list of related disorders[12] resembles the list of disorders reviewed in this chapter; the working hypothesis - food allergy! Diabetes, thryroid disease, purpura, anemia, rheumatoid arthritis, sarcoidosis, vasculitis, lung disease, myositis, eye inflammation, and schizophrenia are all linked to gluten intolerance. The diagnosis of **Celiac disease (Gluten enteropathy)** is made clinically by typical history and confirmed by small intestine mucosal biopsy, which demonstrates atrophy of the absorptive surface. Celiac disease, as defined by the **biopsy** result, probably represents a specific endpoint for gluten reactions; one of many possible patterns of wheat allergy. Despite intensive study, the mechanism of Celiac Disease has not been finally determined. In an comprehensive review, Davidson and Bridges[13] describe the complicated mechanisms by which gluten proteins and/or their digestion products could damage the surface of GIT. While there is no reason to think that a single mechanism is responsible, we prefer the immune-mediated explanations of the disease; a cell-mediated type of allergy is likely involved with a host of complicated consequences, especially **increased permeability of GIT** with more problems downstream. It is too simplistic to think that just removing gluten will solve the whole problem of celiac disease. Comprehensive diet revision is desirable.

Wheat allergy may not show up as intestinal surface damage and a normal biopsy results is often misleading. Far too many patients have been dismissed without proper Diet Revision Therapy when a biopsy is reported as "normal"; they are told: "you do not have celiac disease; eat anything you like". This **diagnostic rigidity** manifests the classic error of **"treating the lab result"** and not the patient. Patients with chronic diarrhea and other symptoms suggestive of celiac disease often benefit from Diet Revision Therapy, regardless of the biopsy result.

Inflammatory Bowel Disease

Allergic Gastroenteritis, Crohn's Disease, and Ulcerative Colitis are all inflammatory diseases of the gastrointestinal tract. Crohn's disease usually begins in young people and tends to involve the end of the small intestine (ileum) in **inflammatory** swelling. Crohn's is associated with European and North American diets and is on the increase. As third world countries adopt our food choices, they report an increasing incidence of Crohn's disease in young people. Most often Crohn's disease is diagnosed after months or years of abdominal symptoms, especially pain, bloating and diarrhea. Early symptoms suggest the food allergy complex and may be first diagnosed as the irritable bowel syndrome. Ulcerative colitis usually presents as bloody diarrhea, containing mucus. Once ulcerated, the colon is slow to heal and this disease is often refractory to treatment; usually cortisone enemas and prolonged ingestion of an aspirin-like drug, asacol.

Crohn's disease is a model of food allergy and process. Patients with this disease usually have many other symptoms which suggest that diagnosis. Once the small intestine is inflamed, it becomes increasingly permeable[14]. This is an example of the "leaky" GIT which produces all the downstream effects of food allergy. Among these whole-body effects are various myalgia and arthritic patterns, brain disturbances and psoriasis.[15]

We are aware of patients with **Crohn's-like GIT disease.** They present with nonspecific, inflammatory symptoms; often diarrhea, pain and tenderness in the right lower quadrant of their abdomen, which suggests Crohn's disease. Fortunately, they often lack the characteristic signs of damage to their small intestine on X-ray or biopsy; and their disease may not progress over many years. These people are likely to have food allergy, plain and simple, and do best on ENFood, followed by the Core Program food reintroduction. By carefully regulating their food supply at a mild stage of the disease, these patients may avoid progression toward the damaged, end-stage inflammatory bowel disease.

Diet revision therapy, rigorously implemented and closely monitored, is essential in inflammatory bowel diseases and has, in our experience, produced clinical remission in responsive patients. Alun Jones and his associates in England demonstrated that specific foods exacerbated GIT symptoms and personalized food exclusion diets were successful in controlling the disease.[16] The use of an **Elemental Nutrient Formula (ENF)** is especially desirable in the management of Crohn's disease. [17] [18] [19] Remission of abdominal pain, diarrhea, and the associated generalized (food allergic) illness can be achieved by replacing food with an ENF with or without prednisone.[20] Once the inflammation is controlled, a slow, careful refeeding, using the Core Program should maintain control of the disease. Many Crohn's patients in remission show increased tolerance to foods after a food months; some take advantage of this, eat carelessly and have another acute episode of inflammatory disease. All relapses are treated the same way. Malabsorption is characteristic of inflammatory gastrointestinal disease and requires adequate nutrient supplementation and careful monitoring of the diet. Seriously ill patients often require prolonged treatment with an elemental nutrient formula and a carefully selected, safe-food list, usually limited to Phase 1 and 2 foods for months or years. Patients with ulcerative colitis do least well with DRT, but should always have the benefit of careful diet revision.

Skin Diseases

The skin expresses food problems in an obvious, eloquent way. Allergic reactions appear as rashes, flushing, bumps, hives, and swellings. The skin surface also accumulates damage and other artifacts. As the years pass, the skin accumulates a track record of ephemeral events. People with chronic, unresolved food allergy show many typical skin changes, especially "bags" under their eyes, dilated blood vessels on their face and trunk, roughened, sand-paper skin on their arms and back, and pigment changes. The following skin conditions are typically related to food allergy:

DIAGNOSIS	SYMPTOMS
Eczema, atopic dermatitis	red thickened itchy
Urticaria	hives, itchy red eruptions
Erythematous rashes	red measles-like eruptions
Acne	pimples,cysts face & back
Pruritus	itching
Nodular eruptions	red bumps in the skin
Flushing	red face, ears, neck
Butterfly rash	rash cheeks and forehead
Contact dermatitis	skin eruptions on contact
Petechia	small skin hemorrhages
Purpura	abnormal bruising
Dermatitis herpetiformis	skin eruptions ; herpes-like
Photosensitivity	sun-triggered rashes, hives
Alopecia	hair loss, baldness
Psoriasis	thickened scaling red skin
Angioedema	swelling, tongue, lips, face
Perianal dermatitis	itching, burning; anus

People with food allergy may itch and squirm with little or no visible skin changes. The skin of the face, upper forearms, and front of the thighs may have a sand-paper surface with fine white to reddish bumps. Technically, these bumps can be called "perifollicular hyperkeratosis". We call them "milk bumps" since they are so common in cow's milk allergy, but they occur with other food allergies as well.

Acne is related to wrong food, not just coffee, chocolate, cheese, and pop; but also milk, wheat, eggs and all the other staple foods. Facial skin eruptions in food allergy are as common as they are diverse; rashes, pimples, and firm, sore, red bumps inside the skin are very common. **Cystic acne** is the most aggressive, disfiguring from of acne, now treated with antibiotics or the toxic vitamin A analogue, Accutane. Core Program diet revision has helped long-term victims of cystic acne and should be attempted along with careful skin cleansing. **Flushing** over many years leaves clusters of dilated blood vessels as permanent reminders of prolonged food allergy. An aggressive version of flushing with vessel and other skin changes is **acne rosacea** which also responds to careful diet revision, but does not always clear completely.

Eczema (atopic dermatitis) is the prototype of food allergic skin disease. Eczema often appears on the face as patches of reddish, scaling skin. As eczema worsens, the skin becomes more itchy, red, thickened, grooved, and may blister, weep, and crack. The typical distribution of eczema is on the face, behind the ears, on the front of the elbows, the back of the knees, the hands, neck, and trunk. Food allergy probably accounts for at least half of eczema; the rest is external allergy, irritants, infection, and injury to the skin through vigorous itching. House dust mite allergy is an important external cause of eczema. Infection with staphylococci is a common cause of suddening worsening of eczema. Eczema can be a severe disease that involves generalized symptoms of food allergy and symptoms from complicating infections; treatment programs should include clearing food antigens on an ENF, antibiotics, and treatment of the immune-mediated inflammation with prednisone. Antihistamines have always been prescribed to reduce itching but are disappointing in controlling the disease process.

Another common allergic reaction, **hives or urticaria**, are itchy, elevated, red blotches of varying size that appear suddenly and disappear mysteriously after hours to days. Hives may be associated with dramatic swelling reactions; swelling of the lips, eyes, and ears can suddenly and grotesquely alter the appearance of an allergy victim. Swelling of the tongue and throat may be life-threatening because of airway obstruction. Other red rashes and skin bumps appear in various patterns during the course of food allergy. Almost any skin eruption can be considered "allergic until proven otherwise". **Psoriasis** responds variably to Diet Revision Therapy and, in several remarkable cases, remission of psoriatic arthritis with clearing of the skin lesions has been achieved, albeit with some difficulty, byrigorousantigen-exclusion diet therapy. **Dermatitis Herpetiformis (DH)**, a less common skin disease, is another manifestation of wheat allergy. In DH, clusters of skin blisters appear which are herpes-like, but do not follow the typical distribution of herpes virus infection.

Food Allergy in Heart, Blood and Circulatory Problems

Fat and cholesterol are clearly related to heart disease and strokes. In relation to coronary artery disease. But what else is going on with the heart, blood, blood pressure and food? Food allergy routinely produces heart symptoms, especially changes in the speed and rhythm of the heart beat. Increased heart rate, often with skipped beats and a pounding sensation in the chest, suggests a "**heart attack**" as immune mediators act on the heart muscle and conduction system. The heart is always involved in asthma with increased heart rate to compensate for decreased oxygenation of the blood. Spasm of the coronary arteries may occur with food allergy, following the migraine mechanism, but leading to alarming chest pain, suggestive of a heart attack. Some patients experience this coronary migraine attack instead of headaches; often waking in the early hours of the morning with chest pain, shortness of breath and panic. Nitroglycerine relieves the pain of coronary spasm, and diet revision will prevent it.

The most dramatic, allergic reaction, **anaphylaxis**, is life-threatening because of damaging effects of allergic mediators on the heart, lungs and blood vessels. Adrenalin and corticosteroid drugs block these effects, but victims may die before these drugs can be administered. Less severe anaphylactic reactions are common among food allergy patients, who report symptoms such as **chest pain**, chest tightness, pounding heart, anxiety or fear, weakness, and dizziness. Often the fear is intense and can be described as a "**panic attack**". Many people have extensive heart investigations to no avail and may also take drugs, long-term, to block **heart rhythm problems**. Sadly, drugs used to slow heart rate and reduce blood pressure, beta-blockers, make the allergic reaction worse; increasing the incidence and severity of both asthma and anaphylaxis.

Cardiovascular problems, related to food allergy:

DIAGNOSIS	SYMPTOMS
Anaphylactic shock	sudden collapse, shock
Tachycardias	fast heart action
Cardiac arrhythmias	irregular heart rhythm
Reynaud's syndrome	white fingers
Edema	water retention - swelling
Hypertension	high blood pressure

Allergens enter the body thru the GIT wall and then interact with blood, en route to damaging target organs. The **circulating immune system** is designed to police the blood. Many of the problems described throughout this book involve skirmishes between food allergens and the reactive system in the blood stream. These reactive mechanisms within include blood-clotting, and cell-damaging molecules called **complement**. Blood cells and platelets act defensively and may be damaged while doing their duty. If the damage is extensive and persistent, loss of blood cells is diagnosed as anemia, or leukopenia; loss of platelets leads to bleeding problems. Several blood conditions can be attributed in part or entirely to food allergy, including:

Blood Problems with Food Allergy

DIAGNOSIS	SYMPTOMS
Hemolytic anemia	red blood cells damaged
Hypoproteinemia	low blood proteins
Hypochromic anemia	iron deficiency anemia
Thrombocytopenia	damaged platelets, bleeding
Eosinophilia	increased eosinophils
Thrombophlebitis	vein inflammation with clots

Early observations of "blood-disease" linked food to immune mechanisms. Henoch and Schonlein described a form of purpura (generalized, spontaneous bruising) associated with abdominal and joint symptoms. The much revered Canadian physician, Sir Wm. Osler documented 50 cases of Henoch-Schonlein purpura in 1914 [21] and suggested that dietary proteins may have been involved. He also noted that patients with purpura often presented with arthritis; a good insight into the more profound possibilities for food allergy and a good introduction to the next section on arthritis.

Food Allergy as Pain in Muscles, Joints, and Spine

Pain, aching, and stiffness are often produced by abnormal immune or biochemical responses to food components, especially proteins. The problem is inflammation in connective tissue, often activated by populations of cells which patrol these tissues. Inflammation may show up diffusely or be localized to tendon or ligament attachments, or may occur in and around joints. A trial of the Core Program may be dramatically successful in alleviating these common pain patterns. Muscle and connective tissue inflammation which may involve food allergy may present as the following conditions:

DIAGNOSIS	SYMPTOMS
Fibromyalgia	aching, stiffness, trigger points
Myalgia	muscle pain, tenderness, weakness
Tendinitis	inflammation tendons; pain and swelling
Bursitis	inflammation in fluid sacs around joints
Arthralgias	joint pain
Arthritis	joint inflammation; swelling, pain,
Spinal arthritis,	chronic back pain, stiffness
Sacroilietis	pain in low back/sacral area;

The diagnoses; **fibrositis, fibromyalgia, fibromyositis, myofacial pain syndrome, idiopathic myalgia,** all point to a pattern of aching and stiffness. Aching is often associated with fatigue and other symptoms which suggest the diagnosis of delayed pattern food allergy. Patients with these diagnoses are usually offered drugs by their physicians; pain-relievers, NSAID's, muscle relaxants, tranquilizers and anti-depressant drugs are all popular. Fibrositis patients often sleep poorly and experience relief by taking the antidepressants, amitriptylene or imipramine at bedtime. In the previous chapter we have already looked at the association of fibromyalgia with "chronic fatigue syndrome" and myalgic encephalitis and suggested that these symptom complexes should be viewed in the wider context of food-related disease. A trial of vigorous diet revision is always indicated to probe the possibility that wrong food choices are responsible for the suffering. More aggressive, severe muscle inflammatory activity occurs in patients with the autoimmune disorders, polymyalgia rheumatica and polymyositis, who require treatment with a corticosteroid, usually prednisone, but also may benefit from diet revision

Arthritis

Allergic arthritis is a definite entity which is often not diagnosed. Typically, a dramatic, acute, painful swelling develops in one or more joints asymmetrically. The joint inflammation is usually brought on by eating a food, either an unusual food eaten for the first time or sometimes a regular food eaten in excess. Drugs can also provoke an inflammatory arthritis. This presentation is similar to, and often confused with, gout. Any food can cause allergic arthritis. Coffee, beef, pork, milk, eggs, and wheat remain the most constant, chief sources of molecular pathogens in arthritis. A wheat gluten-triggered mechanism has been studied in rheumatoid arthritis patients. The clinical observation is that wheat ingestion is followed within hours by increased joint swelling and pain.

Carinini and Brostroff reviewed the concepts of, and evidence for, food-induced arthritis in 1985.[22] They stated:

"Despite an increasing interest in food allergy and the conviction of innumerable patients with joint disease that certain foods exacerbate their symptoms, relatively little scientific attention has been paid to this relationship. Abnormalities of the gastrointestinal tract are commonly found in rheumatic disease...Support for an intestinal origin of antigens comes from studies of patients whose joint symptoms have improved on the avoidance of certain foods antigens, and become worse on consuming them. These have included patients with both intermittent symptoms, palindromic rheumatism and more chronic disease."

In another study, 33 of 45 patients with rheumatoid arthritis improved significantly on a hypoallergenic diet. The authors concluded:[23]

"Increasing numbers of scientific studies suggest that dietary manipulation may help at least some rheumatoid patients and perhaps the greatest need now is for more careful and well-designed research so that preconceptions may be put aside and role of diet, as a specific or even a non-specific adjunctive therapy, may be determined."

In yet another review[24], Dr. R. Panush has stated:

"The observations reviewed support the hypothesis that individualized dietary manipulations may be beneficial for certain, selected patients with rheumatic disease. Further controlled studies are needed to resolve this issue and are underway."

Arthritis is usually treated with salicylates or related anti-inflammatory drugs generally referred to as **NSAID's**. All anti-arthritic medication can produce asthma or chronic rhinitis and a variety of allergic skin rashes. Gastrointestinal surface irritation, bleeding, and ulceration are routine problems of anti-arthritic medication.

A horrible possibility is that the NSAID's make the intestinal tract **more permeable** to large molecules and actually promote the disease mechanism. Does the uses of certain drugs make the arthritis worse in the long run? The use of a prostaglandin E1 analogue (Cytotec) offers some protection against GIT surface bleeding. The avoidance of these drugs and their complications makes DRT a very attractive alternative to drug-therapy.

Arthritis is a common association of inflammatory gastrointestinal disease and further links abnormal GIT function with immune attacks on connective tissue. In all arthritic patients, normal GIT function should be rigorously sought by adaptive dietary adjustments. The function of the colon is critical and food influences on the colon's flora should be carefully considered. **Rheumatoid arthritis** is often considered to be an autoimmune disease and is related to a number of other problems which remain within the food allergy complex.

Autoimmune Diseases

Autoimmune diseases (AD) are terribly destructive examples of immune mediated or hypersensitivity diseases. We can think of these diseases as very bad allergy with additional self-destructive features. All of the symptoms described thus far can occur in AD patients, often in recurrent attacks of illness over many years leaving the victim damaged and despondent. There are several varieties of auto-immune disease; all involve the immune system attacking its own host. This attack means **loss of tolerance** to self-indentifying cell markers. Often **self-tissues are attacked** as if they were transplanted organs being rejected. This terrible mistake must probably has a number of inter-related causes.

Theories of auto-immune diseases must now consider outside causes or chemical triggers in the air, food, and water of victims. The food supply provides abundant opportunity for trigger substances to initiate and then maintain AD activity over many years. Our standard allergenic foods, milk, wheat, eggs, and meat are always the first suspects; but the thousands of chemicals introduced into our food supply make the selection of proper food a complicated issue.

A number of prescription drugs and several industrial chemicals are known to trigger auto-immune disease.[25] In the previous chapter, **Systemic Lupus or SLE** was described as "very bad food allergy"; essentially a disease of circulating **immune complexes**, which fits our model of delayed pattern food allergy (type 3). One of the drugs known to trigger SLE is **hydralazine**, originally marketed for high blood pressure; this drug also occurs in tobacco, smoke, mushrooms and may enter the food supply through contamination with plastics, dyes, and herbicides.

Other food clues have been uncovered. At least one patient with SLE was found to react to **alfalfa** seeds and further investigation of alfalfa in monkeys lead to some remarkable insights into the mechanisms of SLE.[26] A non-nutrient amino acid, **L-canavanine**, found in alfalfa seeds and sprouts, was identified as a trigger of an SLE-like syndrome. The severity of illness produced by canavanine in monkeys is remarkable; an **anemia** from the destruction of red blood cells was a consistent effect. Cooking may remove the problem since canavanine breaks down with heat. Another study of mice[27] demonstrated that removing the milk protein from a standard laboratory diet had a dramatic benefit for SLE mice; 8% of the casein-fed mice survived at 24 months; 100% of the casein-free group survived. This effect ties in with our general understanding of the profound effect of food proteins on the immune system. When the milk protein, casein, is digested, pieces of proteins called **peptides** can have powerful actions in the body. A casein peptide, beta-casomorphin 4-9, stimulates immune cell activity; we think of this as **turning-on immune** responses or creating hypersensitivity. This is another possible mechanism of milk disease; milk proteins creating **hypersensitivity**

All the rules of managing food allergy apply to SLE, but with vigorous adherence to the rules. In SLE patients, control of symptoms is achieved by replacing foods with an **ENF, associated with prednisone,** until inflammation subsides and damaged organs begin to function well again; then careful re-feeding should allow sustained control of the disease.

However, subsequent ingestion of reactive foods proves to be catastrophic, demonstrating lasting hypersensitivity. Prolonged use of an ENF to supply part or all nutrition may be safest course of action. SLE patients, following the Core Program, need to be especially cautious when reintroducing foods and must not eat foods beyond their Core Diet. Staying well proves to be a demanding discipline with little room for error. All higher protein foods may be poorly tolerated and often little or no poultry, fish or meat is tolerated. We always assume that milk and egg proteins are forever forbidden, and probably gluten as well.

Protein can be replaced by free amino acids in an ENF if hypersensitivity remains severe. Reactions to several fruits and vegetables are to be expected. Legumes and nightshades are the least tolerated vegetables. Adequate cooking reduces food problems, presumably because problem molecules like canavanine and lectins are broken down by adequate heating (assume that 100 degrees Celcius for more than 10 minutes is required).

Food Allergy as Genito-Urinary Tract Problems

Whatever comes in must go out. Our urinary system has the job of excreting unwanted, sometime hazardous materials. If problems arise in this system, why not attempt to trace the problems back to body input? A variety of common problems in this system can be related to food allergy:

DIAGNOSIS	SYMPTOMS
Enuresis	bed wetting
Cystitis	bladder inflammation
Orthostatic albuminuria	protein in urine
Nephrotic syndrome	kidney disease with edema
Vaginitis	vaginal itching, burning,
Urethritis	burning, frequency of urination

Bladder and urethral symptoms, especially **urgency and frequency** of and burning on urination, are common symptoms of food allergy. The first diagnosis is infection, but urine cultures will shown not growth of bacteria. Antibiotics may be prescribed, but the problem is self-limiting and clears by itself without antibiotics unless the causative food intake continues unabated. Diet Revision should be considered when symptoms, suggestive of cystitis or urethritis, are recurrent, and not explained by laboratory-documented infections. Some patients with chronic "interstitial cystitis" improve after food intake is replaced by an ENF. Most patients with this disease can safely try an ENF for 10 days or longer to discover if they do "clear."

Women who suffer recurrent **vaginal irritation** or burning on urination (vaginitis, urethritis) may have a food allergy, a local allergy, or infection. Allergens can present both on the surface (e.g. allergy to sex partner's semen) or internally, from circulating allergens. The surfaces of the genitourinary tract should be thought of as similar to the respiratory and gastrointestinal surfaces, with similar allergic reactions. If milk, wheat, and egg allergy can cause rhinitis, they can also result in vaginitis, urethritis, and cystitis!

More serious upper urinary tract problems can be related to food allergy. The kidneys present a large filtering surface to blood contents and are vulnerable to damage by **circulating immune complexes**. These complexes may increase when GIT leaks large molecules into the blood. Again, the food-GIT source of circulating immune complexes (CIC's) has been almost totally neglected in clinical medicine. Doctors will usually think of the most complicated, rare, outrageous things before they will think of the simple, obvious, daily intake of antigenic problems in the food supply!

Transient kidney pain in the flanks signals the presence of CIC's and often imitates an attack of kidney infection or renal colic. Mild, brief versions of this pain are common in people with delayed-pattern food allergy. In the worst case, patients with food allergy may have fever with flank pain and frequency of urination and are often invasively investigated and treated. **Glomerulonephritis** is, a serious form of kidney inflammation, which may sometimes be triggered by CIC's, containing food protein antigens. Kidney inflammation is a serious problem and may lead to hypertension and eventual kidney damage. The recurring triad of transient flank pain, blood or protein in the urine, and the presence of symptoms in other systems should suggest "food allergy" until proven otherwise. Careful diet revision may show benefit in controlling kidney inflammation; an ENF is especially useful in the beginning since all allergenic material is excluded. Patients with existing kidney disease benefit from a low protein diet and will also experience the least demand on diminishing kidney function with an ENF. Close professional supervision is always necessary with serious disease.

---

[1] Knicker, William Immunologically Mediated Reactions to Food: State of the Art. Annals of Allergy. 1987 59:II;60-70

[2] Buscinco L et al. Epidemiology, incidence, and clinical aspects of food allergy. Annals Of Allergy 1984;53:615-622.

[3] Brostroff J, Challacombe SJ. Food allergy and intolerance. Bailliere Tindall, 1987.

[4] Wraith D.G. Food Allergy and Intolerance 486-497; 1987

[5] Pelikan Z., Pelikan-Filpek M., Bronchial response to the food ingestion challenge. Annals of Allergy. 1987; 58:164-172

[6] Heiner D.C., Sears J.W.: Chronic Respiratory Disease associated with multiple circulating precipitans to cow's milk. Am J Dis Child 100:500,1960

[7] Walker-Smith J.A., Ford P.K., Phillips A.D. The Spectrum of Gastrointestinal Allergies to Food. Annal of Allergy. 1984; 53:629-636

[8]Waller SL, Misiewicsz. Prognosis in Irritable Bowel Syndrome. Lancet 1969;ii:753-6.

[9]Nanda R. et al: Food Intolerance and the irritable bowel syndrome. Gut 30:1099,1989.

[10]Pagnelii R. et Al Intestinal Permeability in irritable bowel syndrome... Annals of Allergy 64; 377-380 1990

[11]Bjarnason I., Peters, T. A Persistent defect In Intestinal Permeability in Coeliac Disease... Lancet Feb.12 1983; 323-325

[12]Mulder C.J.J., Tygart G.N.J. Celiac disease and related disorders. Neth J of Med, 31 1987 286-299

[13]Davidson A.G.F., Bridges A.F. Coeliac Disease; a critical review of aetiology and pathogenesis. Clinica Chima Acta, 163 1987 1-40

[14]Olaison, G. Abnormal Intestinal Permeability in Chron's Disease; Scand J Gastroent. 1990,25,321-328

[15]Yates, V, Watkinson G. Kelman A. Further Evidence of an association between psoriasis, Chron's disease and ulcerative colitis. Br Jour Derm 1982;106, 323-330

[16]V. Alun Jones et al: Crohn's Disease maintainence of remission by diet; Lancet July 27 1985 177-180.

[17]Seidman EG, Bouthillier L, Janelli G. et al . Elemental Diet versus prednisone as primary treatment of Chorn's Disease. Gastroenerology 1986, 90:1625A

[18]Saverymuttu S., Hodgson H.J. F., Chadwick V.S. Controlled Trial comparing prednisolone with an elemental diet plus non-absorbable antibiotics in active chron's disease. Gut,1985, 26; 994-998

[19]Belli DC, Seidman A, Bouthillier L, et al. Chronic intermittent elemental diet improves growth failure in children with Chron's disease. Gastroenterology 1988; 94:A37

[20]Teahon K., Bjarnason I., Pearson A.J., Levi A.j. Ten years experience with an elemental diet in the management of chron's diease. Gut,1990,31,1133-1137.

[21]Osler W. The visceral lesions of pupura and allied conditions. Br. Med J. 1,517-525; 1914.

[22]Carinini C, Brostroff J. Gut and joint disease. Annals of Allergy 1985;55:624-625.

[23]Darlington et al. Lancet Feb 1 1986;236-238.

[24]Panush RS. Delayed reactions to foods, food allergy, and rheumatic disease. Annals of Allergy 1986;56:500-503.

[25]Kammuller M.E., Bloksma N., Seinen, W.; . Immune disregulation induced by drugs and chemicals. Autoimmunity and Toxicology; Elsevier Science Publ. 1-34;1989.

[26]Bardana, E.J., Montanaro A., Rene, M. Autoimmune reactions induced by dietary antigens with an emphasis on amino acids. Autoimmunity and Toxicology. Elsevier Science Publ.323-345; 1989.

[27]Carr R.I. et al. Immunomodulation by opioid from dietary casein (exorphins). Ann. N.Y. Acad Sc. 597:374-376.1990.

Chapter 7   Diet Revision for

Nervous System Disturbances

Our mental and emotional status is strongly influenced and sometimes determined by the food and beverages we ingest. The case for food and drink as important determinants of mental states requires full explication, the subject for a separate book. A brief review is presented here to alert the reader to the important opportunities for diet revision in solving mental health problems and associated neurological disease. Our discussion so-far has sketched in the connections between eating behaviors, food selection, addictive problems, and illness. We have recognized that eating is one the most important of human activities, and that attempts to change eating behaviors are usually met with profound emotional and cognitive complications.

Eating is closely related to our emotional life. Neurobiologists refer to the four F's; the basic interests of living creatures and, therefore, the basic functions of the brain. The **four-F's, feeding, fighting, fleeing, and sexual interests** are organized together in the brain and it is not surprising that these interests intermingle; when things go wrong curious and sometimes horrifying short-circuits occur, with fighting and feeding often co-mingled; or sex-feeding-fighting-fleeing jumbled together in bizarre, sometimes destructive behaviors.

Chemical sensors in the nose and tongue allow us to smell and taste. Our chemical sensory systems plays a primary role in determining our four-F behaviors. Immune sensors in the nose, mouth and along the digestive tract also seem to play a regulatory role providing responses and information which interact with information derived from chemical sensors. The smell system begins in the old reptilian part of our brain (limbic system) which has evolved into a system that regulates our moods, emotional life, sexual behavior and at the same time feeds essential information into the neural computers that regulate appetite and eating behaviors.

The **hypothalamus** is a key brain region that integrates body-status information to determine the four-F behaviors. In terms of appetite and fighting behavior, the hypothalamus can be divided into a middle zone which tends to stop eating and inhibit aggression and a lateral zone which tends to turn eating on and excite (predatory) aggression. In animal studies, damage to the medial hypothalamus produces animals who are irritable, eat too much and become obese. Damage to the lateral go-system results in animals who eat little and tend to starve. The hypothalamus is also the brain link to the **hormone system;** regulating the pituitary gland, which in turn regulates the endocrine glands which produce hormones, the blood-born molecules that regulate our day-to-day function. The ingestion, digestive, and metabolism of food is one the chief concerns of the endocrine system.

Both the immune system and the nervous system employ **molecular messengers** to influence events in the body, and some of these messengers; histamine, serotonin, norepinephrine, acetylcholine, endorphins, prostaglandins are common to both systems. Many circuits in the brain have been characterized in terms of specific neurotransmitters used to relay information, and the kind of information in the system. We have described the fight and flight, **sympathetic system** which uses **adrenalin** in the body to recruit emergency responses and noradrenalin in the brain. These chemicals are made from the amino acids, phenylalanine and tryrosine which are first converted into another neurotransmitter, dopamine. An opposing **parasympathetic system** uses **acetylcholine** as the transmitter and is found everywhere in the body, sending signals to muscle cells to contract. In the brain, acetylcholine has arousal functions in the right amounts; but tends to cause depression in overdose. Acetylcholine can be completely synthesized in the body and does not have an essential nutrient precursor, although choline (as lecithin) is often available in the diet, or can be supplemented.

It is interesting to note that many symptoms of food reactions are generated by acetylcholine mechanisms, especially nausea, vomiting, belching, cramps, defecation, sweating, and runny nose. **Nicotine** mimics some the actions of acetylcholine and even veteran smokers who chew nicotine gums for the first time may get a blast of these effects. Drugs which block acetylcholine activity are popular in medicine and have many uses; atropine is the prototype and for years atropine or related compounds have been in medicines to treat upset GIT function; they reduce secretions, and block the pain of cramps; too much and you are dry-mouthed, constipated, and may have troube urinating; you may also have trouble thinking and remembering. In the **lateral hypothalamus,** acetylcholine is the transmitter of **prey-killing,** the necessary pre-condition of feeding behavior in carnivorous animals and atropine tends to block this. This is different from **territorial aggression** which is organized by noradrenalin circuits (fight and flight). Drugs which block this activity (beta-blockers) have found many medical applications including lowering blood pressure, preventing migraine, calming racing hearts, reducing anxiety and aggression.

The **information and control** properties of the immune system are analogues of brain function, with the four major functions of sentience: **Sensing, Deciding, Acting, Remembering.** Important connections between brain-mind-immunity work at a general ambient level of feeling-environment-attitude. Important disturbances of brain function occur during immune activity in the body with the strongest influences on autonomic and mood-emotion circuits. Changes in arousal, mood, sleep-waking patterns, appetite, thirst and temperature regulation are regularly reported by food allergic patients. For example, fatigue, progressing to irresistible sleepiness and/or depression, with sleep disturbances, increased thirst and urination, hot and cold sensations, and attention-memory deficits are routinely reported together in various combinations.

There is significant overlap of immune regulation with the **chemical senses** (taste and smell), and appetite control in the brain. Odors and strong emotions arc likely to influence immune activity, and many patients with food allergy report smell hypersensitivity and strong aversions. Many have been classically conditioned to react to taste and odor stimuli with allergic symptoms and/or emotional responses, including anxiety or panic attacks.

The role of food problems in creating emotionally and mentally disturbed people has been underestimated in our culture. In ancient Greek, Indian, and Chinese medicine, therapy was often based on the understanding of food-body-mind correlations. Mental symptoms were interpreted, along with physical symptoms, as imbalances in the body, triggered by wrong foods and bad environments. Psychic energy was described as Chi and was regulated by the interaction of physical and mental influences. Therapy of disease was directed at balancing Chi. Diet revision was a major mode of therapy. In China, foods were described as "yin or yang", hot or cold, and balance in Chi energy was sought in part by modifying the diet. Seasonal changes in foods and body states were answered by seasonal changes in food selection and recipes. While the Core Program drops many of the colorful metaphors of these ancient traditions and drops the herbs, seasonings and other accessories of the old-ways; it retains the practical intent to regulate body-mind states with food changes and a flexible program of self-regulation.

Yoga and meditation techniques, designed for **clearing the mind,** utilized fasting or food restriction as a basis for reposing in a calm, centered state. It is absurd to think of successful yoga and meditation after drinking 6 cups of coffee, 3 bottles of beer, and eating a pizza. A bowl of rice and glass of water are better brain-inputs for staying calm and clear. It is equally absurd to ignore chaos and confusion in the food supply when people feel and act abnormally. It should be obvious that coffee, tea, alcoholic beverages, junk foods, sugar excesses, chocolate, and imbalanced, deficient diets all play a role in causing mental dysfunction. It is less obvious, but equally true in our experience, that adverse reactions to staple foods such as milk, eggs, wheat and meat also cause mental dysfunction. We need to be concerned about food additives and pesticides. Indeed, we regularly see patients who must exercise exceptional restraint in choosing food and drink to maintain mental clarity and emotional stability. For some, all food intake seems to compromise normal brain function, but living on an elemental nutrient formula allows them to think, feel and behave normally.

We Are One Whole System

We take a strong biological stand and view **mental states** as products of **brain function.** Food is regarded as the input of chemical materials into a body-brain system. Whenever a patient is dysfunctional or sick, his or her brain function is compromised and symptoms include disturbances of sensing, feeling, remembering and acting. We seek to restore orderly, normal functioning by careful **food-input control,** using the Core Program technique of diet revision! We further assume that the majority of psychological or psychogenic explanations of mental illness are little more than gossip about people whose brains are not functioning well.

The mechanisms by which food materials influence brain function are as complex as they are misunderstood. The **brain is a molecular machine** whose first function is to track desirable molecules in the environment and cause them to flow through the body. In Chapter 2 the appetite system was described as a function of the old reptilian brain. This system is designed to establish the most efficient path to reliably available food, then to lock in the behavior and repeat it without further modification. Our appetite system tends to run automatically at this primitive level and defies conscious attempts to alter the program. Any insightful person will be able to track the importance of food searches in their own behavior. If you watch the people around you, you will readily confirm the primacy of feeding behaviors in human social existence.

It is possible to construct a rather elaborate model of brain function in terms of the brain's attempt to regulate the molecular flow of food materials. Feeding behaviors are highly automated and seem to be designed around recursive loops, already discussed under addictive behavior. The old reptilian feeding programs are build into the brain like ROM in computers.

These old programs seem to be based on routines such as *<more sweet (sugar) is better than less; go back for more>* or *<when in trouble, eat more sweet (sugar)>*. If we think of our brains as chemical processors whose first job is to steer us through a chemical soup so that we get the right stuff to function normally, a lot of human behavior makes sense or is more understandable nonsense. We can think:

> *< **If** the brain gets the right signals from the ingested chemical materials **then** we will remain on a stable, adaptive course>*

> *< **If** we get the wrong signals from the ingested chemical materials **then** we will end-up on a wobbly course, unstable and maladaptive>*.

The increased presence of non-nutrient molecules in the food stream in the form of additives, contaminants, toxins, intoxicants and drugs makes brain dysfunction more likely and more difficult to interpret in terms of simple theories or single-substance models. It helps to stand outside familiar behaviors and watch, as if you were an anthropologist viewing a native culture for the first time. In our culture, we socialize at "parties"; one of the principal functions of social networks. If you watch though a window you will see people standing facing each other holding drinks; they talk, laugh and sip intermittently. Someone carries around a food tray and now you observe talk, sip, nibble, laugh routines. Some also add smoking devices to the mix; talk, puff, blow, laugh, sip, nibble.

Would you guess that these creatures are **manipulating their internal body-mind states** by ingesting a variety of chemicals; at the same time observing each others body language and exchanging language-encoded data. Follow sample couples home from the party and watch how the evening develops. You may find that the least stable couples end up doing more sipping, nibbling, puffing, less talking, less laughing, perhaps fighting or fleeing. Would you conclude that social and biological determinants combine in very complex ways to determine how these people behave?

According to neuroscientist, Karl Pribram, **feelings** are the self-referring language of the body system; the inside world. He describes feelings as monitor images which emerge from the core brain as chemical influences are evaluated and regulated. The more effective we are in action, the more stable, less emotional we feel. We get increasingly eniotional (unstable) when our coping strategies fail.

Pribram states[1]:

> "...we construct a World-Within on the basis of our feeling. A great deal is known about one class of feelings which is related to a set of receptors that lie deep in the central core of the brain. This class includes hunger and thirst, sexiness, sleepiness, and mood."

Others have noted that our brain is a "**soggy computer**" steeped in its own chemicals and chemicals arriving from the outside in the form of food, beverages, and drugs. Gas and glue-sniffers remind us that the air is another source of intoxicants. Our feelings and behavior arise spontaneously from an unconscious source. How do we know if it is just my coke and M&M's arguing with your pizza and beer? Or do we really have an authentic dispute? To people who do not think about biological determinants, adding food factors to the behavioral analysis may seem far-fetched. To us, the food factor is bio-logical, and you have to consider it before you will understand human experiences.

Context Dependent Learning

A useful idea in brain science is that the general circumstances or context in which we have experiences influences the way we recall the experiences and also influences how our body responds. **Context-dependency** probably plays a greater role in determining our behavior overall than anyone has appreciated. A context may be as simple as a room at home which assumes the identity of home and cues behavior suitable at home; grown-up children returning to their parents home often experience dramatic shifts in their feelings and behavior as the familiar contexts bring back old programs that were operating during childhood, but faded away in more recent adult contexts. Our appetite and food preferences are context-dependent; we associate different smells, tastes, and feelings with each environment we frequent. If you often had coffee and cake with a friend in a special restaurant, even when you have stopped eating these foods for months or years, meeting that friend again will invoke the stongest desire for coffee and cake; without the food the whole experience will seem odd and different- perhaps not pleasant at all.

The party we just examined is another context; as couples return home from the party the context changes and so does their behavior. On the positive side we tend to have had good experiences which we often try to recreate, paying attantion to the contexts that worked for us in the past. The art of cooking has a lot to do with contexts; the food is less appealing if the restaurant smells odd or the service is bad. The way the food is presented alters its appeal and alters our body response to it. Children, for example, will sometimes insist that food items be separate and are very upset when foods are mixed together; adult-children often retain idiosyncratic preferences for the presentation and combination of foods.

Less obvious contexts are **internal body states**; if I meet a new person when I am feeling dysphoric and anxious, I may on subsequent meetings have difficulty shaking the returning sense of dysphoria his or her appearance invokes, although I do not know why I feel this way; I may project my feelings, blaming the other person; "you were really different the first time I met you." The context idea gets even more interesting when we consider animals who were slowly given increasing doses of morphine. While they remained comfortable in the same cage with the same routine, they tolerated high doses with few ill effects. When they were moved to a new cage, and the drug schedule altered the previously tolerated high dose killed them promptly! Now we have **context-dependent tolerance** for a drug. This is a useful concept when we try to understand allergic processes which also seem to be context-dependent. It is also a useful concept when we try to explain how and why a person will flip-flop, changing states abruptly; acting as if they had two or more personalities.

In children on controlled diets, with parents and teachers monitoring closely, this flip-flop is obvious, and can be related to eating a reactive food. To keep matters simple, we refer to a "food reaction" which triggers behavior change, but we know that many changes are going on at the same time, including a context shift. Think of the **context as a channel** on the TV; when you have a food reaction you also change the channel; you get another program. If you do not like the new channel, you usually have to stop eating the problem and wait for the channel to switch back automatically.

If food intake and the body state it induces is a context which determines the recall of behaviors and feeling states, we can talk about a **personality shift** from a rice and vegetable context to an M&M's and coke context. What is surprising is this shift in food-context can be as dramatic as Dr. Jekyl and Mr. Hyde shift; in the movie Dr. Jekyl swallows a liquid potion (rum and coke) and undergoes a startling metamorphosis. Mr. Hyde is sociopathic and in fits of rage kills innocent people. The children we observe doing **flip-flop food context shifts**, also have fits of rage, and the worst-afflicted display frighteningly aggressive behavior, attacking other children or their parents. These children, if not controlled, soon get the reputation for being "bad" and tend to shift by repeated learning experiences into negative contexts as a relatively permanent feature of their personality. The worst afflicted may end up as some of our more destructive citizens, sometimes in jail .

We know that the same rapid shifts from state A to state B occur in adults, but seldom get to study the phenomena with the same clarity we see in children. Adults report different sets of thoughts in the different states and the more insightful adults will describe distinct personalities. An angry, gloomy side may alternate with a happier, more affectionate, generous personality. Women have been generally more forthcoming in describing their personality shifts. The most obvious **context-switchers** in adults are alcoholic beverages; at low doses the effect may be pleasant and socially useful, at high doses the worst sociopathic, destructive behavior emerges. We are used to thinking of the alcoholic as a split-personality who flip-flops between a sober state and a drunk state; look more closely, and you will find more food-dependent states. A sober, recovering alcoholic may continue flip-flopping by drinking coca cola, or coffee with 3 teaspoons of sugar per cup. Coffee has similar effects to AB's but better concealed effects. Coffee's ability to aggravate or trigger personality and mood shifts, should not be underestimated. The same concern should be recorded for coca cola, teas, and chocolate.

Mind-Body Unity

Experiences with the Core Program path of diet revision have taught us much about the **food-body-brain** connection. Mental, emotional, and behavioral disturbances are meshed with headaches, runny noses, belly aches, joint pains and many other physical disturbances; you cannot readily separate the way you feel in your legs, your abdomen, your heart, and your head. The correlation of physical symptoms, suggesting food allergy, has been helpful in identifying the probable role of the immune system in producing mental disturbances. We have documented thousands of experiences of hundreds of insightful, professionally-trained patients who have discovered that different **foods** and beverages have a **profound influence** on their mental status. The most revealing experiments occur when eating a food shifts the observer from a clear state to a dysfunctional state with changes in clarity of consciousness, memory, and emotional disturbances. We think in terms of '"allergy" when the disturbance has a familiar reactive pattern, combining physical and mental symptoms. The valuable insight that **food reactions trigger mental emotional shifts** can empower an individual to seek a practical remedy for his or her suffering - change body input! This insight reduces both the sense of helplessness or entrapment and the tendency to blame others for internal distress.

For example, an intelligent, resourceful patient who is made ill by many ordinary foods, carefully recorded her struggle to maintain control over chronic food allergic disease. She had experienced depression, panic attacks, and episodes of disturbed thinking that were quite alarming to herself, family and friends. Her medical history strongly suggested allergic disease with many typical physical symptoms over many years. Proof of food allergy came with dramatic clearing of symptoms on the Core Program. She sustained food control for variable periods of time and then would lose control in a fit of binging, becoming quite ill again. This is a standard wobbly process, learning to track normal functioning after living most of her life in ADS. Her symptom list, following a typical "slip", describes the cost of eating her reactive foods: beef, whole wheat bread, cheese, wine, and chocolate. The symptoms emerged sequentially over the course of 3 days and subsided over the next 4 days when she returned to the Phase 1 clearing diet.

The Day I Blew It"

1. Burning sweat on face.	2. Headaches – various.
3. Jittery, jumpy.	4. Out of control, speedy.
5. Compulsive.	6. Gastrointestinal upsets –
7. Acid taste – back of throat.	8. Mucous build-up.
9. Loss of memory – short-term.	10. Very swollen,
11. Muscle weakness.	12. Body itchy all over.
13. Eyes watering and/or puffy.	14. Sinuses stuffed and aching.
15. Ears – painful, swollen.	16. Sore throat, glands swollen.
17. Could not sleep	18. Then nightmares.
19. Clumsy and off balance.	20. Incoherent thinking.
21. Cravings / hunger."	22. Aching joints

Although she feels angry and depressed during a food reaction, she has learned to interpret her distress as a biological problem and does not blame other people, world politics, nor stress for her symptoms or loss of control. She has learned how to recover from the illness by controlling her food intake and is basically confident about regaining self-control. She has learned to apologize when her behavior is inappropriate and takes corrective action. Her biological insight does not give her complete control of her eating choices, nor a symptom-free life. Her insight does give a choice and a sense of imminent control. She is no longer a victim of illness.

Our model of body-brain dysfunction attempts to explain all symptoms as expressions of disturbed body processes. Not a single twitch, itch, pain, or moment of anxiety goes unaccounted. Shifts in mood, changes in concentration, memory, motor control, and sensation are interpreted at the hardware level of **altered brain function**. The incoming food molecules can be thought of as a **chaotic mix**. Various body procedures are called upon to deal with the incoming food materials. The responses may include **alarm** messages which are felt emotionally, and expressed as angry, aggressive behavior. Allergic-immune responses add further chaotic events to disturb brain (and other target organ) function. The association of abdominal symptoms with respiratory congestion, skin itches and eruptions, and mental disorders is understandable if you track the interactions of food molecules from the moment of entry to their final disposition in various tissues of the body. The Core Program is designed to **solve simultaneous problems** in the food supply. Consideration is given to minimizing exposure to food additives, to choosing nourishing, primary, least-allergenic foods as dietary staples, and assuring nutrient adequacy by proper food combining and supplementation. We can summarize our biological point-of-view:

> *The brain is a delicate, precision instrument which is prone to error and requires careful input management. The brain is the first organ to malfunction when body-input is wrong!*

> *Mind-brain-body are one, interacting, whole-system. Disturbances in mental states have physical causes- cellular-biochemical dysfunctions.*

> *Food, as body input, is the molecular substrate of body-mind, the foundation level, which permits or denies healthy function at higher levels of integration. Without a healthy body input mental health is an impossible goal.*

Allergy and the Nervous System

If you have read the descriptions of food allergic disease thus far in the book, you will realize that immune responses often involve mental-emotional symptoms. **Anaphylaxis** victims are said to have **"panic attacks"** if they end up in the psychiatry department. Children with food allergy may have nightmares, tantrums, and fail to learn at school because of **attention deficits.** Some of these children grow into troubled adults with "learning disability". Others remain, hyper, moody, and volatile. Delayed pattern food allergy patients are described as "depressed" or "neurotic". Migraine sufferers may have neurological symptoms that suggest a stroke, or a seizure. The occasional patient will have food-triggered epilepsy. Often changes in sensation, motor control, balance, and vision accompany food allergy and suggest the diagnosis of a serious neurological disease like multiple sclerosis.

In the next section, the emotional responses to changes in diet are described in detail. Everywhere we look in the food business there are emotional disturbances to consider and **symptoms of brain dysfunction**, ranging in severity from minor anxiety to disabling disease. Different interpretations, different names for the same events, and a great deal of dogmatic misunderstanding has obscured the truth of the food-allergy brain connection. Dr. Walter Alvarez, a well-known physician of the Mayo clinic and medical writer, gave us a personal perspective on food-mind interactions, twenty years ago, in his introduction to the text "Allergy of the Nervous System":

> "For years I knew I was highly sensitive to chicken fat, I suffered from what I called "dumb Monday," when I was too dull to do much constructive work like writing. Finally, I discovered that bad Mondays were due to the Alvarez family's habit of having chicken for Sunday dinner... My most remarkable personal experience with brain dulling due to food allergy came many years ago when... I ate a whole broiled chicken. Next day I had severe diarrhea and with this I became so dulled I could not read with comfort. And that night I had a hallucination of sight, such as I had never had before and haven't had since."

Dr. Alvarez, and other astute physicians, knew about food allergy and its mental effects for many years.[2] [3] [4] Allergy was implicated in depression, anxiety, hyperactivity in children, epilepsy, migraine, Meniere's syndrome, multiple sclerosis, and Guillain-Barre Syndrome. Unfortunately, this clinical wisdom, shared by many prominent physicians for many years, has somehow been lost to subsequent generations of physicians, and needs to be renewed. Dr. Alvarez' problem with chicken may alarm readers who find chicken breast as a food choice in Phase 1 of the Core Program. Chicken can be a problem to some people, but remains a workable "meat" choice, when a meat is desirable. The use of smaller portions of breast meat, well-cooked, with fat removed, reduces the frequency and severity of chicken problems. We are always alert to remaining problems with any Core Program food, and are ready to discontinue eating chicken, in favor of another food. A complete vegetarian version of the Core Program is possible and, from many points of view, desirable.

Was it a quirk of history that placed **psychosomatic theories** in the place of the theory of allergic disease? Many have suggested that psychosomatic notions are obsolete. An insightful psychiatrist, Z. Lipovski, suggested:[5]

> "...the concept of psychogenesis of organic disease is as reductionistic as the germ theory of it, against which pioneers in psychosomatic medicine inveighed...To distinguish a class of diseases as 'psychosomatic disorders' and to propound generalizations about 'psychosomatic patients' is misleading and redundant. Concepts of single causes and of unilinear causal sequences – for example, from psyche to soma and visa versa – are simplistic and obsolete."

Psychosomatic theories, in our opinion, are basically wrong. What is really going on is the other way around. Body-brain events produce mental events. Real, physical, practical things, especially materials entering the body and reaching the brain through the mouth, are important in determining mental events. This is "**Somatopsychics.**" One of our clinical psychologist colleagues, Chuck Bates, wrote frankly about his experiences in an instruction manual he provided to his clients. His remarks are worth considering: [6]

"My own case history exemplifies many of the fundamental principles (of Diet Revision Therapy). This technology did more for my mental health than all of the clinical psychology I have learned. As a boy I was diagnosed as having spring pollen and house dust allergies. I sniffled and sneezed continuously, and years of desensitizing injections didn't seem to help. I continued to have attacks into adulthood.I was a moody and irritable teenager, experiencing great difficulty concentrating on my studies. My marks disappointed those aware of my high I.Q. In my late teens I experienced severe clinical depression. As an adult, my depression moderated considerably, but took other forms. I experienced frequent fatigue attacks. Typically I would retire to bed right after work. I experienced muddied, clouded consciousness a good percent of the time, and often sat there in a daze barely able to participate in conversations. I frequently became irritable and snapped at my wife for petty reasons. I had frequent food cravings and was always at least 20 pounds overweight despite constant dieting. I went on pizza binges, washed down with quarts of milk. Every morning I coughed up mucus. I had insomnia and nightmares. I usually felt jumpy and impatient. I experienced constant flatulence, heartburn, gas pains, indigestion of every sort, and diarrhea. None of these things were regarded as symptoms of anything at all. At most I attributed my moodiness to being a spoiled child, and beyond that I had no awareness that anything was amiss.

"Using (Diet Revision Therapy) technology... a new me emerged. All my symptoms disappeared. I experienced a previously unknown mental clarity and ability to concentrate. My moods, especially my irritability disappeared, and the proof is my spouse's testimony. My wife is even more certain of this than I am."

Few food-provoked symptoms are "psychological". Adverse reactions to foods or "food allergy" have a physiological basis, and can be explained by proper insightful medical biology.

Dr. Aas, a Norwegian allergist and researcher, remarked at the Marabou symposium on "Food Sensitivity"[7]:

> "In my institute I am the only experimental monkey that we have and from several passive transfer experiments on myself, with occasional rather severe reactions, I am the first to admit that allergic reactions are accompanied with intellectual and emotional disturbances. If you have not experienced that, I ask you to be a volunteer in my laboratory."

The concept of allergy - reacting defensively to foreign materials with damage to ourselves - can be extended to our nervous system which also reacts to world events with defensive procedures. Both immune and nervous systems interact when things go wrong at the level of molecules and cells. The molecular-cellular mechanisms are monitored (but not controlled!) at the level of consciousness. The experience of symptoms, is the **monitor image** in consciousness of problems at the molecular-cellular level. In technical terms, we can speak of information and noise in the system of person and environment. **Information noise** is the disorder and chaos in experience that confuses or interferes with a successful relationship with our environment, the achievement of our goals with associated peace of mind. **Molecular noise** is the disorder or chaos created by substances flowing through our body-brain. At certain levels in us information noise is equivalent to molecular noise. At the level of equivalence we cannot tell the difference between a molecular problem and a personal problem. As noise increases, the system becomes more unstable or hypersensitive. We feel this instability as emotional disturbance and physical symptoms.

We are very aware of long-suffering patients who are **hypersensitive** in all departments; they react to food, air, drugs, smells, people, ideas, feelings in an exaggerated, often harmful manner. Their physical symptoms are made of the same biological stuff as their mental and emotional symptoms. The hypersensitive person requires more protection from adverse foods and environments than their more robust peers. The hypersensitive has a great deal to offer by way of ideas, insights, feelings, and when many hypersensitive people get ill from food and environmental problems they warn us the rest are soon to follow.

Migraine and Other Headaches

It has been estimated that 10-20% of the population will consult physicians with headache as their primary symptom. The principle task facing the doctor is usually to rule out the more serious causes of headache. Almost everyone with a chronic, persistent headache fears a brain tumor. Physicians are generally alert to the clinical patterns and some of the physical signs associated with serious problems, and make an effort to sort common, benign headaches from the more sinister variety. Brain tumors are rare; headaches are very common; most investigations designed to rule out this diagnosis prove to be negative.

Among the chemical causes which are familiar to us as headache triggers, we must consider a range of substances which are native to foods, as well as additives, collaring agents, and contaminants. From an allergy point of view, any headache response is seen as part of a complex of untoward events following the food ingestion. Most of the allergic mechanisms which produce headache are not of the immediate type, and, therefore, are not immediately obvious.

When headache is thought to be of the tension or migraine type, diet revision can be tried as the first and principle mode of therapy. A practical method of approaching the problem of diagnosing and treating headache is to begin with a Core Program clearing sequence. If the headache does not go away, further investigation of its cause should be undertaken. Headache is a withdrawal symptom for the first several days of any clearing effort, so that 10 days is an appropriate decision point. The regular ingestion of coffee produces tolerance not only to the drug effects of caffeine, but also to the toxic effects of the numerous other chemicals in coffee. The sudden cessation of regular coffee intake is followed by a typical withdrawal headache, which may be severe. Often, the coffee drinker is caught in a vicious cycle, where continuing ingestion of coffee is necessary to prevent the withdrawal headache. This is an addictive pattern.

Migraine Headaches

Migraine is a fascinating set of food allergic problems which allow us to examine the link between food, the circulating immune system, and brain disturbances. While pain is the main event, many other symptoms which occur before, during, and after a headache can only be explained as a food allergy mechanism. The pain of migraine arises from blood vessels, supplying blood to the brain. Some brain disturbance are stroke-like, originating from reduced blood flow to the brain; this transient cerebral ischemia is most likely to occur before the headache occurs; blood vessels are constricting at this time, reducing blood flow. The vascular mechanism of headache, including most of the migraine variants, may have both allergic and biochemical triggers. Typically, a migraine sufferer will follow a rhythmic or cyclic pattern. The underlying biorhythms and changes in tolerance for trigger substances will vary the response to ingestion of certain foods. This variability has confused researchers to date. The only solution to a frequently-occurring migraine headache is to alter the food intake while attending to the reduction of other trigger factors. In cyclic migraine, as in the menstrual cycle pattern, underlying hormonal changes will set the stage for food triggers to act.

In addition to ingested substances triggering headaches, there are a variety of airborne or environmental causes. Numerous chemicals in our home, office and industrial environments are capable of producing headache. We have mentioned the ubiquitous nitrates. Many people find that they are sensitive to the aromatic substances in the air, which can range from paint solvents and industrial chemicals to the perfuming ingredients in for cosmetic purposes. Many of the strongly-smelling, volatile substances act indirectly on pain-sensitive structures and others act through a complex mechanism of mediator release to produce pain. The effect of inhaled substances and ingested substances often act synergistically. This means that if you overload your body's defence mechanisms by both ingesting and inhaling trigger substances, a pain pattern will be produced. Other inhaled toxins which typically produce headache include cigarette smoke, carbon monoxide, and air pollution gases, NO_2 and SO_2. Some people are reactive to propane and natural gas leaking from stoves and heaters. Formaldehyde is another substance which can produce headache; it is found typically in plywoods, press board furniture, carpets, and air contaminated by cigarette smoke. Patients who have typical airborne allergies, reacting to pollens, dust and moulds, often experience headaches. These problems are easier to diagnose because they are associated with obvious localized signs, which include nose and sinus congestion, sore throat, cough, and irritated eyes.

The dietary advice that has been most often repeated with respect to migraine prevention is the avoidance of tyramines. Tyramines are amino acid-like chemicals present in highly fermented foods, such as red wine and cheddar cheese. Other tyramine substances, which collectively are known as amines, include the drug phenylethylamine, which is found in chocolate. Tyramine ingested in excess has a variety of untoward effects, usually involving changes in brain function. Experiments using tyramine alone have failed to substantiate its primary role in causing migraine headaches. The problem with many food-headache studies has been an overly simplistic view of the pain-causing sequence. In general, any food that has the property of imitating or releasing mediator substances in the bloodstream may produce   pain.   Any food that is capable of producing an allergic response can cause headache. Any combination of food which overloads detoxifying and clearing mechanisms may cause headache. Often the real dietary solution to a headache problem involves complete diet revision   and not simply the exclusion of one or two substances.

Migraine headaches are most clearly caused by food allergy. In an   English headache study[8], the authors state:

> "The diagnosis of migraine is based on clinical criteria and should not depend on mechanism or aetiology. Migraine is a multifactorial disease which may be induced through the ingestion of large amounts of chemical mediators in some individuals, or through an allergic reaction to foods in others. In the latter group, the exact mechanism by which foods cause the migrainous attacks is not clear. Some food-allergic reactions arise through an immune–complex–mediated mechanism – that is, a form of serum sickness triggered by a type–I hypersensitivity reaction in the gut. In these circumstances, the composition of the immune complex or the mediators released govern the damaging capacity.

A century of reports of the food-migraine connection often go ignored in the medical management of migraine. Dr. Munro has reviewed the history of reports of food provocation of headache. [9] The drug bias is so strong in medicine that   most "news" reports regarding migraine announce yet another drug, better than the last for reducing headaches. The drug approach to migraine has varied from the atrocious to the interesting. The atrocious side of drug treatment is the over-prescription of narcotic and sedative drugs, including barbiturates, valium and related compounds. A wide variety of drugs may reduce the severity of migraine; the diverse mechanisms by which these drugs act point to the multistage, complex mediator pattern of migraine. Aspirin or ASA remains one of the best drugs if taken in the first few minutes of an attack; related anti-inflammatory drugs work by the same ASA mechanism of blocking the production of prostaglandins, mediators generated in the first stage of a migraine response. In later stages blood platelets release serotonin, and other blood components come into play; when the attack is well-underway our best immune-suppressant agent, prednisone, can abort the late stages of the attack. Better than drugs, why not remove the original cause?!

To make a complicated problem simpler, we assume that at least two thirds of migraine headaches comes through the mouth. Migraine sufferers are likely to have true food allergy and are likely to respond well to adequate diet revision. It is usually not adequate just to eliminate a few things from the diet. Too much coffee, chocolate, junk foods, and alcoholic beverages are a common cause of migraine; but normal food components; milk, wheat, barley, rye, oats, corn, eggs, peanuts, soy, almonds, cashews, oranges, and salmon, are all headache triggers. While all the details of migraine's mechanisms are not yet understood, it is likely that many headaches are triggered by food antigens interacting with blood cells and blood-vessel walls. The circulation to the brain is disturbed with important but transient mental and emotional consequences. In migraine's more serious forms, active constriction and, later, inflammation of the arteries, supplying blood to the brain, severely compromise brain blood flow and lead to symptoms suggestive of stroke. Emotional and cognitive disturbances are common among migraine sufferers and indicate the profound impact of this disease mechanism on brain function.

Many patients we see have mixed headache patterns, with common or "tension" headaches occurring more frequently than their sick, migraine headaches. "Tension headaches" or generalized head-pain, associated with increased neck, scalp, and facial muscle tone and tenderness and often associated with subtle impairment of cognitive function, are also often caused by ingested substances and not "stress" or "tension". The muscle tension and soreness associated with these headaches is often an effect of the underlying biochemical cause of the pain and not a cause of it! Alcoholic beverages, coffee, tea, food additives, cereal grains, dairy products and milk are the more obvious foods strongly correlated with "tension" headaches.

In a study of children with migraine and other serious disturbances, excellent results were produced by dietary therapy. [10] A summary of their results follows:

> "93% of 88 children with severe frequent migraine recovered on oligoantigenic diets;
> the causative foods were identified by foods provoking migraine was established by a
> double-blind controlled trial in 40 of the children. Most patients responded to several
> foods. Many foods were involved, suggesting an allergic rather than an idiosyncratic
> (metabolic) pathogenesis. Associated symptoms which improved in addition to
> headache included abdominal pain, behavior disorder, fits, asthma, and eczema. In
> most of the patients in whom migraine was provoked by non-specific factors, such as
> blows to the head, exercise, and flashing lights, this provocation no longer occurred
> while they were on the diet. Introduction of cheese, chocolate, and red wine
> sometimes provoked migraine, allegedly owing to an idiosyncratic response to a
> pharmacologically active substance, tyramine. This response is perhaps due to

monoamine oxidase deficiency... Double-blind administration of tyramine to patients
who benefited from a low-tyramine diet did not provoke attacks of migraine... In this
study, children with severe migraine were given an oligoantigenic diet and in those
who improved the causative foods were identified by open reintroduction; responses
were confirmed by a double-blind controlled trial of reintroduction of the causative
foods."

Effective management of headaches depends on a multi-factorial plan. The ingested and
inhaled chemical and allergenic triggers are eliminated as much as possible through a
series of progressive steps. Physical measures are instituted as the principal means of
relieving pain. The use of strong analgesic medications, tranquilizers, and other drugs can
generally be minimized or avoided if appropriate dietary and physical therapies are put
into place. The simplest pain relievers are used when necessary. There is great concern
to avoid dependency on narcotic drugs or dependency on tranquilizers or muscle
relaxants.

Disorders of Mood, Arousal and Consciousness

Fight and flight arousal, triggered by allergic reactions, is a dramatic example of
abnormal arousal states. **Anxiety, fear and panic** are hyper-arousal emotions associated
with food, drug, and airborne allergy. More subtle and complicated problems occur
within the arousal systems of the brain to influence our state of consciousness, our ability
to concentrate, complete tasks and remember what we have done. Once conscious, we
need attention or the ability to focus on tasks to accomplish tasks. The **attention system** in
our brain is unstable and many chemical influences will spoil our ability to pay attention.
More depression of the arousal system and we feel tired, exhausted and/or fall asleep
when we should be awake. The arousal-attention system is closely linked with the system
that controls **mood** and regulates **appetite, thirst and temperature.** We are not surprised
to hear a patients report that they feel tired, cannot concentrate, and at the same time feel
anxious, angry, thirsty, cold and crave foods. This is dysfunction in the limbic-hypothamic
circuits of the brain and it is often associated with other symptoms which suggest food
allergy.

Patients have difficulty describing the daily changes in the clarity of their **consciousness.**
We do have good words for consciousness clarity, and patients use descriptions like
"blurred, foggy, spacey, dizzy, dopey, stoned" to indicate the problem. Some will compare
food-induced dysfunction to intoxication with alcohol or drugs. Some food reactions will
act more like hypnotic drugs or anesthetics, putting the person to sleep. Sleep attacks are
so severe in some patients that they cannot work, drive, or carry out normal daily routines.

Arousal disorders interfere with organized activity, concentration and memory. In children, we refer to "**Attention Deficit Disorder**"[11] and attribute learning disabilities to this dysfunction. Some of these children are hyperactive and have major behavioral problems which grow into life-long psychosocial disturbances. In adults with arousal disorders, we note shifting energy and mood levels. **Hyperactivity** and attention deficits continue in some adults, as long as they eat the wrong foods and drink the wrong drinks. Their arousal disturbance may often be associated with social withdrawal, disinterest, disorganization, failure to complete work tasks, failure to honor personal commitments and low self-esteem. In the worst case the arousal disorder is disabling.

Arousal disturbances are often **bipolar,** with rising and falling mood and energy. In children and adults, we observe sudden, dramatic shifts in mood and behavior as a food reacts. Often, the initial response to a dose of reactive food is temporary relief, with increased energy; followed in 1-3 hours by a crash into a tired, despondent, dysfunctional state. Cravings and compulsive eating seem to accompany mental and emotional disturbances, and perpetuate the eating-reaction loop.

Depression

Depression is a major problem in many of our patients. The term "depression" is merely **descriptive** and does not point to one discrete disorder, but a common failure mode of the human animal. Often in medical literature depression is treated as a *something* which causes other problems; but depression is not a entity and not a cause. Depression is a description of the effects of biological causes which act on the brain. Depression means brain dysfunction.

Often the meaning is turned upside-down; for example, a radio report described a study of smokers which found that depressed smokers get more cancer than "normal" smokers; the conclusion was that depression is a contributing cause of cancer? But **depression is a collection of effects, not a cause!** The symptoms of depression are caused by the chemicals in cigarette smoke itself; and also by associated eating and drinking habits. Smokers who also drink coffee, drink alcoholic beverages, and eat bad food combine addictive habits with the common properties: (i) disturbing brain function and (ii) promoting cancer.

Patients who are told that "depression causes your physical symptoms" should look for another physician. The body-mind states we call "depression" are an expression of underlying biological problems. Our depressed patients are often pleasantly surprised when their suffering can be alleviated by changes in their diet.

The term "depression" is a rather trivial description of suffering that can be both profound and life-threatening. William Styron in his book "Darkness Visible"[12], describes his depressive experience as a "howling tempest in the brain". He recounts a history of alcoholic beverage abuse, and suggests that depression comes from a mix of bad chemistry, genetics and adverse experiences. He underestimates the primary significance of bad food and drink in disturbing brain function to the point of a "...poisonous fog bank rolling in ". Styron discounts psychotherapy, and expresses concerns about psychotropic drugs, so freely prescribed, often not helpful, and sometimes harmful. A depressed person, serious about getting better, must stop smoking, stop drinking and do diet revision until their body intake produces a normally-functioning brain. Occasionally, carefully selected drugs, at low doses, are useful adjuncts to this recovery process.

Depression is an **arousal-mood disorder** and begins with fatigue, loss of interest, and loss of pleasure. As depression worsens, emotions blacken, tears flow, anger increases, all pleasures and interests vanish. Death thoughts become attractive. **Thinking** is usually disturbed, with reduced attention span, distractability, and increased difficulty in remembering recent events. Depressed moods may fluctuate and in some people high and low moods alternate in a pattern referred to as "bipolar affective disorder". Often eating patterns fluctuate with the mood in a **complex 4-F interaction**. It is not obvious that changes in food selection precede the mood change until the patient has cleared all symptoms and then re-introduces food.

With mood changes, thinking shifts, sometimes dramatically. The **cognitive styles** and structures attached to different moods may be so distinct and dissociated from other cognitive structures that different personalities seem to emerge in the same person. Splitting of the personality is often reported by insightful patients, most of whom would otherwise be thought of as ordinary, sane people. Many patients describe an abrupt "Jekyl and Hyde" transformation. This **flip-flop**, abrupt style of mood transition is typical of food reactions. The surprising fact is that different foods have a profound impact on mood cognitive styles, and personality. The mood and behavioral style of entire populations may be influenced by their food supply!

We often use color metaphors to describe moods; black seems naturally suited to the negative moods, associated with night, anxiety, fear, and death. Happy moods are not white, but light colors; the purest sky blue is chosen in Tibetan symbolism to represent the clear, untroubled mind. The sense of not-being-well is "dysphoria". The sense of all-being-well is "euphoria". If a high energy state is modulated by dysphoric signals, suffering is the result - dread, despair, doom. If the same high energy state is modulated by euphoric signals, the "high" experience of bliss, oneness, ecstasy is the reward.

As with all our brain functions, mood signals can intermodulate in a jumble of confused feelings; agitated depression may occur, or a hyperactive, manic state with high energy and overly-optimistic interpretations, but with dysphoric feelings spoiling the manic high.

Patients often describe **paradoxical emotional states**, combining depression with irritability or restless, disorganized activity. They may be hyperactive, loud, and aggressive while failing to complete tasks, relate to others, or feel pleasure. This paradoxical arousal state is unstable and often explodes in an inappropriate burst of anger and other irrational, behaviors. At the other end of the mood spectrum, they may collapse with fatigue and dysphoria, consumed with negative, critical thinking, hopelessness and inconsolable self-doubt.

The effect of erratic brain function is chaos. Two people living together with erratic brain function increase chaos by more than a factor of two; more people interacting erratically increase chaos exponentially until family structures, community structures, and national structures fall apart. **Bad chemicals** entering brains from wrong foods, alcoholic beverages, legal and illegal drugs are surely the best prescription for a society's dysphoric collapse. The folly of "fighting a drug war" has been demonstrated by recent U.S. experiences. The **demon lives at home**. A total solution involves a community clearing its chaotic brains of "bad chemicals" in one sweep of enlightened self-interest.

Unfortunately the "drug sellers" are on every street corner and penetrate almost every household; we must be smart enough to see the connections among food materials which influence brain function: alcoholic beverages, tobacco, teas, coffee, chocolate, spices, food additives, sugar excess, wheat, milk, eggs, prescription drugs and street drugs. An addicted society will tolerate the diseases caused by tobacco smoke, alcoholic beverages, air pollution and food contamination but displaces its dysphoric energy in a "drug war" against cocaine, a single problem among many. (Recall that displacement is one of the basic properties of the reptilian brain).

Mood determination is closely linked to brain procedures which regulate all body functions, and it is not surprising to observe close relationships between food, mood-arousal disorders, digestive and immune dysfunctions. A continuous flow of proper nutrients is essential to normal brain function. Just as important is the absence of interference with proper brain function by avoidance of the inappropriate input of problematic molecular species. Coffee, tea, alcoholic beverages, chocolate are among the more obvious food problems, but even "healthy" diets cause major mental problems because of food allergy mechanisms, or other abnormal procedures - metabolic problems, nutrient disproportion, or food toxicity.

As long as we assume that mood disorders are the result of physically-induced brain dysfunction, we look for practical, effective solutions and not waste so much time gossiping about the look and behavior of the depressed person. It is not helpful to discuss the contents of a depressed mood.

Depression can be thought of as a black container which collects negative thoughts; the thought content is not really interesting and can be acknowledged and then dropped. When the mood improves, the black container, full of negative thoughts, is put on the shelf as a souvenir; the depressed thoughts are no longer functional, no longer relevant. Our attention should be focused on the many possible causes of brain interference entering the body through the nose and mouth, not on the abnormal thought processes.

The confusion and despair of depression leads to suicide in the most seriously afflicted. Bad food and the abuse of alcoholic beverages and other drugs are most effective in setting the stage for suicide. Patients with depression are now told that their suffering comes from a "chemical imbalance in the brain"; drugs are prescribed, allegedly to "correct this imbalance". Patients are not told that **the chemical imbalance comes from the wrong chemical input to the brain through the mouth!** Adding prescription drugs to a bad chemical mix entering the body is hardly a rational solution to the problem.

The Core Program encourages a return to **adaptive self-regulation.** We are aware that self-regulation is easily sabotaged by other people, by circumstances, and by years of bad habits which seem to be written into the brain in indelible ink. Self-regulation can only occur if chaotic elements in a person's life are brought under control. In families this is only possible if everyone cooperates and everyone succeeds at getting better. A tall order. Self-regulation can only occur if the molecular flow into the brain is rational, coherent, consistent and free of the wrong-stuff!

> *Changing the chemical input to the brain by careful control of ingested materials can reduce or correct depression. Often the negative, angry, critical thinking and sleepless nights vanish on Phase 1 of the Core Program, but not before these disturbances intensify during withdrawal. Mental fogginess, difficulty concentrating, memory- loss, and confusion clear along with improvement of physical symptoms.*

Mechanisms of Brain Disturbances

There are many complex ideas which link food ingestion to brain states, by considering the operation of different systems of the body. The following discussion is intended to expand the reader's ideas about what sort of explanations might be considered. While we are most interested in the many possible interactions of immune system and nerovous system, basic biochemistry has much to offer. Biological psychiatry has focused on the biochemistry of neurotransmitters, as revealed by drug action in experimental animals. Chemical theories of depression, for example, are often over-simplications, based on observations of altered neurotransmitter synthesis and function in the brains of mice and rats. The brain activity of antidepressant drugs has provided elementary understanding of the different brain systems involved in creating and regulating psychic energy.

Nutritional influences brain function in a variety of ways. The brain disturbances of an alcoholic, unstable diabetic, pellagra victim, or elderly patient with vitamin B12 or folic acid deficiency are all recognized examples of nutritional mental illnesses. **Vitamin deficiency** is always a concern with brain dysfunction, and the risk of deficiency increases as mental disorder increases. Vitamin-mineral supplementation is always a desirable component of nutritional therapy, although high doses of individual nutrients are seldom required. The B-vitamins play a critical role in brain function. The supplement levels recommended in the Core Program instructions will usually provide adequate nutrient intake. Most food-input problems can be avoided by using an elemental nutrient formula during the clearing period. We can expect brain function to settle into a normal baseline mode after 10-14 days on an ENF even in very disturbed patients.

Sodium, potassium, calcium and magnesium are the key mineral ions in the brain and must be maintained in critical balance. Low calcium levels produce tetany, painful muscle contractions with dizziness, confusion, and even seizures. Hyperventilation causes a sudden drop in blood calcium levels and produces tetany. Magnesium can reduce brain irritation and block seizures in alcohol withdrawal and toxemia of pregnancy. Extra calcium and magnesium tend to have a calming effect and are safe to take in supplemental form. Potassium intake is often deficient and routine addition of potassium salt to food is recommended on the Core Program. Sugar is not added to food, and sodium salt is used in moderation.

As we now know, food has many more interactions with body-brain than nutrient status alone can predict. Other abnormal food-body interactions may underlie many modern mental disorders. There are many different mechanisms for problems to occur in food-body-brain interactions. A quick summary of the more important brain problems in our food supply allows one to run through a check list in solving problems:

Nutrient Deficiencies	Nutrient Excesses
Nutrient Disproportion	Toxic Effects
Metabolic Abnormalities	Food Allergy
Proteins and Peptides	Drug Effects
Colon Metabolites	Carcinogens

Acetylcholine, Drugs and Pesticides

Our principle brain arousal network uses **acetylcholine (Ach)** as the transmitter. Increasing Ach activity arouses our thinking, memory, and computational abilities, but too much may make us feel depressed. Most **antidepressant drugs** block acetylcholine circuits, and, if taken in overdose, produce stupor and coma by Ach blockade. In this drug-overdose mode, the same Ach drug, physostigmine, awakens the comatose patient immediately, although the effect is short-lived and must be repeated. Physostigmine improves thinking and memory in patients with Alzheimer's disease; loss of Ach production and destruction of Ach-using neurons characterize this disease. The administration of choline, the Ach precursor, to improve memory may also produce fatigue or depression.

Smoking increases nicotine levels in the brain with initial stimulation of Ach circuits and later blockade. This dual action produces the typical biphasic response of an addictive drug with initial psychomotor stimulation followed by depression. The drive to smoke is essentially a drive to maintain brain nicotine levels. The nicotine is accompanied by a complex of toxic chemicals including carbon monoxide and benzene which can seriously depress brain function. Smokers cannot expect to have clarity of consciousness, nor stable moods. Heavy smokers develop tolerance to toxic effects but slowly deteriorate by all measures of biological competence.

Common **pesticides** (Malathion, Parathion, EPN, Schradan), which contaminate our food supply and poison farm-workers, are related to "nerve gases" (Saran, Soman), which all act on the Ach system. They block the breakdown of Ach, so that it accumulates and prevents further Ach messages to get through. The result is respiratory failure and convulsions, quickly fatal if the dose is high enough. The role of pesticide residues in our food supply in causing mental and emotion symptoms is unknown, but anyone who doubts a possible connection should review their neurochemistry.

The Role of Amino Acids

The **neurotransmitters** serotonin, norepinephrine, and dopamine, are involved in the regulation of our moods. These transmitters are made from amino acids, supplied as proteins in foods. Serotonin is made from tryptophan. Phenylalanine and tyrosine become norepinephrine, epinephrine, and dopamine. **L-Dopa** is synthesized within brain cells and is not considered to be a nutrient, but is used to treat patients with **Parkinson's disease** who have deficient dopamine. Parkinson's victims experience fatigue, depression, and slowing of all movements along with the characteristic pill-rolling, resting tremor. L-dopa must be given with an enzyme inhibitor which reduces the liver's ability to breakdown the amino acid in order for increased amounts to reach the brain. Increased brain uptake of L-dopa promotes the synthesis of dopamine, the deficient neurotransmitter.

Many problems are associated with L-dopa use, especially marked fluctuations of motor performance during the day. Dr. Pincus and colleagues at Yale University demonstrated that food choices were relevant to patients on L-dopa. They reduced protein content of the diet with smoothing of motor performance and decreased need for L-dopa. High protein snacks would induce immobility in sensitive patients within 45 minutes. Our perception of all attempted amino acid therapies follows this observation: you must change the whole input recipe in order to succeed! Indeed it is likely the agents which damage neurons in this disease enter via the mouth on a regular basis. We would be inclined to start every newly-diagnosed Parkinson's patient on an ENF for a rather prolonged trial of clearing and then slowly, very carefully reintroduce Core Program foods, watching closely for changes in symptoms. Unfortunately, an oxidation product of dopamine, is a potent, selective toxin for dopamine neurons in the brain; the production of damaging 6-hydroxy dopamine could increase with high protein diets and with the administration of L-Dopa. Reducing proteins, avoiding L-dopa, and increasing intake of antioxidants (vitamin C, E, selenium) may be helpful.

Rather simple theories have linked the ingestion of foods containing more or less of the amino acids: tryptophan, phenylalanine, and tyrosine with mood changes. These amino acids, taken orally, are not powerful antidepressants, but may contribute a well thought-out neurochemical recipe.

When we work with pure nutrients, in an elemental nutrient formula, amino acid considerations are most important; one possibility for nutritional programming is to experiment with different amino acid proportions in an ENF to improve brain function in disturbed individuals. This technology would seem to offer an alternative or adjunct to psychotropic drugs. When you deal with real food, in complex combinations, you are no longer just dealing with amino acid proportions and another, more complicated story emerges.

Clues to the **amino-acid-neurotransmitter** relationships have been studied by Richard Wurtman and his associates at MIT. They showed, for example, that the uptake of tryptophan was enhanced by sugar and decreased by competition with other amino acids. **Tryptophan** is converted to **serotonin** in the brain and Dr. Wurtman suggested that serotonin deficiency caused depression and was helped by eating high carbohydrate foods (increasing trytophan intake). Drugs that increase serotonin levels have differing effects; fenfluramine, for example, has been studied for many years as an appetite suppressant with disappointing results in our patients, especially the binge eaters. Some antidepresants which boost serotonin levels increase appetite and may lead to progressive weight gain. A new antidepressant drug, prozac seems to be different and decreases appetite. Antidepressants of the MAO-inhibitor group (parnate, nardil) increase norepinephrine levels but not serotonin and have been moderately helpful in over-eating patients.

According to Dr. Judith Wurtman, food-induced changes in energy and mood can be explained by the effect of foods on neurotransmitter levels. She suggests choosing foods on the basis of their content of principle amino acids and **carbohydrate/protein ratios**. The basic idea might be that high protein foods are "stimulating" because they increase the synthesis of norepinephrine from phenylalanine and tyrosine; "carbohydrate" foods are sedative because they increase the synthesis of serotonin from tryptophan. Trytophan uptake in the brain is enhanced if it is ingested alone along with sugar. In Wurtman's book "Managing Your Mind Through Food" [13]we are encouraged to eat high protein foods "...when your brain's supply of dopamine and norepinephrine is beginning to run short..." Suggested meals include whole-grain bread, skim milk, cottage cheese, and eggs. Other suggestions include drinking coffee in the morning for its arousal effect.

Our clinical **experience** is often just the **opposite** of Dr. Wurtman's predictions. High carbohydrate foods such as breads, buns, crackers are strongly sedative in some patients; induce cravings and compulsive eating; and are associated with symptoms of food allergy. Clearly the effect of a food is far more complex than simple theories make it seem. Milk, and eggs are strongly allergenic; their proteins may adversely affect brain function through immune-mediated mechanisms, before their content of amino acids has any relevance! In reference to SLE in the previous chapter, the role of **immune-modulating peptides** was mentioned; milk protein can act both as an allergen but also can stimulate the immune response. [14] We had known that pieces of milk and wheat proteins (peptides) could act like the body's own endorphins and were described by Zioudro, Streaty and Klee as "**exorphins**" in 1979.[15] The exorphin mechanism might explain some the symptoms and the addictive properties of these allergenic foods. Several effects could occur in sequence, making the interpretation of milk and wheat disease very difficult.

Many food allergic people would be sedated, or disabled with poor concentration, and decreased memory by milk, eggs, meat, and fish. Some would be paradoxically restless, irritable, or anxious. Very few would be alert, oriented, or happy. Milk and wheat disease regularly disrupt arousal, attention and mood. Coffee is also a bad offender; regular brew leaves you aroused (perhaps to the point of irritability, tremor, or anxiety) but with reduced mental acuity and probable memory deficits, the **Coffee Users Fog (CUF)**. De-caffeinated coffee has less arousal effect but CUF remains a problem because the some of the other 500 chemicals in coffee, including pesticides, remain neurotoxic. Teas and chocolate are similarly implicated in arousal disorders with an addictive profile. These common substances play a major role in the psychopathology of daily life, but are so concealed in the fabric of "normal" existence that hardly anyone notices.

The high carbohydrate intake of depressed patients, especially in the **winter** months may not be related to brain tryptophan and brain serotonin levels but to the more complex brain effects of gluten proteins, food allergic mechanisms, and/or light-deprivation changes in hormone regulators such as melatonin. This "**seasonal affective disorder**" could be another food allergic disease, increased by increased and altered food intake in the winter, not just a light-dependent hormonal change. Most depressed, over-eating patients we see have obvious symptoms of food allergy and improve when they try the clearing diet which is high in carbohydrate but relatively free of allergenic effects. Eating wheat-containing foods triggers a typical craving, compulsive-eating cycle, following a typical addiction pattern.

We have to expand our view of food-caused brain dysfunction to include many complex mechanisms. Food can be viewed as the input to the **multi-dimensional body-brain matrix** involving many body systems. Problems in the food supply impinge on brain function, disturbing perceptual, cognitive, and behavioral processes. The critical role of the food supply is evaluated by strategies of diet revision. Within the complex of dysfunctional patterns, food allergy has emerged as a unifying concept of the origin of many dysfunctional patterns. The newer models of food allergy postulate several overlapping problems, including the wrong entry of large molecules into the blood stream, through the intestinal wall. This wrong entry triggers immune responses and otherwise disorders metabolic and biochemical processing in target organs, including the brain.

> *We are convinced that food allergy mechanisms can and do cause*
> *serious mood or affective disorders, and refer to this form of*
> *depression as "Immune Mediated Affective Disorder" (IMAD).*

The food allergy model also postulates that foods immunize us against a very large number of antigens. This vast and continuously changing immunity produces, by a variety of mechanisms, dysfunction and disease, including brain dysfunction. Brain dysfunction is expressed as disordered thinking, feeling, behaving, and remembering. The food allergy illness patterns in children and adults involve typical clusters of digestive, respiratory, skin, and behavioral disturbances. The illness patterns occasionally involve inhalant allergies, defined in the usual way by skin and blood tests, but can operate independently through other, more complex immune mechanisms.

The Major Neurological Diseases

Our interest in explaining major brain diseases is perked almost daily by patients who have obvious **food allergy** and at the same time symptoms suggestive of one or more of the major neurological diseases: **Multiple Sclerosis, Parkinson's, Alzheimer's, and Schizophrenia.** Some patients with food allergy eventually cross the boundary between mild to moderate manifestation and overt disease with permanent disability. We wonder how many years does it take to develop full-blown Alzheimer's after the first symptoms of decreased concentration, memory loss, and disorganization sets in?

There are many clues to these neurological diseases which point to the food supply. A fascinating example of food toxicity and neurological disease occurred on the Pacific Island of **Guam**; flour made from the seeds of the **cyad plant,** a staple food during the second world war has been implicated in causing a mixed neurological disease, combining features of three major degenerative diseases; Alzheimer's, Parkinson's and Lou Gehrig's disease (amyotrophic lateral sclerosis). The effects of the toxic food seemed to be delayed many years. Leonard Kurland of the Mayo clinic remained convinced that cyad seeds were responsible and with Peter Spencer of the Albert Einstein College of Medicine was able to show that nerve cell damage was probably caused by BMAA, a non-nutrient amino acid in the seed.

Another food-toxin clue to **Alzheimer's disease** was a permanent memory loss suffered by people who had ingested toxic Atlantic mussels in 1987. The toxin, **demoic acid**, appeared to be a product of algae eaten by the muscles during an unusual algae bloom. Demoic acid is similar to kainic acid, a metabolite which occurs naturally in the brain; it seems to damage cells in the **hippocampus**, an area of the brain essential for recent memory function.

Yet another clue to Alzheimer's disease is the neurological damage caused by **aluminum salts** in patients undergoing kidney dialysis, and by accidental poisoning. Residents of an English village, Cameford, were exposed to high levels of aluminum in their drinking water, after a truck driver dumped aluminum sulfate into the water supply by mistake. Many residents presented to their physicians in the following weeks with a symptom complex that sounds familiar: burning mouths, abdominal pains, diarrhea, itchy rashes, and mouth ulcers. Fatigue, aching and stiffness appeared along with memory loss and personality changes. These symptoms fit the general pattern of food allergy and could also fit the CFIDS or myalgic encephalitis description. Dr. D. McLaughlin of the University of Toronto has associated Alzheimer's disease with increased brain levels of aluminum. Acid rain increases the bioavalability of aluminum in soils. High levels of aluminum are found in some foods, especially corn bread, processed cheese, cake, pancake and icing mixes, baking powders, fast-food hamburgers; tooth pastes also contain aluminum salts; (Crest is the highest and Aqua-fresh the lowest). Many common antacids are made of aluminum salts. With high exposure to packaged foods, toothpastes and antacids high aluminum intake is to be expected.

Dr. Pat McGeer at the University of British Columbia has found evidence of chronic **inflammation** in the brains of patients dying with Alzheimer's disease. Infiltration of brain tissues by lymphocytes suggests an immune-mediated or allergic disease. Perhaps aluminum salts (and other agents) make the blood brain barrier more permeable to food antigens, turning mild to moderate food allergy into a disabling disease. Of the staple foods, milk, egg and gluten proteins are the most common causes of depression with chronic fatigue, concentration difficulties, memory impairment and sleep disturbances. Basic foods as well as chemical additives and toxic contaminants may be implicated in all the neurological diseases.

Schizophrenia

Neurologists have never taken care of schizophrenic patients even though they have profound disturbances of brain function; perhaps they were too disruptive and bizarre. These patients went to mental hospitals and psychiatrists took over their care. The schizophrenic patient has yet to receive medical care appropriate for someone with an acute, disabling brain disease. An acute episode of schizophrenia should be treated as a medical emergency in an intensive care unit with continuous brain monitoring. The disease process is damaging to the brain and unless it is controlled early in the illness, permanent disability in the form of dementia is likely. Schizophrenia may be another immune-mediated disease with immune cells attacking brain cells; or it may be a viral or neurotoxic disease. Again the food supply of a victim looks very suspicious.

Control of acute disease should include replacing food with an ENF, fortified with higher than usual intake of vitamins especially B1, B3, B6, B12 and Vm.E. Mineral intake needs to be carefully regulated and much thought should be given to fatty acid intake; increased amounts of EPA and GLA look attractive, but no-one knows how to correctly regulate these nutrients; some safe experimentation in a controlled environment would be highly desirable. Some schizophrenics may have defects in the handling of amino acids, and this, in theory, may be regulated by adjusting the amino acid values of an ENF. The only general rule is that increased dopamine activity makes schizophrenia worse; decreasing intake of tyrosine and phenylalanine would be the first logical experiment; other biochemical theories suggest that reducing methionine might help since this amino acid contributes the methyl groups which convert other amino acids from normal brain molecules to hallucinogens. Other measures appropriate to the control of allergic disease are also required - clean air and water are essential.

An acute schizophrenic attack so disturbs information processing in the brain that a schizophrenic needs information protection; only simple information and minimal stimuli will be properly interpreted. Spontaneous brain activity increases as well, so that thinking and dreaming become hallucinations and delusions. This mind activity is an abnormal artifact and, while often interesting (as dreams are interesting), has no value to the interpretation or treatment of the illness. Arousal disturbances in schizophrenics may be the same processes we see in food allergic children and adults with mood swings, episodes of irritability, hyperactivity, attention and memory deficits. Food control should alleviate these disturbances within the schizophrenia complex even if an underlying disease process remains intact.

Dr.F. Dohan has consistently advocated a gluten-schizophrenia link.[16][17] He states:

> "Many diseases are caused by genetically–deficient utilization of specific food substances. Perhaps the best studied example is phenylketonuria...far more common disorders, for example, atherosclerosis, and coronary heart disease, are strongly suspected of being due to genetically defective utilization of certain food constituents. Similarly, considerable evidence indicates that the major cause of schizophrenia is the inborn inability to process certain digestion products of some food proteins, especially cereal grain glutens..."

Among Dr. Dohan's interesting recommendations is the **"gluten tolerance test"**. A gluten tolerance test could be initiated with routine evaluations before and after ingestion of grain foods. More sophisticated versions would measure gluten proteins and derived peptides in the blood, and would track the path of these molecules into organs, especially the brain. Finally, the impact of these molecules would be evaluated by monitoring the function of the target organ in real-time. Real-time monitoring of brain activity, topologically-computed in gluten-sensitive patients would be of great interest. These patients report changes in their level of psychic energy, cognitive abilities, and emotional states. The problem of adverse brain effects of molecules derived from food is under-recognized. These and other clues to mysterious and threatening neurological diseases suggest that any prudent person, suffering early brain-dysfunction symptoms, would be wise to pursue vigorous, thorough diet revision at the earliest opportunity.

We expect during the next decade, a new level of awareness from physicians, psychiatrists, and psychologists. Profession ignorance of the food-illness-mental-state connection is no longer acceptable. Professional therapists must be able to deal with the day-to-day practical necessities of good biological functioning, expressed as the daily choices of food and drink - body input. They must also recognize that smoking, airborne chemical exposure, and other adverse environments affect brain function and adversely influence mental status.

---

[1]Pribram K.H. Languages of the Brain. Prentice Hall; 183; 1971

[2]Alvarez, W.C. Ways of discovering foods that are causing distress. Proc Staff Meet Mayo Clin, 7:443,1932

[3]Davison, H.M. Allergy of the nervous system. Quart Rev allergy 6:157,1952

[4]Randolph, T.G. Ecological mental illness – levels of central nervous system reactions. Third World Congress Psychiat Montreal June 1961.

[5] Lipowski ZJ. Psychosomatic Medicine in the Seventies.1977. Am Jour. Psych.134:233-244

[6] Bates C. Personal communication. 1985. See also Bates C. Essential Fatty Acids & Immunity In Mental Health. Life Sciences Press, Tacoma WA 1987.

[7] Aas K. General Discussion. Nutr Rev 1984;42(3)119.

[8] Monro, J.; Carini, C.; Brostoff, J. Migraine is a Food-Allergic Disease. Lancet. Sep 29, 1984. Vol. II. pp 719-721.]

[9] Monro J, Brostoff J, Carini C, Zilkha K. Food allergy in migraine: A study of dietary exclusion and RAST. Lancet 1980; ii: 1-4.

Munro J. Food-induced Migraine. Food Allergy and Intolerance. 633-665 Balliere Tindall 1987

[10] Egger,J.; Carter, C. M.; Wilson, J.; Turner, M. W.; Soothill, J. F. Institute of Child Health, London. Is Migraine Food Allergy? A Double-blind Controlled Trial of Oligoantigenic Diet Treatment.The Lancet.1983.Vol.II. 866-869.

[11] Gislason S.J. Food, Learning, Behavior. Chpt 14; Core Diet For Kids 1989 PerSona Publ. Vancouver BC; Canada V6R 1P2; 205-232

[12] Styron W. Darkness Visible A Memoir of Madness Random House NY 1990.

[13] Wurtman J.J Managing Your Mind Through Food. 1988 Harper & Row, N.Y.

[14] Carr R.I Immunomodulation by Opioids from Dietary Casein(exorphins) New York Acad Sc. 597; 374-376:1990.

[15] Zioudrou,C.,Streaty R.A., Klee W.A. 1979. J. Biol. Chem.254:244-6.

[16] Dohan FC. Cereals and schizophrenia: data and hypothesis. Acta Psychiatr Scand 1966;42:125-42.

[17] Dohan FC. More on celiac disease as a model for schizophrenia. Biol Psychiatry 1983;18:561-4.

Chapter 8

Patterns of Illness and Case Histories

There are many biological possibilities for things to go wrong after eating food. Few patients have simple, single problems. Each person tends to have a collection of disturbances in different body systems, which emerges, in complicated sequences over time. We allow each patient to have several problems, in any combination, in any order of frequency, severity, and timing. We allow more that 10 symptoms to occur simultaneously without deciding that the patient is neurotic or hypochondriac. We allow different patterns of food allergy to coexist with eating disorders, metabolic problems, diabetes or whatever other food-related illness wants to join the party. We allow the symptoms to be intermittent or inconsistent, because the human body is not a simple linear machine, but a complicated, changing, wavey device, like the weather or the sea. We accept the concept that illness is an expression of chaotic events and do not get upset when symptom patterns do not fit our preconceived notions. We permit a great deal of uncertainty about the mechanism of the problems and focus on the likely source of the disturbance and a likely solution. We accept that diet revision, properly conducted, will resolve a great number of problems simultaneously. Even if we are not sure why the patient got better; we are happy with the good outcome, nevertheless.

We are not inventing something weird and new. Consider an apt description of food allergy in the writings of the ancient Greek physician, Hippocrates, 2000 years ago. [1] This description fits contemporary patients we see every day:

> "But there are persons who cannot readily change their diet with impunity; and if they make any alteration in it for one day, or even a part of a day, are greatly injured thereby. Such persons, provided they take dinner when it is not their wont, immediately become heavy and inactive, both in mind and body, and are weighed down with yawning, slumbering, and thirst; and if they take supper in addition, they are seized with flatulence, tormina, and diarrhoea, and to many this has been the commencement of serious disease, when they have merely taken twice in a day the same food which they have been in the custom of taking once.

> "And thus, also, if one who has been accustomed to dine, and this rule agrees with him, should not dine at the accustomed hour, he will straightway feel great loss of strength, trembling, and want of spirits; the eyes of such a person will become more

pallid, his urine thick and hot, his mouth bitter; his bowels will seem, as it were, to
hang loose; he will suffer from vertigo, lowness of spirit, and inactivity...If he should
attempt to take at supper the same food which he was wont to partake of at
dinner...these things, passing downwards, with tormina and rumbling, burn up his
bowels; he experiences insomnolency or troubled and disturbed dreams; and to
many of them these symptoms are the commencement of some disease."

Hippocrates described a disorder with many symptoms; dysfunction of the gastrointestinal
tract is associated with disturbances of mood, energy, and sleep. He noted that these
symptoms may herald the onset of more serious disease. He was aware of the fascinating
phenomena of addiction to the allergenic food, marked by withdrawal dysphoria if the
food is not eaten regularly. This withdrawal phenomenon has been variously
misconstrued, especially as "hypoglycemic reactions". The frequent occurrence of cravings
for the allergenic foods, and marked withdrawal discomforts, make investigation and
treatment of food allergy a complicated business. We can conclude from Hippocrates'
clinical description that the ancient Greek patient and the contemporary-world patient
have much in common.

Typical Case Histories

The following patient descriptions illustrate common patterns of food-related illness,
especially the delayed patterns of food allergy. Notice how the individual problems,
described in the previous chapters are distributed through the case histories in different
patterns and combinations; each person illustrates the inter-relatedness of common
health problems. Chronic **fatigue** and/or **depression** are among the most prevalent
features of the illness patterns. We can think of layers of problems which emerge over
time. More obvious allergy problems such as asthma, eczema, or migraine headaches may
dominate the foreground, with fatigue, digestive, emotional and cognitive disturbances
lurking in the background.

Traditional diagnostic methods tries to separate each problem into individual named
boxes. While this analytic, sorting procedure helps us deal with complexity, it has distinct
limitations and may mislead us. An alternative, often complementary, method of
analyzing health problems is to use a **whole-system's approach** to problem-solving. We try
to understand how different problems are expressions of a common, underlying disease
processes.   Each patient has a collection of symptoms in different body systems. We
assume that a **dysfunctional matrix** underlies the illness, not a single mechanism or cause.
We often ask where was the original problem? how did it get in? how was it distributed?
how long did it take to act? and so-on. We ask - did the problem originate in the food

supply? A rational problem-solving approach might assume that the original problem might have been in the food supply and set about to change body input in a methodical manner; do the Diet Revision experiment. DRT tends to succeed even when other interventions fail. The following case histories present the initial problem description and all may conclude with the statement: with appropriate Diet Revision Therapy, using techniques to remove foods contributing to food allergy; behavioral modification to ensure stability of new, more successful eating patterns; and nutritional methods to resolve metabolic problems and to ensure adequate nutrition, **these illness patterns tend to resolve.**

Chronic Fatigue, Rhinitis, Headache

A 32 year old woman presented with several health problems which included:

Nose congestion　　　　　　*Flu-like illnesses*
Chronic cough　　　　　　　*Fatigue*
Insomnia　　　　　　　　　*Headache*

She described a "flu" syndrome, dragging on for many months, with nose congestion, increased throat mucous and digestive disturbances, indigestion and bloating. She generally felt tired and listless. Repeated medical investigations had revealed no clues to the problem and she had been told that "nothing is wrong". She was seeing a chiropractor weekly for manipulation therapy of her neck for headaches without lasting benefits. Her diet was unrestrained. By her own admission, she ate poorly. She lived alone, did shift work, and ate most of her meals in restaurants. She preferred sandwiches, cheese, pasta, and snack foods in general. She drank 4 cups of tea per day, and 48 ounces of red and white wine per week. She was not aware of any food intolerances. The pattern of a complex, polysymptomatic, multisystem disorder is consistent with the diagnosis of food allergy.

Fatigue, Pain, Mental Fogginess

A 28 year old professional man presented with a several problems, including:

Fatigue　　　　　　　　*Abdominal pain*
Chest pains　　　　　　　*Generalized aching*
Mental fogginess　　　　　*Dizziness*
Disorientation　　　　　　*Reduced efficiency*

He stated that he caught a virus a year and a half ago, with only partial recovery, and recurrence within the past year - "...I totally ran out of gas...". While growing more tired and weak, he experienced increasing epigastric pain and generalized aching with daily indigestion, burping, and heartburn. Any exertion seemed to aggravate both muscle pain and fatigue. He noted that he felt better when he ate less food. On his worst days, he stopped eating altogether and felt better. He had bouts of diarrhea, passing 3-4 watery bowel movements during the day, often 30-60 minutes after eating. Repeated blood tests, and X-rays were not helpful in revealing the cause. Muscle relaxants were prescribed, but made him more "dopey". His diet included large amounts of milk, whole-wheat bread, pasta, beef, and packaged foods, especially cereals, soup mixes, and quick dinners; a third of his meals were eaten in restaurants. He admitted that his diet was disorganized and inconsistent. Digestive symptoms cleared promptly on Phase 1 of the Core Program and he slowly recovered energy and stamina over a 3 month period. He frequently had symptoms when he returned to restaurant food; his most demanding adaptation was to learn to prepare his own meals.

Asthma, Panic Attacks, Abdominal Pain Asthma

A 41 year old career woman presented with a complex history of illness:

Asthma.	*Abdominal bloating*
flatulence	*Abdominal pain*
Chronic fatigue	*Insomnia*
Itching	*Panic attacks*

She described a slowly progressive, chronic illness. Asthma was a major problem; she required three asthma medications, Beclovent and Ventolin 3 or 4 times daily, with theophylline tablets. Her digestive symptoms were becoming increasingly severe, with daily abdominal distension, belching, heartburn, and episodes of acute abdominal pain with diarrhea. All GIT investigations were negative. She was always tired and sometimes depressed. She had withdrawn from all social and recreational activities in the past 2 years, but continued to work. Occasionally, she would experience unprovoked panic attacks with fast irregular heart action, flushing, sweating and tremor. These attacks were so distressing that she avoided driving and going out alone, fearing a disabling attack. Her diet included moderate intake of bread, muffins, pasta, occasional eggs, some yogurt and cheese (but no milk), poultry, beef, salads (but few cooked vegetables), and fruit, mostly citrus. She drank coffee (2 cups), occasional tea and hot chocolate but avoided alcoholic beverages, knowing they made her feel sick. She chose to clear on an ENF, and by day 5 was beginning to improve. She continued to complete recovery within 6 weeks on the Core Program. She experienced several food reactions during Phases 2 and 3, but accurately identified the problems, and emerged well. She found that rice caused persisting fatigue and had to omit it. Most fruits were better tolerated cooked. Her "panic attacks" did not recur and her asthma was 80% cleared with food control; 20% remained an airborne problem. Her prescription drug use dropped dramatically.

Depression, Drinking, and Night Sweats

A 38 year mill-worker presented with life-long depression and many associated and chronic symptoms, including:

Nose congestion	*Cough*
Abdominal Bloating	*Fatigue*
Insomnia	*Night sweats*

This hard-working family man described years of moodiness with a tendency to withdraw, remain silent, and lose interest in all recreational activities. He would become inexplicably irritable and lose his temper at his children and wife unreasonably. He worked hard and had little energy left in the evenings, often falling asleep in front of the TV. He never slept well and often woke feeling anxious, hot, and sweaty; his wife had preferred to sleep separately for several years and they seldom had sex. His nose had been congested since early childhood, and he had cough with shortness of breath and chest pains increasingly. He drank 6-8 cups of coffee per day, and at least 2 bottles of beer every evening. On the weekends he drank beer at home alone and with his friends probably having 8-12 bottles on an average weekend. He described compulsive drinking and thought it was a problem but never had tried to stop. He preferred "meat and potatoes", and ate a lot of bread, cheese, eggs, processed meats, packaged cookies, and "junk food". He avoided milk but "loved ice cream". Improvement on an ENF occurred within 10 days, after major withdrawal symptoms, and he was remarkably compliant on the Core Program for several months, feeling and acting dramatically better. He received little support, however, from his friends and work-buddies, and began a relapsing course of "falling-off-the-wagon" for weeks and then returning to his Core Diet with reliable improvement. Despite his relapses, he remained convinced of the benefits of food control, and seemed determined to keep trying.

Edema, Bloating, Fatigue, Excess Sleep

A 42 year old woman presented with a history of chronic illness, progressive over the last 15 years. She was most troubled by:

Generalized edema	*Leg swelling*
Abdominal bloating	*Chronic fatigue*
Extreme sleepiness	*Nose congestion*
Headaches	

She had suffered a great deal over the years and had sought help from a number of physicians who failed to contribute to her recovery. She had accepted the advice of several nutritionists and described many trials of diet change with partial success in controlling her symptoms. In the past year, she had excluded all dairy products, with some improvement and then stopped eating yeast-containing foods, and followed a "rotation diet" after skin tests showed some food reactivity; she ate a number of grains, including oatmeal, rye bread, and barley in soups; she also took a generous amount of vitamins and minerals, herbal preparations, and drank herbal teas. She had, however, remained tired and congested, with episodes of marked abdominal distension, often beginning 30 minutes after eating. She was often overwhelmed with the need to sleep and this interfered with work, socializing, and driving. She retained water intermittently and often had marked ankle edema. She cleared after 6 days on the Core Program, sleeping for the first 2 days, and remained virtually asymptomatic through a 3 month follow-up. Her maintainence diet included the following foods: Breakfast, rice, peaches, pears, pumpkin seeds; Lunch, rice, cod, carrots, beans, zucchini, peaches; Dinner, rice, turkey, carrots, cauliflower, yams, spinach, pears.

Generalized Pain, Chronic Fatigue

A 35 year old woman presented with a complex of clinical problems, including:

Muscle pain	*Joint pain*
Abdominal bloating	*Abdominal pain*
Constipation	*Nose congestion*
Chronic fatigue	*Weakness*

She had several investigations to try and identify the origin of her multiple complaints. Two gallstones were noted, and other investigations were normal. She had generalized muscular tenderness, particularly over the neck, shoulder, and interscapular muscles. Her diet consisted of milk and whole wheat bread, with daily potato intake and some beef. She often made milkshake meals with milk, bananas, eggs, and engevita yeast. The clinical diagnosis was fibromyositis, associated with GIT dysfunction and fatigue. This syndrome is very often a manifestation of delayed pattern food allergy. She chose to clear on the elemental nutrient formula, and cleared all symptoms by Day 8. This demonstration of dramatic symptom remission cancels speculation that the illness is "psychosomatic", or caused by "stress".

Heartburn, Anger, Hyperactivity

A 28 year old mechanic presented with severe prolonged indigestion, often with heartburn, excess gas, and abdominal distension. He had several investigations and many drugs with little benefit. He took 4-8 ounces of antacid per day. He ate poorly, with high bread, beef and dairy intake. He craved milk and consumed at least 2 quarts per day. He stated that he had had milk allergy as an infant with eczema, colic, and was a hyperactive child, who did not do well in school. He admitted to extreme moodiness, irritability, with frequent outbursts of inappropriate anger. He had trouble keeping friends and jobs. His marriage ended after 4 years. His wife left him with their 2 year old son because he was angry and abusive. He regretted his behavior and stated that he often felt out-of-control, restless, with outbursts of aimless, hyperactive behavior. He seldom slept well. His nose was congested, lymph nodes enlarged, and he had a pustular rash covering his back. On the Core Program he cleared remarkably. With normal GIT function restored, he reported feeling calmer, clearer and more in control.

Arthritis, Chest Pain, Heart Palpations

A 52 year old professional man presented with unexplained chest pain and attacks of fast, irregular heart action, associated with a number of chronic complaints, including:

Arthritis	*Carpal Tunnel Syndrome*
Bloating	*Diarrhea attacks*
Fatigue	*Depression*

He complained of declining health, but medical investigations had not determined the source of his multiple complaints and treatments had not been effective. He had a long history of intermittent digestive problem with excess gas, distension and regular bouts of diarrhea. He had joint pains of many years duration especially in his wrists, knees and ankles, wrist swelling had produced pressure on the median nerves (carpal tunnel syndrome) with numbness and tingling in his index and middle fingers and loss of grip strength; surgery was planned. In the past 2 years he has had several attacks of chest pain with fast irregular heart action and associated panic feeling; thorough investigation excluded coronary artery disease and he was advised to take a long vacation and a drug, inderal, to slow his heart. The inderal had made him impotent, tired, and he complained of decreased ability to concentrate. He often had headaches, occasionally of the migraine variety. He had suffered mild depressions for many years, usually in the winter.

He enjoyed eating, and prided himself on knowledge of wines and gourmet cooking. He ate a great deal of meat, whole-grain breads, pasta, aged cheeses, and drank 3-4 cups of coffee, 2-3 glasses of wine and usually 2-3 ounces of whiskey per day. He followed the Core Program, at first reluctantly, and then with obvious benefit and eventually became a convert to "Asian cooking". His digestive problems disappeared as did the heart problems without inderal. He boasted of weight loss, increased energy and was surprised to find that joint pain subsiding, flaring occasionally after wrong meals, eaten in restaurants. The heart palpitations returned briefly after one such meal, featuring red wine, coffee, and a chocolate dessert.

Chronic Fatigue, Aching, Dizziness

A 30 year old woman   was "very sick" for over 18 months. Her problem list included:

Extreme fatigue	*Dizziness*
Ear Ringing	*Pneumonia, recurrent*
Muscle Pain	*Headaches*
Fevers	*Memory loss*

She described a progressive illness over 2 years duration which became disabling 18 months previously, forcing her to quit her job. Her illness had been characterized by exhaustion, lymph node swelling, recurrent low grade fevers, muscle aching, stiffness, and episodes of coughing and chest congestion, diagnosed as "pneumonia", but not improved with antibiotics. Blood tests had been negative. She recalled earlier, less severe symptoms and had had chronic rhinitis most of her life. Her hearing was now impaired with loud ringing in both ears and attacks of dizziness which kept her in bed. Her son had milk allergy in infancy, and subsequently had chronic rhinitis, ear "infections", and was hyperactive with attention deficits. She suffered decreased ability to concentrate, mental fogginess and lapses of memory. Her food intake consisted of bread, pasta, cereals, eggs, milk and dairy products, beef with some fruit and vegetables; 2 cups of coffee and 5 cups of tea per day, with no alcoholic beverages. Diet revision permitted complete recovery, but symptoms recurred promptly if she ate foods containing wheat, milk, or eggs.

Asthma, Colitis, Fuzzy-head

A 35 year old professional man described a life-long history of allergic disease with childhood hay fever, asthma, hives and dramatic reactions to foods. His current problems included:

Chronic rhinitis, sneezing	*Sore throats*
Swallowing difficulties	*Chronic cough*
Muscle aching	*Abdominal bloating*
Diarrhea with blood	*Fatigue*
Impaired Concentration	*Memory problems*

His history of allergy followed a typical atopic pattern for many years with asthma, eczema, and hives occurring in rather obvious ways to specific stimuli like grass pollen or animal exposure. A more chronic progressive illness, however had emerged slowly in the adult years with persisting digestive problems, congestion in his nose and throat, excessive weight gain and increasing experiences with fatigue and "fuzzy-headed" episodes which interfered with his work. On his worst days he had difficulty concentrating, remembering, and would sometimes feel woozy or light-headed. His two young children had early onset of similar symptoms; one son had obvious milk allergy as an infant and went on to develop chronic rhinitis, digestive problems and asthma. Family diet revision produce symptom remission in all three patients.

Eczema, Abdominal Pain, Depression

A 34 year old career woman presented with a complex of clinical problems, which included the following:

Eczema	*Depression*
Chronic fatigue	*Headaches*
Abdominal bloating	*Nose congestion*
Obesity	

She had often experienced symptoms after eating, especially abdominal bloating, fatigue or sleepiness and headache. She had had a weight problem, with a range over the past 12 years of 148-242 pounds, and was currently 210 pounds. She had undertaken several diets, mostly within the Weight Watchers program, and had lost up to 90 pounds in one 8 month session. She had regained 70 lbs in the ensuing three years. She craved a number of foods, including pasta, chocolate, and baked goods, and binged on chocolate chip cookies, or chocolate ice cream. Her diet included large amounts of cereal grain foods and dairy products, especially cheddar cheese. She had trouble organizing meals at home, as she did shift work. As a result, her eating patterns were disorganized and food selection was poor. Her bloating response to some foods is an indicator of digestive problems, which leads to whole-body problems, probably arising from absorption of the "wrong stuff". Eczema is food allergy until proven otherwise.

She spent two weeks clearing her initial symptoms, and arrived at a simple list of Core Program foods which seemed to work well. She required assistance in developing a behavioral modification program, directed at changing food choices, food shopping, cooking methods, and avoidance of tempting social situations.

Diarrhea, Depression, Binging

A 38 year old woman presented with a complex of problems, which included:

Diarrhea	*Abdominal pain*
Depression	*Weight gain*
Cravings	*Compulsive eating*
Cold extremities	*White fingers*

This woman described a pattern of recurrent illness with episodes of abdominal pain, bloating, and diarrhea. Depression and headache accompanied her GIT disturbances. She took Lomotil for diarrhea; Salazopyrin (a drug usually prescribed for ulcerative colitis); and an antidepressant. While on the antidepressant, her appetite increased and she gained 20 pounds. Her weight gain was associated with increased cravings for bread, pastries, and cookies which she ate in excess with increased abdominal bloating and diarrhea. She avoided milk, but ate cheese, yogurt and ice cream. A physician had advised her to increase her yogurt intake. The complex of irritable bowel syndrome, depression, and systemic illness suggests delayed pattern food allergy. Her high intake of cereal grains and dairy products suggests these foods are the main culprits. GIT surface reactivity is felt as pain, bloating and diarrhea, and the systemic illness emerges as a result of the the "wrong stuff" entering her blood stream. Reynaud's phenomenon consists of fingers and/or toes which turn chalk white and numb after cold exposure and is often associated with circulating immune complexes, one of the chief mechanisms of food allergy. Her cravings and compulsive eating posed a compliance problem, but she did rather well on the Core Program, with complete symptom remission during phase 1 which she extended for 3 weeks. Three weeks after symptom remission was achieved, the antidepressant drug was slowly withdrawn.

Diarrhea ,Weight Gain, Irritable bowel

A 29 year old designer was disabled by a chronic illness of 5 years duration. The features of the illness included:

Extreme fatigue   *Chronic diarrhea*
Weight loss   *Depression*
Inability to concentrate   *Lymph node swelling*

This talented young man experienced a slowly progressive illness that defied diagnosis and treatment. He had become too ill to work 2 years previously and was on a government disability pension. He first became ill with a viral-like illness with lymph node swelling of his neck and diarrhea. He lost weight slowly and progressively and became profoundly depressed. A psychiatrist prescribed an antidepressant drug that made him feel like a "zombie". In a fit of despair he took an overdose of this drug and was critically ill in intensive care. Blood tests for EB and HIV virus were negative on 3 occasions. He complained bitterly of mental fogginess, inability to concentrate and poor memory. His brain dysfunction blocked any efforts to work, study, or carry on with his social life. He withdrew to a relatively impoverished life, spending a great deal of time sleeping.

His "sick diet" included canned soups, bread, processed cheese, kraft dinner, milk, beef and potatoes. He cleared dramatically on an ENF, which he required for several months because of low tolerance, even to Phase 1 foods. Eventually a simple, basic Core Diet of Phase 1 and 2 foods was established. He gained weight and slowly resumed a normal living pattern .

Weight Gain, Rhinitis, Migraine

A 29 year old career woman presented with the following problems:

Chronic nose congestion   *Cough*
Chronic fatigue   *General malaise*
Excessive weight gain   *Migraine headaches*

She had had chronic upper respiratory symptoms for over ten years. During the past year, she had felt generally unwell, with reduced energy, reduced enthusiasm, and lack of stamina. Frequent migraine headaches often disabled her for 2-3 days at a time. She took most of the drugs offered to migraine sufferers with little benefit. She had had skin tests for allergy done four years previously, and reported positive reactions to cats, dogs, grasses, trees, and dust pollen. Beconase nasal spray and oral Sinutabs offered some symptomatic relief for a while. She saw a chiropractor twice a week for a year after he diagnosed a "slipped vertebra" in her neck. Her dentist had suggested some expensive oral splinting for temporo-mandibular joint (TMJ) problems which he claimed were responsible for her headaches.

During the past two years, she had gained weight excessively. She attended a weight loss clinic and found that she maintained her weight on 800 kcalories per day. Her diet was otherwise unconstrained, although she described herself as a "fussy eater". She avoided most meat, and was very selective about which vegetables she ate. She stated that she "loved cheese" and consumed a large amount of dairy products in general. She tended to eat a majority of her meals in restaurants, and indulged in snack foods freely. Her staple foods were whole grains, poultry, uncooked vegetables, fruit, and dairy products. She supplemented her diet with multi-vitamins, minerals, vitamin C 500-1000 mg/day, and calcium 500 mg/day. After 5 days of withdrawal symptoms and reluctance to eat rice and vegetables, she began to clear, admitting 2 weeks later that she actually enjoyed Phase 1 foods. She continued to enjoy headache and congestion free weight loss over the next several months.

Headaches, Eczema, Diarrhea

A 35 year old professional man presented with an ill-defined illness of several years' duration. His chief complaint was a daily, relentless headache. He described several pain patterns, the most prominent being a throbbing pain in his right forehead and temple and sharp pains behind his right eye, extending into his right cheek. A more generalized right-sided pressure pain often began in his shoulder or neck and extended forward to involve the entire right side of his head. In association with the pain problem, he had a long list of other complaints, which included:

Itching, eczema and hives	*Difficulty concentrating*
Muscle pain	*Abdominal pain*
Fast irregular heart action	*Diarrhea*

He had undergone frequent, extensive investigations, including a CAT scan, and several gastrointestinal investigations. He had received many forms of therapy, from exercise, stress reduction, massage, and chiropractic manipulation, to ointments, drugs, dental attention for TMJ problems, and psychotherapy. He felt "...disturbed most of the time, but I manage to function nevertheless." We could make several diagnoses, which would include migraine, fibromyositis, atopic dermatitis, urticaria, and irritable bowel syndrome. Delayed pattern food allergy is the correct diagnosis. Compulsive habits, including drinking, smoking cigarettes, and disorganized eating posed major compliance problems. Many people in this chronic dysfunctional state need close professional supervision and support in habit modification.

Panic Attacks, Insomnia, Abdominal Pain

A 22 year old woman presented with:

Panic attacks	*Restless sleep*
Nightmares.	*Abdominal pain, bloating*
Diarrhea.	*Chronic fatigue*

She described a lifelong ill-defined illness, beginning with attacks of limb and abdominal pain in childhood. A pattern of recurrent flu-like illnesses with abdominal pain and bloating, nausea, headache, joint pain, ear pain, hearing loss, and episodes of dizziness began in early adolescence. Her adolescent years were characterized by daytime sleepiness, mental "fogginess", and episodes of restless agitation. Many doctors were consulted, and her parents were often told that she was "attention-seeking". Her frequent illnesses interfered with school performance and she often felt inferior to her more robust peers.

She had been admitted to hospital on three occasions with severe abdominal pain. After one hospital admission, she was treated with heavy doses of Demerol for 6 days, and was then discharged abruptly with no explanation or treatment plan from the hospital when test results were "negative"; a very distressing narcotic withdrawal followed her discharge. She was often distressed by frequent attacks of agitation with fast heart action, flushing, dizziness, often associated with generalized itching, and hives. She was not aware of specific food reactions, but she avoided coffee, tomatoes, milk, and red meat. Her staple foods were whole wheat bread, cheese, eggs, corn products, vegetables, and fruit. She experienced sugar and chocolate cravings, and her favorite reward foods were chocolate brownies or banana cream pie.

This young woman's history illustrates the ongoing misunderstandings facing some patients with food allergy. Much suffering can be avoided by timely, intelligent Diet Revision Therapy. Food allergy is a lifelong illness which evolves over time and leaves a trail of physical, emotional, and social problems. Often patients with food allergy are admitted to hospital with acute abdominal pain. X-rays and blood tests seldom reveal the problem and treatment is often inappropriate.

Headaches, Aching, Poor Concentration

A 32 year old woman presented with a history of chronic headaches with several associated problems:

Abdominal pain	*Diarrhea*
Nose congestion	*Itchy red eyes*
Aching with joint pain	*Chronic fatigue*
Difficulty concentrating	*Memory loss*

She described headaches of over 10 years duration in varied patterns, mostly pressure sensations involving her whole head. During the most severe headaches she felt groggy and disoriented.   She complained that she had not experienced a "clear head" for months. Associated symptoms had grown progressively worse during the past year, especially the gastrointestinal disturbances, congestion, aching and stiffness.   Her food intake included milk, dairy products, bananas, citrus, bread, and six to eight cups of coffee per day. She cleared promptly on an ENF and experienced minor symptom recurrence on Phase 1 and 2 foods. She remained on these foods for over 2 months before trying Phase 3 and 4 foods, because she felt so well.

Abdominal pain, Joint Pains, Headaches

A 28 year woman presented with a history of chronic symptoms which included:

Abdominal pain, bloating	*Diarrhea*
Nose congestion	*Cough*
Red itchy eyes	*Aching muscles*
Migraine headaches	*Fatigue*
Poor Concentration	*Joint pains*

She described a slowly progressive illness of 10 years duration. Repeated tests were not helpful in revealing the nature or origin of her suffering. She failed to improve with several medications, including pain-relievers, tranquilizers, antihistamines, and anti-depressants. She first developed hayfever 10 years ago and had positive skin reactions to pollens and took shots for a while. The shots reduced her seasonal allergy in the first 2 years, but later, she developed more generalized, continuous symptoms, with year-round nasal congestion, eye irritation, aching and fatigue. She frequently "had coughing spells, often at night. These disturbances slowly increased, and she stopped the shots, thinking they were making her worse. Bouts of abdominal pain and diarrhea led to several X-rays, stool tests, and drug trials with no diagnosis and no treatment benefits. She had a history of milk allergy since infancy and generally avoided milk but consumed dairy products and "loved cheese". Her diet was high in intake of cereal grains, bread and baked products, meat and fruit. She drank at least three cups of coffee and three cups of tea per day but avoided alcoholic beverages. She cleared uneventfully on Phase 1 foods and continued to do well with Core Program food re-introduction.

Congestion, Migraine, Fatigue

A 23 year old woman presented with an illness that emerged over the past year. She felt chronically ill with:

Nose congestion	*Hearing loss*
Migraine headaches	*Flushing, facial rashes*
Aching and stiffness	*Extreme fatigue*

She described a history of hayfever in her teens with spring nose congestion and sneezing. She had positive skin reactions to dust, pollens but not foods. In the past year, she had developed continuous nose and sinus congestion which did not improve with antihistamines. She stated that she used to have surplus energy but now had difficulty completing ordinary activities. She was aware of food reactivity and noted that ice cream and chocolate triggered flushing, increased throat mucus and bloating. She was tired through the day and had episodes of extreme fatigue, often an hour after eating. She required extra sleep and had stopped most physical activities. On her worst days, she ached and felt stiff..." I feel 80 years old". Her face flushed, beet-red, and often broke out in a pimply rash. She had daily headaches, and 2-3 days per week, the pain became increasingly severe with throbbing, nausea, blurring of vision, and mental fogginess or confusion, lasting several hours.

Her diet consisted of cereals, bread, pasta crackers, cheese, fruit, and some meat. She drank 3 cups of coffee, occasional wine, and treated herself with desserts (cheese cake, cinnamon buns) 2-3 days per week. She cleared promptly on phase 1 foods, and had little difficulty establishing her own Core Diet. Prompt symptom recurrence, after eating non-Core Program foods, convinced her that she had food allergy.

Depression, Abdominal Pain, Dizziness

A 41 year old professional woman presented with a long history of a polysymptomatic, multisystem disorder, which included the following clinical problems:

Chronic fatigue	*Depression.*
Abdominal pain	*Chronic rhinitis.*
Neck and back pain	*Headache.*
Dizziness	*Ringing in ears.*

She was most distressed by chronic fatigue and recurring depression. She received treatment from Dr. ... which involved "desensitization drops" and testing with a machine. She thought initially she had some benefit from drops and vitamins but after several months and several hundred dollars she had a major relapse and decided the therapy was of no value. Her food-intake-symptom record showed a very complex pattern of food selection, based on a rotation plan (not at all hypoallergenic) with recurring daily symptoms. She continued to eat many grains, nuts, wheat, eggs, and several odd foods that she had not eaten before, including quinoa, herbal teas, and soya-based products. She required an organized, practical, and sensible approach to her food-related illness and responded well to the food choices on the Core Program.

Obesity, Fever, Depression

A 36 year old woman presented with a complex of chronic problems including:

Obesity	*Chronic Rhinitis*
Flushing	*Psoriasis*
Abdominal pain	*Bloating*
Fatigue	*Headaches*

This professional woman described chronic symptoms and problems with excessive weight most of her life. Her symptoms had been chronic and slowly progressive with nose and throat congestion, flushing and digestive problems as daily disturbances for several years. She was troubled by fatigue with increasing depression; feelings of disinterest, sometimes despair, irritability and irrational outbursts of anger. Despite a hysterectomy, she remained aware of menstrual cycling with mid-cycle ovulation pain and premenstrual accentuation of her symptoms, especially headaches and depression. Psoriasis appeared on her scalp, elbows and knees in her early 20's and often flared with itching and disfiguring, thickened red skin. She was also aware that some foods bothered her, especially whole milk and creamy sauces and chocolate. She described attacks of flushing, fever and sweating after eating chocolate confections, alcoholic beverages and ice cream. Her maximum weight was 235. She craved chocolate and described compulsive eating, especially of bread, buns, and crackers with cheese. When she overate wheat-containing foods, she experienced dramatic abdominal bloating with fatigue and mental fogginess. She experienced dramatic remission on Phase 1 of the Core Program and chose to remain on these foods for 3 weeks before slowly adding Phase 2 foods.

Chronic Fatigue, Migraine

This 26 year old secretary presented with an illness of over six months duration with a complex of symptoms, which included:

Touch aversion	*Migraine headaches*
Flushing and acne	*Aching and stiffness*
Extreme fatigue	*Sleepiness*

She stated that she declined from a high energy athlete to a tired, despondent state. Her relationship was on the rocks because she was disinterested in going-out, had lost her sex drive, and was generally irritable and easily annoyed. She described a strong "don't touch me" aversion, even to affectionate touching. She had difficulty completing ordinary activities and required extra sleep, during the evening and on weekends. On her worst days, she felt too tired to go to work, and often stayed in bed with generalized aching and stiffness, sleeping 12 -16 hours per day. Her throat was sore, and her neck lymph nodes were enlarged and tender. She had severe, sick headaches at least once a week, lasting all day, often with nausea, occasional vomiting, and light intolerance.

 Medical investigation had been largely negative, including negative allergy skin tests. She was told she had chronic EB virus infection. She was aware of food reactivity and noted that dairy products triggered bloating and a dopey, tired feeling. She had stopped drinking any alcoholic beverages because they made her very ill with immediate flushing, quick intoxication, and a heavy hang-over that lasted at least 2 days.

She thought she had a good diet with a high intake of whole wheat cereals, muffins, pastas, milk, cheese, salads, and she drank 3 cups of coffee per day and about 12 ounces of white wine per week. She chose to clear on an ENF, reporting dramatic improvement of all symptoms by day 8, and a sustained remission on Phase 1 and 2 of the Core Program.

Abdominal Pain, Depression, Anxiety

A 68 year-old widow presented with several problems, including:

Abdominal pain   *Depression*
Hypertension   *Anxiety and tremors*

She described a history of "irritable colon" for over 30 years. She was particularly troubled by fatigue, as well as depression, associated with digestive complaints. She lived alone and prepared her own meals. Her diet had been unconstrained until recently, with a preference for whole grain cereal foods, moderate consumption of poultry, eggs, and vegetables, and a high consumption of fruit. She was less interested in food since her husband's death two years ago, and often settled for a sandwich, or crackers and cheese. During the past year, she increased her milk intake, hoping to obtain calcium, and improve her general nutrition. Unfortunately, her general health   deteriorated. She stopped drinking milk and eating dairy products on the advice of a health-food store nutritionist, and noted improvement in her digestive complaints and general status. She took a full range of vitamin and mineral supplements, in addition to digestive aids. Complete symptom remission was achieved on the Core Program.

Depression, Edema, Abdominal Bloating

A 43 year-old nurse presented with the following problems:

Depression   *Insomnia*
Premenstrual tension *Aching and stiffness*
Abdominal bloating   *Periodic edema*

She described emotional instability, with outbursts of inappropriate anger. These disturbances increased during her premenstrual week. She had evidence that her diet altered her emotional status. On a weight reduction diet, consisting mostly of vegetables, fruit, and poultry, for 3 months, she felt much better. Her physical symptoms improved, and she felt more stable emotionally. Her usual diet was nutritionally well-balanced but she favored whole grains, beginning with 7-grain cereal in the morning, whole wheat bread for lunch, and, often, whole wheat pastas for dinner. Her favorite snack was bran muffins, and she often only ate muffins at work in the hospital. She was aware of specific food reactivity with diarrhea, following cheesecake ingestion; and chocolate cravings, with headaches as a usual consequence of eating too much chocolate or drinking hot chocolate milk. Her digestive tract symptoms included abdominal distension, almost daily, and she complained of a coated tongue and bad breath.

Fatigue, Aching, Dysphoria

A 52 year-old businessman presented with the following problems:

Chronic fatigue   *Aching and stiffness*
Cognitive dysfunction   *Memory loss*
Depression

He reported a long struggle with moodiness, progressive mental "fogginess" with memory loss, and disorganization. He was tired most days, and experienced generalized aching and stiffness which curtailed his physical activity. He was concerned about his work performance and had passed up an opportunity for major promotion, since he believed that his deteriorating mental activity would impair his performance. Several medical investigations revealed no abnormality. A neurological investigation, a year before, included an EEG and a CAT scan which were normal. He was advised to "reduce stress", but a two week vacation left him feeling worse. Subsequently, a psychiatrist prescribed antidepressant medication and a sleeping pill. He dropped the antidepressant medication because of intolerable side-effects, but continued to use the sleeping pill intermittently. He had attempted several dietary changes, and abstained from alcoholic beverages, coffee, and tea with only slight benefit. His diet was unrestrained, with a high intake of bread, pasta, beef, cheese, snack foods, ice cream, and yogurt, 10-12 ounces of wine per week, and 2-3 cups of coffee per day. He ate in restaurants at least 5 times per week and preferred Italian or French cuisine. He was eager to try any diet revision that offered benefit and, after two weeks of basic exclusions, went on an ENF exclusively for 10 days. He reported dramatic improvement after 6 days on the ENF, stating that his mental clarity and energy was better than he could ever remember.

Diarrhea, Weight loss, Disability

A 44 year old woman had become disabled by an progressive illness of several years duration. She developed GIT problems in her early 30s with bloating, and bouts of abdominal pain and diarrhea. She was repeatedly investigated for Crohn's disease, and treated symptomatically with little benefit. Since there was no evidence of intestinal damage or infection, she was told that there was no serious problem and to eat whatever she liked. She declined slowly with weight loss, increasing fatigue and difficulty concentrating on her work. Many foods triggered her symptoms and she began avoiding foods to avoid the disturbances they caused. She lost more weight and strength. Her family physician accused her of anorexia and demanded that she eat fortified, milk-containing supplements. She complied and grew worse, with increasing episodes of exhaustion, fever, weakness, abdominal bloating and pain. She was a bright, conscientious woman, who was very distressed by her declining health, and alarmed by the bad advice she was receiving from MDs. She sought help from other advisors; a naturopath, dietician, nutritionist, who all provided conflicting advice and she remained ill. When she was unable to work, an insurance company disputed her claim of a physical illness and she was referred to a psychiatric unit, where she received the worst treatment to date; they rejected all her claims of food reactivity, refused her a suitable diet and treated all her symptom reports as evidence of a mental disorder! The psychiatric diagnosis was "somatization disorder". Fortunately, she finally came to the proper diagnosis and treatment of food allergy, improving dramatically on an ENF.

Cystitis, Weight Gain, Fatigue

This 32 year old mother of 4 children presented with an interesting complex of problems, especially interstitial cystitis of over 10 years duration. She stated that her symptoms began a year after her last pregnancy with increased frequency of urination and urgency. She underwent several investigations and treatments over the 10 year period without benefit. She described progressive increase in pelvic and urethral pain during the past two years and was quite distressed by her deteriorating health. She avoided drinking water to reduce the discomfort of urination.

Associated problems included excessive weight gain, fatigue, cognitive dysfunction, and anxiety. She gained weight excessively to her maximum weight of 200 pounds. She was chronically tired and experienced episodes of agitation and anxiety with difficulty concentrating. She had followed some diet revision advice in a book on cystitis, mostly an avoidance of acid foods and amine reduction.

There were clues in her history, pointing to the diagnosis of food allergy and she tried an elemental nutrient formula for 10 days with dramatic improvement. She reported that she slept through the night for the first time in years without waking up to urinate. We were encouraged and began slow food introduction and she reported continuing improvement with tolerance of the early foods re-introduced. It is "bio-logical" to think that urinary tract inflammation can be caused or influenced by the food supply since immunologically the bladder surface is related to GIT and many ingested molecules exit via the urine.

Diarrhea, High Blood Pressure

This 29 year old professional man described a history of progressive gastrointestinal symptoms, especially frequent episodes of crampy abdominal pain with uncontrollable diarrhea. Associated symptoms included:

Weight gain   *Hay fever*
Flushing   *Rashes*
High blood pressure   *Insomnia*

Most of his problems were diet-related and included elevated cholesterol. He had typical spring hay fever to grass and tree pollens, with positive skin tests to pollens but not foods. His history suggested food allergy with GIT problems and increasing evidence of whole body problems, including flushing, rashes, fatigue, sleep disturbances and high blood pressure. His father had had a history of high blood pressure and died in his late 50's of a heart attack. He felt better during Phase 1 of the Core Program but then relapsed over Christmas, eating everything. He was depressed by the return of all his symptoms and made a new year's resolution to clear again. After 3 months on the Core Program, he had lost 20 pounds, his blood pressure had dropped from a high of 180/110 to 140/85 without medication, his cholesterol had dropped to within normal range and his GIT problems had subsided.

Hives, Migraine, Arthritis, Indigestion

A 64 year old woman presented with the problem of hives (urticaria) of seven months' duration, associated with generalized swelling. This most recent expression of allergic disease was associated with a history of other problems, which included:

Migraine headaches   *Indigestion*
Aching, with joint pains   *Hearing loss*

She first developed hives when she was travelling in England. The eruptions continued on a daily basis when she came home. Increased upper GIT disturbance, fatigue, and cold symptoms, particularly recurring laryngitis, were associated with recurrent eruptions of hives. She developed alarming symptoms occasionally, with swelling of her lips and face. She was fortunate not to have breathing problems. Apparently, she saw Dr... who did skin tests, found no skin test reactions, and made no significant recommendations for therapy other than taking an oral antihistamine which did not help. Hives, with associated swelling reactions, are best explained as ingested allergy. Allergens, usually in the food supply, find their way into the circulation, and excite a variety of immune responses. Allergen encounters with sensitized mast cells in the skin and mucous membranes, for example, can trigger the swelling and itchy, red eruptions. Aching and joint pain often accompany hives, since the reaction is internal, as well as on the skin surface, and can be attributed to food allergy. She followed the Core Program and within three weeks cleared remarkably; all her major symptoms remitted with no further occurrence of hives. She felt best on Phase 1 and 2 foods.

---

[1]Hippocrates, On Ancient Medicine. Adams 1886.

SECTION 2

Core Program
A Complete Instruction
Set for Diet Revision

Core Program Foods

Rice, converted	Carrots	Rice cakes	Rosemary
Rice cereal	Broccoli	Peaches	Basil
Rice flour	Peas	Pears	Thyme
Yams	Olive oil	Turkey	Parsley
Zucchini	Flax oil	Chicken	Oregano
Squash	Safflower oil	Pepper	Vitamins
Green beans	Sunflower oil	Salt	Minerals

Celery	Cauliflower	Applesauce	Watermelon
Lettuce	Asparagus	Honeydew	Cantaloupe
Turnip	Cucumber	Plums	Apples
Spinach	Onions	Strawberries	Raspberries
Brus. Sprouts	Bok Choy	Blueberries	Avocado
Mushrooms	Chives	Nori	Water chessnuts
Mung B. Sprouts	Sui Choy	Kelp	Bamboo Shoots
Rice noodles	Basmati rice	Sole	Lamb
Arrowoot flour	Rice bread	Cod, Snapper	Beef
Brown rice	Rice pancakes	Halibut	Tuna
Tapioca Starch	Sweet Rice	Other white fish	

Celery	Lima beans	Vanilla	Carob
Leeks	Peanuts	Ketsup	Sesame
Daikon	Apricots	Vinegar	Currie
Radish	Cranberries	Sugar	Garlic
Lotus Roots	Nectarines	Honey	Ginger
Yellow wax beans	Mango	Wasabi	Marjoram
Azuki Beans	Grapes	Miso	Mustard
White beans	Blackberries	Tofu	Tofu products
Chickpeas	Papaya	Tofu ice cream	Soy infant formula
Kidney beans	Lemon–lime	Soya beans	Soy Milk
Lentils	Buckwheat	Soya flour	Soy sauce
Split peas	Millet		

Cabbage	Cornstarch	Orange	Lobster
Tomatoes	Corn	Currants	Trout
Artichokes	Pumpkin	Pineapple	Salmon
Kale	Chard	Prunes	Shrimp
Parsnip	Potatoes	Cherries	Crab
Kohlrabi	Garlic	Coconut	Abalone
Beets	Mint	Prawns	

Chapter 9 The Core Program

Stages of Transformation

The Core Program is a personal transformation technique, using diet revision as the vehicle for change. Diet revision involves major, important changes in your biological function, with great potential for improvements in physical and mental health. This is an organized approach to re-designing a custom-fitted, healthy approach to food selection and eating behavior. Most diet advice suggests that changes in your food choices are easy and straight-forward. All our experience suggests otherwise. Meaningful, lasting changes in food selection are difficult to make; several obstacles will block your path. The food lists are deceptively simple; the experience of change is profound. Good information, planning, and perseverance will help you seek better health. The Core Program, has been organized into five phases which correspond to stages along a transformation path.

The **5 phases** of the Core Program can be thought of as a series of transformations which progress logically from the simple to the more complex. The Core Program can be thought of as the technical foundation of a **healing process** which might involve other healing processes such as exercise, massage, mediation, yoga, dance, exercise, sports, and learning better self-caring strategies. All major transformations require a well-informed, well-motivated participant. The better you understand the stages of transformation, the more successful you will be.

The first step is to **simplify** a complex situation. You begin by eating only basic, staple foods with a low risk of problems. You intend to clear all your current symptoms. You intend to interrupt all behavior loops which previously regulated your eating behavior as an automatic program. You intend to make deliberate decisions about what foods you are going to eat in the future, based on how you feel right now.

The design of the core program was based on experience solving the problems of food allergies. All foods are considered to have a reactive potential, and are to be evaluated as you reintroduce them to your newly emergent diet. Manufactured and processed food containing food additives have been eliminated. Many of the foods containing allergenic proteins have been eliminated, especially milk, egg, and wheat proteins. The first foods not only have a low-allergy profile, but also are highly desirable from a nutritional point-of-view. Other desirable foods are then added progressively, slowly enough to note which foods provoke recurrent symptoms. This method of diet revision proves to be successful with many types of food problems, not just allergy.

The goal of Core Program food selection policy is to develop a healthy diet of simple, carefully selected, natural foods. Fresh or frozen vegetables, rice and rice products (or alternatives), fruit, poultry, and fish and other seafoods are the basic food choices. These are primary foods that allow us to reconstruct daily menus, with confidence of good nutrition, and stable life-long eating habits. A shift to meals featuring cooked vegetables is the most important change for most people. You can select a vegetarian option and not eat poultry or red meat. If you are already a devoted vegetarian, you can eat well from the rice, vegetable and fruit list. Legumes and tofu are usually reserved for later introduction in Phase 3, but can be introduced sooner as a vegetarian option. Built into both the food selection and the meal-planning rules are the basic precepts of nutrition, including recommendations to reduce fat, salt, added sugar, and to increase fibre.

Preparation, Timing and Pace of Change

You begin with identification of your **need for diet revision.** The preceding chapters have reviewed the many reasons for doing diet revision. If you have identified a need for you to change, you then tentatively prepare, often going through a period of doubt, or trials of minor changes. You should reread chapters of this book until you understand the concepts and methods of proper diet revision. You probably have discussed your options with family, friends and professional advisers, and have collected different, often contradictory opinions. Finally you decide to go-for-it.

Compare the experience of diet revision to going on a **trip of discovery.** Adopting a new cuisine is similar to travelling to a foreign country, or camping in the woods. You study the map (this book). You buy the supplies you will need. You pack away the food you will not need. You set the departure date. You inform family, friends, and co-workers that you are going on a "trip"; you are moving from your present state; you are going to change the way you eat, the way you look, the way you act, and certainly the way you relate to other people about food.

Choose Your Method of Clearing

You begin diet revision by choosing among three methods method of clearing. This is the most difficult part of your transformation. You first experience withdrawal symptoms, an intensification of old symptoms, often with cravings, fatigue, depression, headaches, restless sleep and other disturbances, especially during the first 4 days, then clearing of symptoms begins with increased well-being within the first 10 days. Your clearing choices are described in detail in the next chapter. Stand back and review your options carefully.

Progressive Food Re-introduction

Feeling better, you proceed to **Phase 2** food reintroductions: a slow, progressive addition of specified foods. We expect the occasional recurrence of symptoms, and you make decisions to delete specific foods from your emerging Core Diet food list. Patience, good self-monitoring, and decisions about the acceptability of each food are required. As you improve, you will seek to reward yourself; if the choice is a non-Core Program food, you may suffer recurrent symptoms and have to wait for a few days to clear again. These improvised "challenge" experiments help you to define the new limits of your tolerance.

If things are going well, you progress to **Phase 3,** a period of stabilization of your Core Diet. You cope with the consequences of change, attempting to stay on course. You resolve some of the emotional responses to change and get better at explaining your new habits to family, friends, co-workers, waiters and waitresses. You practice a problem-solving approach to symptom recurrence, striving for a reliable, healthy, asymptomatic state. You add food items slowly, especially flavorings, soya products and legumes, if everything is going well.

When you are stable and well-adjusted, you reward yourself with another round of food introduction, entering **Phase 4** or expansion of your basic Core Diet. Further food introductions are designed to increase the variety of food choices, and palatability of meals. Often, new cooking methods and the use of substitutions (eg. baking with non-wheat flours) are important activities. A nutrient intake evaluation is desirable to aid decisions about long-term vitamin-mineral supplementation, and to assure optimal nutrient intake.

Long-Term Maintainence

After 3 months or more of a stable, new eating pattern, you make a longer term commitment to your Core Diet with adjustments, and fine-tuning of your program, entering **Phase 5** or long-term maintenance. Your individualized Core Diet becomes a strategy of self-maintenance, intended to serve you for years to come.

Your **long-term strategy** requires you to deal successfully with relapses. Inevitably, you will eat reactive foods. Deviations from your Core Diet may trigger major symptom recurrence, often with renewed cravings for and compulsive eating of problematic foods. A rest and recuperation strategy, retreating to Phase 1 foods or to ENFood 1 for several days, is implemented to clear recurrent or new disturbances. The art of self-monitoring and self-management is practised and perfected by those who successfully maintain good health.

Emotional Adjustments

Changes in food intake often shift body functions in major important ways, and are associated with emotional disturbances. Emotional adjustments to the Core Program are complicated. We expect **resistance** to diet change of this magnitude. The more severe the illness, the more motivation there is for change. The longer one has suffered, the more patient and enduring is the motivation to change.

We often overestimate our ability to decide change by some thought procedure or act of will. **Eating behaviors** and food selection are highly **automated** procedures in us and do not change easily. Often we have to reprogram our basic assumptions, learn about our options, and then wait for the necessary changes in our thought patterns and motivation to occur. Food changes, to be successful, must work on a purely functional basis, and also must be acceptable to your self-image and to your family, and friends. There are many reasons why a major change needs to be postponed or the pace of change prolonged.

Just think of suffering migraine headaches for 20 years. You become a migraine person; your family and friends know all about your disability and learn to accommodate for it. You get some sympathy and attention. You pay for the concern by lost social opportunity and the distancing-effect which all illness and disability produces in those around you. You have spent untold days lying by yourself in misery, with pain. You have taken many drugs at great cost, with many side effects, seen many doctors, tried many other therapies with little benefit, and you are reconciled to your fate. If you go on an ENF and/or Phase 1 foods and clear, not only headaches, but also your abdominal pain and bloating, fatigue and generalized aching in two weeks, it may be difficult for you and your family to accept. It is hard to believe that the real solution was always immediately available, but you never knew about it. You may have trouble adjusting to the idea that you are no longer the disabled, prematurely aged, migraine-sufferer. Deep down inside, you are afraid that the recovery is only transient and all the trouble will soon begin again. You have cognitive dissonance; how could all the doctors and other therapists have misled you for so long - they couldn't all be wrong!? You find yourself denying that recovery has taken place. The wise therapist reassures you to persevere a little longer, to continue self-monitoring, to stop eating anything that seems to produce symptoms, even if your short food list shrinks a little more. We encourage slow-recovering patients to restore a healthy identity in all aspects of their life. Family and friends now look for recovery and are pleased when you gradually emerge better and more functional.

The Path of Change, A More Detailed View

The Core Program reveals important but poorly understood body-mind shifts, as food input is changed. We have carefully mapped the terrain and know the successes and the difficulties of diet revision. There are typical experiences as patients follow the Core Program, with a range of individual variations and adjustments to the experiences. The remainder of this chapter introduces you to the typical terrain in the territory of diet revision.

The Core Program includes a map with territories such as; *addictive loops, withdrawal, clearing, denial, acceptance, advance, and retreat.* This vocabulary allows us to talk easily about typical experiences that people have as they move through the stages of transformation.

Many Core Program instructions are in the form; **if you do this, then expect to experience that.** You will not fully understand the instructions or the meaning of the map until you have gone on the journey of diet revision! We are not aware of any other text which clearly describes the common experiences of food-related symptoms and the experiences of diet-revision. The following discussions further describe the stages of transformation; the Core Program experience.

Starting Point

There are many starting points for the Core Program. If you have identified a symptomatic and dysfunctional state, you assume there is a **mismatch** between the biological properties of your body and the kind of food and environment you live with everyday. The mismatch may seem trivial or inconsequential; coffee and muffins for breakfast every morning seem pleasant and familiar but may leave you in a dysfunctional state. The mismatch may be obvious and difficult to change: you may have the fast-food habit or snack on chocolate bars, chips, crackers and cheese or salami; you may be drinking beer or whiskey, and smoking cigarettes instead of eating proper meals. Often, the role of food choices in producing your dysfunction has not been appreciated and you may have doubts about your need and motivation for change. We get **lost in our habitual states** and often do not realize how dysfunctional we have become. Most people have lost track of how much better they could function and feel.

If your illness is not so severe or you are pursuing an optional diet revision plan, you can approach the Core Program in gradual steps. You may try to reduce coffee consumption first or reduce intake of alcoholic beverages. You may eat more dinners with foods on the Phase 1 and 2 food lists, slowly adapting to Core Diet meal plans. You may negotiate with family and friends to gain their support for your proposed change in eating habits. You may seek professional opinions or try potions from the health food store first. You may read this book frequently and eventually schedule the beginning of Phase 1. You may search for other books and try other techniques that seem easier. If you have serious addictive patterns, or are uncertain and uncommitted, or have questionable support systems, we recommend professional assistance and a more gradual transition toward the Core Program.

We are convinced that each person, sooner or later, needs to   **clear**, using a **Phase 1** technique, and then reintroduce foods to design a unique, custom-fitted Core Diet. While this technique may be the most demanding you will encounter, it is the best. Once you are aware of the strategy, it is just a matter of time until you decide to do a proper, complete job of diet revision. We expect a **withdrawal crisis** in Phase 1 of at least a few days duration.   The "cold-turkey", quick change, approach is actually the most effective transformation path. Rapid change may be shocking, but merciful in the long run.

The **timing and pace** of change are important variables in human affairs. We often encounter patients who are not yet ready to commit to major diet change, even if the benefits are obvious and desirable. A 26 year-old man, for example presented with obvious food reactions, including digestive disturbances, skin eruptions, and episodes of sleepiness or exhaustion after eating certain foods, especially wheat and dairy foods. He spent a week on the clearing diet and improved dramatically, but dropped out of the program; returning a year later at day 23 on the Core Program doing well. He explained that he had to get over the sense of deprivation he felt when he started the program. During the elapsed year, he thought about his eating behaviors, observed his symptoms with detached interest, and finally felt empowered to "do something constructive for myself." He described a spontaneous moment of decision, arriving at the checkout counter of the local supermarket with Core Program foods in his basket, finally ready to pursue a lasting solution to his health problems.

Preparation For Clearing

The ideal setting for clearing would be a comfortable **retreat** environment where you can be quiet, protected, and helped by knowledgeable persons. This is a healing transformation and should be associated with all the good influences that you can muster on your behalf. There may be too few opportunities for a pleasant and successful retreat to make this a good option for you. If we were a more enlightened society, we would quickly trade in some of our restaurants, bars, resorts, hotel and hospital rooms for supportive "health" environments where bad habits might be shed, clearing undertaken to interrupt dysfunctional food habits, and remedial diet and exercise programs begun.

Supportive retreat centers may be available in your area and may consider going through the clearing week as a healing vacation away from work and home. Retreat environments must offer clean air and water, refuge for those suffering inhalant allergies and chemical sensitivities. It is disappointing to attempt clearing of food-related problem but to remain symptomatic because of exposure to chemicals, wood or tobacco smoke, airborne allergens, or air pollution. We desire, and often require, clean air and water to clear completely.

If you smoke and choose not to stop, you will still benefit from food changes. Carry on with diet revision, but acknowledge that you will not get completely better; your symptoms will not completely go away as long as you continue smoking. Limit the amount you smoke, and consider writing down a schedule for slowly decreasing your cigarette intake. You may consider the challenge of food changes equal to the challenge of stopping smoking and decide to seek complete, total reformation in one sweeping session. Often patients report hypersensitivity to smoke as they clear food problems and want to quit because each cigarette makes them feel conspicuously sick.

If a supportive retreat is not available to help you cope with the initial demands of change, then create comfort and support in your own surroundings. Remember our idea that diet revision is similar to going on a major trip; act as if you are going on retreat for the first week, and make all the necessary preparations to have only the right food, to be restful, comfortable, and supported by family or at least one friend. During withdrawal, you may feel like crawling into bed and staying there for a couple of days; this is often the best approach.

Our Bodies Are Self-Cleansing

Clearing is a modern biological concept and has different implications than the old-fashioned concepts of "cleansing", or getting rid of toxins. Many popular diet, fasting, and "cleansing" programs encourage the use of laxatives, enemas, herbal mixtures, clays, charcoal, and other bizarre self-ministrations. Clearing need not be associated with purging by laxatives or enemas, nor the ingestion of any exotic or questionable substances. Purging is often harmful; herbs may be allergenic or have toxic side effects, and efforts to alter the bacterial flora in the colon are ineffectual at best, hazardous at worst. You do not need to clean out your colon; the bowel is self-cleansing if we put only the correct food into it. It is sufficient to stop the input of problems and wait for your body to find its own balance point. We abandon the false idea that dumping things into the body will make it better; **less is more**. Clean air, clean water, simple food, clear thoughts - these are the ingredients of a healthy, sane life.

Obstacles to Beginning

Adaptation to the dysfunctional state involves many hidden adjustments and compensations, inside your body, and outside in your social behavior and expectations. Any worsening trend in the way we feel may motivate us to change. But, we may not be prepared for the degree of change required to fully recover. Therapeutic change disrupts the adaptations made thus far and is resisted, at first, by well-established, adaptive mechanisms. We should, therefore, expect some difficulties in changing ourselves and prepare intelligently to cope with the problems encountered.

Eating and drinking patterns tend to be well-established, automatic procedures in our brain which defy intentional modification. Casual changes in food selection tend to be short-term and relapses to old, destructive eating-patterns are common, even among people who get quite ill and are otherwise highly-motivated to do the right thing. We often miss or deny the evidence that the coffee and muffin breakfast, or the lasagna and cheese lunch may perpetuate unhappy days of irritability, abdominal bloating, and afternoon fatigue; perhaps interfering with learning, work, and intimate relationships.

Addiction

Dysfunctional eating-drinking patterns can be so powerful and disturbances so severe, that a rational decision to change cannot be sustained. The alcoholic, for example, has a serious problem and requires a profound, whole-life solution. He/she must get professional help, join Alcoholics Anonymous, abandon old social habits, say goodbye to old drinking friends, familiar clubs, and bars. A new self-image, new friends, new interests and activities are among the prerequisites for long-term success. We understand addictive behavior as the drive to obtain and ingest specific substances which influence brain function adversely. Chemical triggers that activate uncontrollable appetites are addictive.

We assume, in diet revision practice, that specific foods and beverages, especially alcoholic beverages, coffee, tea, chocolate, milk, wheat and egg proteins and some sugars will trigger cravings and compulsive eating and drinking. Incoming "addictive" molecules set up **recursive behavior loops** that are resistant to change. You know you are in such a loop when you feel strong cravings, and tend to compulsively eat or drink specific foods and beverages. The drive to ingest addictive materials is stronger than healthier drive and often exceed our ability to control our behavior.

Compulsive eating behaviors overwhelm any conscious intent not to indulge even in foods that can make you ill and more compulsive.

Many patients with food allergy crave and compulsively eat the foods that make them ill. Everyone experiences some **cravings and loss of control** after eating **trigger foods**. This cruel paradox of craving the foods that may you ill makes recovery especially difficult for some people. All addictive food-beverage molecules need to be eliminated before the cycle is broken. Complete abstinence is required. **Abstinence** applies equally to alcoholic beverages, drugs, chocolate, coffee, crackers, cookies, cakes, donuts, bread, milk, cheese, ice cream, peanuts, potato chips, and soda crackers; any incoming substance that triggers cravings and compulsions.

Remember that illness states are chaotic. To get better, you are trying to renew orderly biological function, clarify your mental state, and reorganize your behavior by returning to a basic, simple set of foods, eaten regularly and reliably, without exception. **Custodial support** or a buddy-system is helpful to people who consistently fail to interrupt recursive behavior loops. The buddy or custodian may be a relative or friend, or a self-help group or a program like Alcoholics Anonymous, Weight Watchers, or Overeaters Anonymous. Additional professional help, social and psychological counselling, fitness programs, sports, meditation, and yoga are all positive strategies. Hospitalization may be required (as the last resort) for people with major illness, disorganized lives, and poor social support. Diet revision remains the foundation of constructive change and must not be forgotten when seeking supportive networks. The Core Program has proven to be helpful for people with addictive eating and drinking disorders.

Resistance From Others

We frequently encounter **saboteurs** who resist well-intentioned efforts to follow the Core Program. Unfortunately, resistance often originates from family, friends; and even from physicians, other professionals, and eating-disorders treatment programs. You may encounter a surprising degree of negativity and ignorance, even denial of food-related illness. There are many reasons for this denial and often we are surprised with the passion and hostility that underlies the saboteur's efforts to prevent you from doing better. You will encounter even casual acquaintances with strong opinions and prejudices about food and illness who will challenge your confidence and methods or offer suggestions for faster, easier remedies. Some recovering patients express the insight that the entire society conspires to sabotage their effort to get better; fast food outlets, convenience stores, drug stores, bars, restaurants, TV commercials, magazines all preach the doctrine of no restraint; indulge in everything, and everything will be OK. It is probably easier to say no to the impersonal temptations offered by a consumer society running amok, than to resist the constant persuasion of a friend or intimate person.

Needless to say, one of the criteria for selecting a **support system** is to locate people who are knowledgeable about your food-related problems and are supportive of your efforts to get better and stay well. You do not have to cater to, or support the denial of others. Denial is a common strategy of the addict who gets angry with the mere suggestion of a food or drinking problem. Bad advice is plentiful. It is better to concentrate on your own truth. Find out what works for you. Believe your own evidence as you do diet revision. Expect, and insist on care and concern for your well-being when you order, buy, share, and accept foods from others.

Some patients are disappointed with physicians who fail to diagnosis food-related problems; and worse, fail to understand or support proper Diet Revision Therapy. Food allergic disease patterns are serious, disabling, and occasionally life-threatening illnesses that require careful management. Insist on an appropriate level of safety, care and consideration. If you encounter professional ignorance, it is not your fault. Do not accept criticism or blame. Find professionals who are educated about food-body interactions, understand food allergy, and can assist you in your endeavor to get better. Do not accept professional denial of your problems, or the dismal of your suffering as something you invented or as a "second-class" problem.

Emotional Adjustments

The different stages of the Core Program are associated with typical emotional experiences mentioned above. We can use **transactional analysis** and notice that the personality splits which typically occur with attempted diet revision. Transactional analysis suggests that we operate with three interacting personalities; the **adult, parent and child**. We prefer to operate from the adult level, making rational decisions about our food, our habits, and values. Your adult reads this book with understanding, identifies the need for change, and plans the diet revision strategy. The first internal conflict is experienced as your pleasure-oriented child confronts your adult decision to make a deliberate change in habits. Your child does not want to change and is impulsive, pleasure-seeking, easily frustrated, often petulant and cries when he/she does not get the desired treat. Addictive loops thrive in your child and sabotage your adult personality.

When we deal with real relationship of children and parents the interactions are common, with the child often challenging the parent, acting-out, and sometimes resorting to "crime" to get forbidden foods. Prohibition does not work. If the parent is too strict, the child is most likely to resort to lying, cheating, and stealing food. Some family dynamics get hopelessly complicated when adult parents operate from their three personalities, confront each other and their real children as well; the number of real and virtual personalities interacting at different times increases beyond anyone's ability to keep up.

As the **parent** aspect of your personality attempts to mediate internal conflict, you may punish your child and make your adult feel guilty. Your **child** argues strongly that it is not true that your food is hurting you; you can eat cake, pie, ice cream, pizza; forget the Doctor's advice; he is some sort of quack; forget the whole thing and carry on as before. In the worst case, if your child wins through pleasure-seeking, impulsivity, and denial; you fail to achieve lasting change. You drop back into old patterns and remain dysfunctional. Your parent continues to make you feel guilty; your adult drops the issue of change and decides that your illness has nothing to do with food and takes more pills to suppress symptoms! Your adult may project your guilt and other bad feelings onto the world outside. Others are to blame for your suffering; your relationships are faulty, your work is inferior, your world-view is pessimistic, and the Core Program is a doubtful technology.

The answer to this endless potential for conflict and confusion is for one **courageous adult** to establish " **law and order**"; a Core Program **food policy** and a written menu plan for the whole family. The law is permissive and kind; offering good food for dinner, reducing temptations by keeping the kitchen clear of unwanted foods, and offering rewards (not food) for good compliance. Both the real parent, dealing with real children and the adult, dealing with their internal parent and child personalities can use the same strategies.

If, in the best case, your impulsive child responds to adult reasoning, adult planning, and adult support, your transformation proceeds. The adult position confirms that you will be making a sustained effort to change your eating pattern, and this effort will affect a surprising number of transactions with other people. You inform your friends, spouse, lovers, neighbors, relatives, co-workers that you are going on the Core Program. Reassure those close to you that you have important health goals and a rational plan. Ask for their cooperation and support. Good information and clearly stated intentions are the best defense against anger and resentment. Share the information in this book with your intimates and close friends

Grieving the Loss of Familiar Foods

The pursuit of diet revision involves a paradoxical emotional experience. One might feel overjoyed that the solution to a major health problem is as simple as changing food. But often, patients express sadness and dismay as they improve; they have a large investment in familiar food choices and eating habits. The prospect of long-term changes hits us at a deep emotional level. We sometimes interpret the emotional responses you may experience as part of a mini-grieving process. We recognize the **four stages of grief** as successful patients move away from old, dysfunctional habits to new, more successful eating patterns:

Anger that I have to make an effort to be well that others find unnecessary; or that I have been sick so long. Why didn't anyone help me before; or anger at a spouse who is not as helpful as you would like. It is a basic healthy response to get angry and express it. The truth is not always to our liking, and nature is not always kind. It is best to quickly express anger and get on with the job of getting better.

Denial that there really is anything wrong with me, or that it could be related to food. Denial is one of the trickiest stages since it takes so many forms. Some patients become convinced, once they are well, that their initial problem was not all that bad, and that further food control is unnecessary; the same patients often deny the reappearance of symptoms or claim that they have the "flu", a "cold", or that "stress" is getting to them. While other causes of dysfunction and disease may contribute, our problem-solving assumption, that *a food did it until proven otherwise*, should avoid this form of denial. A more typical and understandable denial takes the form of questioning the diagnosis of "food allergy", or looking for quick fixes; solutions you can buy from the health food store or from one of the many phoney therapists who perform "tests" for food allergy and prescribe expensive drops or other potions. There is no quick fix.

Negotiation is a positive stage of dealing with the problem and the difficulties of the solution. We all want the best possible deal, which translates into the most foods with the least symptoms. The biggest question at this point is, "Why do I have to avoid all the foods eliminated on the Core Program? What if I'm not allergic to bread or cheese or potatoes?" The best answer is that you should follow a **food selection policy** that tends to work, just as you should buy stocks that tend go up in value.

The Core Program involves a food selection policy, based on the success of a large number of people with problems and needs similar to your own. You use the proven, general **policy first**, and then, gradually **custom-fit foods** and daily menus to your own specifications. "Negotiation" turns out to be a dialogue with yourself; as in the transaction model just discussed; or more precisely, a negotiation between the **biological rules** you are now discovering (adult) and the **pleasure-principle** approach to eating (child). This negotiation between your emerging biological insight (adult) and the pleasure-principle (child) will be ongoing for the rest of your life.

Acceptance is the happy result of health emotional adjustment to change. You finally accept the new food selection, find pleasure in eating Core Program foods, and deal effectively with the problems of eating out, and feel comfortable answering the questions and challenges of family and friends. You are grateful to be better, and are determined to maintain your health by careful food management. Renewed energy and vigor allow you to be more physically active and more productive at work and play. The outlook for the rest of your life is much improved; the prospect of chronic degenerative disease is reduced as is the probability of suffering cancer, heart attacks, and strokes.

Withdrawal and Clearing

The Core Program begins with a concerted effort to stop ingesting any and all problems, to "clear" symptoms. Clearing means that you feel better, often dramatically better. Your body undergoes a major change as problems "washout". Withdrawal symptoms usually increase in the first 3 days and then subside.

Clearing occurs rapidly for most people after a week on the Phase 1 clearing diet. With clearing, there are some surprising responses. The obvious response is " I feel great. I can't believe it!" A small, but significant, minority of people are slow to clear, or are reluctant to clear, or reluctant to admit improvement. Other people will have biological problems which require resolution with expert professional help. We regularly manage patients who take several weeks to clear on an ENF and then have difficulty tolerating food reintroduction. We often have to wait several months for their hypersensitivity to subside and tolerance for Phase 1 and 2 foods to return. Often medication is required to suppress their allergic reactivity. Patience is a great asset in the beginning, if things do not improve as rapidly as we would like.

There are many reasons for slow recovery and failure to recover. Obviously, there are many other biological problems, unrelated to food supply. There are environmental problems, metabolic problems, infections, hormonal problems, autoimmune diseases and so-on. The Core Program approach to medical diagnosis and treatment simply gives priority to solving food-related problems. With problem reduction, diet simplification, and slow diet reconstruction, other problems tend to diminish or become more apparent, and may be more easily solved. Sometimes we are disappointed.

A successful problem-solving method requires that each problem is identified and corrected as it arises. It is your task to keep a record of the changes you make, the problems you have, and the decisions you make to reduce your symptoms.

Post-Clearing High Sensitivity

The path of transformation, as people navigate the Core Program, involves a major journey, sometimes of heroic proportions. Often the closer you get to your goal of restored good-health, the more difficult and demanding the journey becomes. During clearing, you begin to experience decreasing tolerance to foods and environmental stressors. Decreasing tolerance is the same as increasing sensitivity. The term "hypersensitivity phase" describes this early change in your reactivity, appearing as foods are withdrawn. Hypersensitivity often persists for many weeks or months.

During the hypersensitivity phase, wrong food ingestion is more likely to produce an acute reaction: abdominal pain, sudden joint pain or headache, immediate sore throat and mucus flow or hoarseness are typical examples. It is as if low-grade chronic symptoms have been traded for acute dramatic symptoms of short duration. This newly emergent reactivity of a person in the hypersensitivity phase is most convincing of an immunological mechanism, underlying the pre-existing disorder. It is likely that suppressed allergic mechanisms start operating again at higher gain. These mechanisms were probably suppressed by sustained doses of food antigens.

Hypersensitivity is a useful phase, since reactive foods are now more readily identified when they are reintroduced. It is sometimes alarming to people who are beginning to feel well and indulge in a small treat, like a sandwich or chocolate bar, only to develop acute abdominal pain, headache, or similar symptom. Heightened smell awareness appears with hypersensitivity and is associated with **decreased tolerance** for airborne chemical stressors; smoke, automotive exhaust, household chemicals, and perfumes become more noxious. The decreased tolerance adds to the social burdens of the recovering person, since many environments and some people now become unmistakably obnoxious. The emerging **avoidance behavior** in the recovering person triggers another round of misunderstanding and resentment.

Hypersensitivity is a perfectly valid, fascinating biological phenomenon which needs detailed study. It is not "psychosomatic" or "neurotic". Appropriate, **responsible adult behavior** is characterized by selectivity, **discriminating awareness,** and sufficient self-assertion to protect oneself against unpleasant, undesirable, and harmful people and environments. A newly emerging social awareness will support this appropriate self-protective behavior.

Hypersensitivity tends to stabilize after a few weeks and slowly increasing tolerance for more foods is experienced by many patients during the first year. A smaller number of people experience progressively decreasing tolerance in the first year. This is a difficult problem which requires expert management. There are many strategies to try to improve tolerance, but often a limited food list, supplemented by an ENF are the supports needed to stay well. The concurrent solution of environmental problems may also be required. Drugs that block various components of the immune response may be required in the most hypersensitive patients.

Phases 2 to 4: Progressive Addition Plan

The food introduction sequence is based on the incidence of symptom occurrence from least to most. The methods of preparing the food are intended to reduce problems and to improve digestibility. A food, eaten in combination with others, may act differently than when eaten alone. You will do better if you are consistent with food purchases and preparation. Your emerging Core Diet remains free of most grains, dairy products, excessive sugar, nuts, coffee, tea, chocolate, snack foods, and all processed or manufactured meats. Abstinence from all alcoholic beverages is required at least for the first three months. When symptoms are reduced, foods may be added back in an orderly manner to determine the limits of your tolerance. By monitoring your progress, you can identify recurring problems, and change the food selection to avoid them. If symptoms recur, you retreat to an early stage of the diet, even to the initial Phase 1 foods, for several days, to allow the disturbance to clear. The strategy is to custom-fit a diet plan to your own individual needs.

Fast or Slow Track:

Slow, careful food introduction is biologically ideal. We are interested in reiterating infant food introductions, watching each food carefully for adverse reactions for 3-7 days before introducing another. The **"slow track"** of the Core Program is often required for serious illness and is made possible by the use of **an elemental nutrient formula (ENF)** which supplies problem-free nutrition as food is slowly introduced. For major problems, Phase 1 begins with **ENFood** alone for 7-10 days Then ENFood is continued to supply a portion of the required daily nutrients as foods are gradually reintroduced. ENFood acts like mother's milk or a safe formula in infant feeding, supporting nutrition as a brand-new solid food diet is created. The pace of food introduction varies with the illness and state of tolerance; when we are resolving major, chronic health problems it may take 3-6 months to create a new, safe, nutritionally complete food list..

This plan is **a workable compromise** between reasonable menus and ideal biological food selection. The relatively fast pace of food introduction (1-2 foods per day) in the Fast Track Core Program is based on the impatience of many people to resume eating full menus and may compromise efforts to identify problems as you reintroduce food. We often start out on a fast track, but need to slow down when any symptoms recur. People with little evidence of food allergic reactivity will do best on the fast track.

Chapter 10

Core Program Food Choices

The Core Program is a sequential, diet-revision path, designed to restructure the diets of both children and adults; a method of developing a long-term, healthy eating-strategy. We refer to the food selection and meal-plans emerging from the Core Program as a "Core Diet". The term "diet" refers to each person's typical selection of foods and eating habits; not a temporary weight-loss program.

Immediate Goals Of The Core Program

* to achieve safe, superior nutrition
* to alleviate food allergy and other illnesses
* to resolve abnormal eating behaviors
* to prevent common diseases
* to aid weight control programs

Food selection is directed toward solving personal health problems, but at the same time serves ecological and environmental needs. Healthy personal choices tend to produce healthy community choice, and healthy outcomes for planet earth as a whole. Our food choices must become locally and personally correct. Dietary recommendations for the prevention and treatment of many diseases tend to converge on several common food choices. The Core Diet Program has been designed to solve several problems simultaneously. Regional variation in food quality is to be expected, influencing your food tolerances. Reports from other countries suggest that the Core Program food list is generally correct and adaptable to most modern citizens.

The success of the Core Program involves **regulating body intake** and minimizing opportunities for biochemical confusion. To **simplify** the task of food selection, the Core Program suggests avoiding packaged or processed foods in bottles, cans, and boxes. There are, of course, exceptions: Core Diet Program recipes may include canned fruit (sugar-free), tuna (packed in water), herbs, and carefully chosen jams, jellies, and sauces. Frozen vegetables, fruit, fish, and poultry are recommended.

The Core Program is suitable for the following dietary needs:

Hypoallergenic	Weight Reduction
Milk and Dairy-Free	Additive-Free
Gluten-Free	High Vegetable Fiber
Low Fat	Low Cholesterol
Low Sugar	Low Sodium
High Complex Carbohydrate	Moderate Protein

The Core Program begins with Phase 1, a hypoallergenic diet, designed to remove the most common food problems. This means the **complete exclusion** of dairy products, eggs, cereal grains, processed and packaged foods, and other common allergenic foods; peanut butter, nuts, seafoods, citrus fruits, and bananas. Coffee, teas, herbal teas, alcoholic beverages are also missing. Poultry, fish, and meat options are included in the Core Program but are not essential. A complete vegetarian version of the Core Diet is readily achieved by selecting only the rice, vegetable, and fruit options from the food lists. Meat portions are, in any case, much reduced from North American averages. From all points of view, red meat consumption should be reduced, and poultry and fish, carefully selected, are preferred high-protein foods.

Vegetable diversity is a key to the success of your own Core Diet, and one of the clearest, emerging dietary recommendations from many scientific studies. Increased vegetable intake reduces obesity, coronary artery disease, strokes, cancer, and probably diabetes. Vegetable foods should account for **60-70% of daily calories**. Complete, if not superior, nutrition is possible with vegetable foods alone. Many people are unaware that vegetable foods have enough protein to maintain athletic body-building. The only trick is to **combine vegetable foods** so that the set of nine essential amino acids is complete. If you mix four vegetables from different botanical families (eg. carrots, peas, broccoli, squash), you tend to get complete amino acid sets. The combination of rice and a legume (peas or beans) is an easy method of completing vegetable protein. Core Program policy is to combine 3-4 vegetables per meal. If you wish, the addition of small portions of poultry, fish, or red meat easily completes the daily requirement for protein

Four Food Groups; Obsolete

The Core Program replaces the "four food groups" method of meal planning with a more appropriate, modern, flexible meal-planning strategy. The four food groups include cereal grains, dairy products, and meats which are not suitable or desirable for everyone to eat. Food allergy and other food-related illnesses change body-input rules, often eliminating one or more of the four food groups. Vegetables and fruits are lumped together as one food group and their importance tends to be diminished in four-group meal plans. This four-group concept is based historically on agricultural practice and preferences, economics, politics, not any cogent biological information. If experience of the 20th century has taught us anything about nutrition, it is that the four-food group concept is fundamentally misleading and needs to be changed.

The exclusion of dairy products, egg whites, and the cereal grains is a firm rule of the Core Diet Program plan in the first 2-3 months at least. Milk substitutes may include infant soy milk formulas, as well as other soy milk and tofu products (including ice cream substitutes) Soya products are usually not introduced until phase 3.

The Core Program is **Gluten-Free.** Gluten is a name given to the protein fraction of the cereal grains (wheat, rye, oats, barley) which gives them their sticky elastic properties. Exclusion of wheat, rye, barley, oats is necessary in the initial stages of the Core Program. Durham flour, triticale, and bulgar are all excluded. The bran of these cereals is also excluded. Our packaged, fast-food, and restaurant food industries rely heavily on wheat flour to produce their products. Pasta is made with high gluten flour and is off our list of Core Program foods. Gluten exclusion also means no malt, a barley product, and no malt-containing beverages; Postum, Ovaltine, beers, and ales. Bread is the most desired wheat product, and is, unfortunately, the hardest food to duplicate with non-grain flours, since gluten elasticity is important for the texture of breads. The exclusion of cereal grains significantly alters vegetarian regimens, dependent on grains. **Corn** is related to cereal grains and often produces similar allergic reactions. Corn is less tolerated than rice, and is introduced in Phase 4 of the Core Program in limited amounts, not as a staple food. Corn ingestion in susceptible people may produce dramatic undesirable behavioral changes, and this effect must not be missed, even in the absence of the more explicit symptoms like abdominal gas, pain, or diarrhea. Corn appears in a multitude of products, including snack foods, oils, margarine, and cereals. **Corn syrup** and other corn carbohydrates (eg. maltodextrin) usually do not have allergic properties and can be introduced. Corn sugar is mostly fructose, and has replaced cane sugar (sucrose) in a multitude of manufactured food products and beverages. Fructose intolerance occurs with about 5% frequency and may present as true hypoglycemia following ingestion of fruit, corn syrup or other high fructose foods. Infant soya formulas with corn sugars and/or carbohydrate solids may not be a problem, even in people with high corn sensitivity. The allergy problem is connected to the protein fraction of the corn.

Rice is the staple food chosen for the Core Diet Program because it has low allergenicity, is versatile, is widely available, and provides a carbohydrate caloric base to the diet. Rice comes in many varieties, and originates in many parts of the world. Texas, Arkansas and California rices are readily available; Thai rices have been inexpensive imports with interesting taste and texture variety. Rice is a staple food in Japan with special status. Japanese rice production is carefully protected by the government; rice prices in Japan have been up to six times the world price despite $6.3 billion per year in direct subsidies to farmers. The Japanese idea is to remain completely self-sufficient in providing a staple food, no matter what the cost.

Converted white rice is preferred at the start of the Core Program. Brown rice may have slightly more nutrients, and some prefer it by taste and texture; however, the husk also contains more potential problems. Rice-eating peoples generally polish their rice, removing the husk. Brown rice may cause increased digestive difficulties and should be introduced only after tolerance for converted white rice is established. Regular white rice is second choice to converted rice; wash bulk rice in hot water before cooking. Rice can be utilized in a variety of forms, including rice cereals, rice pablum, puffed rice, rice cakes, rice noodles, rice vermicelli, and rice flour (starch). All foods, including rice, have the potential to be allergenic, however. The most common symptoms of rice intolerance are fatigue, constipation, bloating and feeling cold.

Buckwheat is an interesting grain-like food to add, especially if rice is not acceptable. Buckwheat is not a grain, but belongs to the Polygonaceae family which includes sorrel, rhubarb, and dock. Buckwheat is a seed, however, and resembles the grains in having a starchy endosperm; it can be ground into a flour, cooked as a cereal, or prepared as rice. Buckwheat flour is disappointing for baking since it lacks gluten, the elastic, chewy component of bread. **Cassava**, a root vegetable, is ground into arrowroot flour; Tapioca is made by heating and moistening arrowroot. Flour is also made from Taro, a Japanese tuber, common in Hawaii where Poi is a food paste made from Taro roots. Soybeans are versatile and highly nutritious seeds which can be ground and utilized as a flour as well. Other flours such amaranth, quinoa, kamut, spelt, chickpea, and other legume flours are options but may not be well-tolerated by people with food allergy.

We often see patients treated for food allergy with very **odd, exotic food choices** and a series of new food products of doubtful safety. Nut milks, for example, made of cashews or almonds should never be eaten on a regular basis. Soya milks with many additives, including gums, flavors, preservatives may not be well-tolerated. Exotic legume products, herbal teas, new flours, nut mixtures, dried fruits, and a host of new snack foods are all put on our ??? list; we are not sure what these products will do to you, so eat them with caution; stop if you get symptoms; back to basic foods, if you are not sure. Studying food-related illness, we are constantly reminded that even the most wholesome-appearing food may be harmful to those with allergies, digestive, or metabolic abnormalities.

Food Additives And Contaminants

Food additives are chemicals used at home or by the food industry to improve the taste, color, texture, and longevity of food. Food preservation with salt, smoke, spices, and sugars is the origin of food additive technology. Commercial food additives are regulated in the U.S.A. by the Federal Food, Drug, and Cosmetic Act. Food additives tend to receive the most detailed scientific attention because of regulatory scrutiny. We know less about the chemicals intrinsic to food than we know about additives.[1,2] A brief discussion of the more popular additives will serve to illustrate their problems.

Sulphites are used as bleaching, antioxidant, and preserving additives in food. Sulphites have been implicated as allergens. A typical sulphite reaction involves flushing, dizziness, shortness of breath or wheezing. Asthmatic attacks can be provoked by sulphites and a few deaths have been attributed to them. Sulphite sprays have been widely used on fresh produce in stores and restaurants to prevent browning with air exposure. French-fried potatoes are also treated this way. As preservatives, sulphites were found in processed food, alcoholic beverages (wines and beer), and drugs. Even aerosols used to treat asthmatics contained sulphites as preservatives! The increased notoriety of sulphites in 1985 has led new regulations limiting their use. The FDA has banned the use of six sulphite preservatives in fresh fruit and vegetables The ban still permits manufacturers of processed foods, dried fruits, wines and beer to use sulphites, although, if these manufacturers are prudent, they will voluntarily restrain or curtail sulphite use.

Nitrites, usually sodium salts, have been used widely as preservatives, especially in bacon and other processed meats. Saltpeter is the best known nitrite with its undeserved reputation as the sex-drive inhibitor. Nitrites also occur naturally in foods. The chief concern is the ability of nitrites to combine with amino acids in GIT to form **nitrosamines**, potentially carcinogenic molecules. Vitamin C inhibits nitrosamine formation and is thought to protect against GIT cancer. Vitamin C is an antioxidant preservative, and can replace less desirable preservatives in some foods. Tobacco smoke is the major source of human exposure to nitrosamines.[3]

Acetylsalicylic acid (ASA), or aspirin, is one of the most popular and useful drugs of all times. Other **salicylates** are common in vegetables and fruit; the first medicinal salicylates came from plant sources like willow bark. Methylsalicylate has been rubbed on many cold-stricken chests and inhaled freely by coughing children, with all the conviction of mothers' best medicine. In its prime, ASA was found in hundreds of over-the-counter medications and was associated with pain relief more than any other drug in history. ASA is an effective drug, with diverse benefits, but it routinely causes GIT irritation and bleeding. It is a good allergen, and causes many rashes and hives. Salicylates occasionally trigger asthma . The implication of ASA in **Reye's Syndrome,** a rare, but sometimes fatal, allergic-type reaction following viral illnesses, has led to widespread substitution of acetaminophen as a pain-reliever, with fever-reducing characteristics. Dr. Feingold postulated that salicylates and food dyes produced **hyperactivity** in children, and popularized low salicylate diets. These chemicals have not proven to be the most important causes of children's behavioral disorders, although they remain a potential problem and must be considered whenever food problems present. Feingold recommended avoiding foods that contained natural salicylates or chemically similar substances. His lists excluded such foods as peaches and cucumber, for example, which are low in our list of symptom-producing foods.

Food colors and preservatives have been suspected of producing allergic reactions, and behavioral disturbance. Their exclusion was part of Dr. Feignedly program for treating hyperactive children. Food colors are used liberally in all commercial food manufacture and have been popular in home use. The yellow dye, **tartrazine,** is definitely associated with **hives** (urticaria), as is the preservative, **benzoate**. In the study of hyperactive children by Egger et al, tartrazine and benzoate were the most common substances to provoke abnormal behavior in children, although they were never the only cause of behavioral problems. Tartrazine is a yellow food color, common in a wide variety of manufactured food products. Tartrazine produces symptoms typically within 90 minutes of eating producing a variety of symptoms, including asthma, hives, generalized swelling, headache, and behavior change, usually hyperactivity. Colors derived from natural plant and animal sources are usually exempt from FDA control and are **generally recognized as safe (GRAS)**. Beet pigment, beta-carotene, grape skin extract, paprika, saffron, turmeric, and vegetable juice are example of GRAS colors. While these substances are not known to be toxic, nor carcinogenic, there is no assurance that they are not allergenic, or otherwise troublesome to some people. Certified colors are approved by the Food Drug and Cosmetic act and bear the certification name FD&C Red No. 2 and so on. Tartrazine is FD&C Yellow No. 15. Of the nine colors currently certified, seven may be used in amounts consistent with good manufacturing practice.

Monosodium Glutamate, well-known as MSG, is perhaps the most vilified of additives. MSG is blamed for almost everything that goes wrong in a Chinese restaurant, and many people scan food   product labels, rejecting any bold enough to display MSG. It is likely that MSG is a victim of the single ingredient fallacy, discussed in earlier chapters. Ironically, glutamate is a perfectly respectable, normal amino acid, continuously present in all our cells, and always available in the blood. One possibility for MSG to act in a negative fashion would occur with the sudden absorption of a large amount. A rapid rise in blood glutamate may activate receptors which ring alarms, causing the headache and shooting pains that are associated with MSG. A variety of other symptoms are commonly reported, including flushing, numbness and tingling, chest pains, fast heart action, abdominal pains and behavior changes, including irritability, hyperactivity, and angry outbursts. In pure form, we would not expect MSG to trigger allergic effects. MSG products may contain allergenic contaminants from the vegetable source including corn, beets, and wheat.

Often MSG is mixed with an enzyme in commercial food enhancers like "Accent". The most common enzyme is **Papain,** derived from Papaya. Papain is a protein allergen. It is possible that MSG is often blamed for the allergenicity of papain. Papain may be injected into ruptured intervertebral discs as an alternative to back surgery. The injection is potentially dangerous if the patient has been previously sensitized to papain by ingestion of it in food. This risk illustrates the immune principle that ingestion of an allergen may sensitize the whole body to its effects.

Aspartame

The popular artificial sweetener, aspartame, contains two normal amino acids: **phenylalanine** and **aspartic acid.** The sweetness of this combination was a surprise discovery. The ingestion of this substance should pose little or no problem to most people except those with known phenylalanine intolerance or a family history suggesting and intolerance. Excess phenylalanine, would affect brain function, usually increasing excitability of brain cells, in the worse case, promoting seizures. Epileptics should consider carefully the use of aspartame and refrain form ingesting too many aspartame-containing products. There may be some benefits of extra phenylalanine in normal people and the use of aspartame should not be automatically discounted. Occasional reports of "allergic" reactions to aspartame are surprising since this molecule should not act as an antigen - more information is needed about his possibility.

Pesticides, Contaminants and Carcinogens

Let us consider one of the alarming facts of the late 20th century. Our food supply is contaminated by a variety of agricultural chemicals, water and air pollutants. We have been told that we must live with a degree of chemical contamination, since our industrialized, agricultural industry depends on chemical technology to feed us. The replacement of long-lived with shorter-lived chemicals is in our favor, but hardly reassures us when we become ill with ill-defined-illness.

The diagnosis of any form of food-related illness always raises the question of food contaminants. The problem is that we never know what role contaminants play, and we have no technology readily available to find out. The postulate that **Agent X in** the food supply is causing the problem, or promoting the problem, is always viable. The neglect of imponderable factors in our food supply is surely one of the contributors to ignorance about, and denial of, ill-defined illnesses in contemporary populations.

Surveillance may detect chemical contamination before the food reaches consumers, but it is unrealistic to expect that government monitoring alone can assure an uncontaminated food supply. It is also unrealistic to believe official reports that the incidence of contamination-related illness is very low, since the majority of the potential problem is concealed from official view.

Systematic population studies, relating illness patterns to food selection, to tissue levels of different environmental contaminants, are needed to assess the prevalence of contaminant illness. **The major contaminants in our food supply are:**

  * Pesticides, herbicides, and fungicides
  * Antibiotics and hormones in animal tissues
  * Environmental contaminants, including toxic heavy
  * Metals - lead and mercury
  * Radioactive isotopes
  * Organic acids,
  * Hydrocarbon residues (from fuel combustion)
  * Processing, refining contaminants, detergents,

* Bleaching agents, solvent residues, waxes, dyes
* Biological contaminants - endotoxins
* Insect and parasite eggs, rodent feces
* Bacteria, fungi, and viruses
* Contaminants from shipping and storage containers

Coping with Dangers of Agricultural Chemicals

David Steinman reviews some of the food contamination is issues in "Diet For A Poisoned Planet"[4]. He rated foods by their content of pesticide residues in green, orange and red categories; basing his ratings on 1982-86 measurements carried out by the USA FDA. In the FDA "Total Diet Study", food samples from four geographic regions in the U.S.A. were analyzed for up to 100 chemical contaminants.[5] Steinman's best vegetables and fruit ("green light") are Core Program food choices, although they are distributed through the four phases of the program because of other considerations. Steinman points out that pesticide contamination of fresh fruits is often alarmingly high. Canned produce is often less contaminated than fresh! Canned peaches and pears have low pesticide residues and have been the best tolerated fruits in our experience; fresh peaches did not do as well in the FDA analysis with up to 97 chemicals residues; fresh pears had 79. Phase 1 vegetables on Steerman's moderately contaminated food list include broccoli, parsley, sweet potato, and winter squash. You should by these vegetables from an organic source if possible; thorough washing and complete cooking are essential safety measures. Phase 2 foods on the moderate list include blueberries, cantaloupe, celery, cucumbers, lettuce, plums, spinach, turnips and strawberries. Steinman recommends avoiding peanuts and raisins.

Rice receives high marks with low concentrations of chemicals. Malathion is the most likely contaminant. Cereal grains have more contaminants; pesticide residues in breakfast cereals and bread were in the 30-50 range. Wheat and other grains were contaminated during the 80's with **ethylene bromide** a fumigant used to retard grain spoilage in storage and transport. This chemical may have contributed substantially to the apparent increase in wheat disease in the past decade. Ironically, **fungal contamination** of grains is an equal threat to the chemicals used to control it. **Aflatoxins** may be produced by fungi, and the **ergot** fungi produce a host of neurotoxic alkaloids, closely related to LSD.

Lowest Pesticide Residue Core Program Foods, Listed by Phase & Number of Pesticide Residues

Core Program Food Choices	Phase	Pest			Phase	Pest
Applesauce	2	13		Guavas	4	2
Asparagus	2	4		Lentils	3	0
Adzuki Beans	3	0		Limes	3	1
Bananas	4	0		Mushrooms	3	31
Bean Sprouts	4	0		Onions	2	0
Beets	4	4-6		Papayas	4	0
Brussel Sprouts	2	3		Peaches canned	1	14
Carrots	1	8		Pears	1	1
Cabbage	4	7		Peas	1	12
Cauliflower	1	3		Pineapple	4	0
Chives	3	0		Sunflower seeds	3	0
Corn	4	1-2		Tomatoes canned	4	13
Cranberry juice	4	0		Watercress	3	0
Dates	2	0		Watermelon	2	1
Grape Juice	2	16				
Green beans	1	12				

These values are out of date (pre '86 measurements) but give us an idea of the problems in the food supply. Measurements of food need to be routine, both to inform us about best food choices, but more importantly to encourage food producers to make changes in their methods to reduce our exposure. Contact your local health department and ask for up-to-date information on pesticide levels in the food you buy. If this information is not available, begin political action to get better information and better protection.

What does the presence of industrial and agricultural chemicals in our tissues mean? If you have a toxin in your body, which should not be there, what assumption are you going to make? These chemicals are good metabolic poisons, and so you are going to assume that they will in some way alter the way your body works. Agricultural chemical residues in the body mean increased risk of illness until proven otherwise. The people who deny the problem (until proven otherwise) are not credible. Pesticides have a special proclivity to alter the way our brain works and, therefore, the way we think, feel, remember, and act. The same chemicals may be carcinogen and you are going to assume that you have a higher risk of cancer. Rather than despairing, there are practical steps to be taken individually and collectively to reduce the pollution hazard.

Alar is a chemical (daminozide) sprayed on apple orchards to keep ripening apples on the trees and to improve appearance of the apple after picking. The U.S. Environmental Protection Agency proposed a ban on Alar which was subsequently withdrawn - they had evidence of a cancer-causing effect of a breakdown product UDMH. Apple juice was especially suspect because the heat used in juice production created UDMH. Shortly after Consumer Reports published an article on Alar[6] its manufacturer, Uniroyal, withdrew it from the market. The article states: "Consumers, especially parents, should not accept Alar in the apple juice and should not be required to rely on industry promises that aren't always kept...it's the governments job to protect all consumers. The EPA should ban daminozide sooner rather than later."

Heavy Metals

Lead is the major heavy-metal contaminant to find its way into our food supply in increasing amounts. US industry consumes 1.3 million metric tons of lead annually, releasing half of it into the environment each year. Leaded fuels contribute 90% to air lead pollution, and have increased the agricultural burden of lead. Soils contaminated by airborne lead accumulate the mineral, and plants absorb it from the soil. Increasing acidity of soils from fertilizers and acid rain increase the solubility of heavy metals like lead. Animals grazing on leaded plants concentrate the mineral in their bones. People eating leaded plants, eating soups made with boiled bones, or supplementing their calcium intake with bone meal increase their lead intake. Lead poisoning from food ingestion alone is seldom apparent, but will contribute to the body burden of problems. Lead also appears in ground water supplies and dissolves from solder in water-pipe solder joints, especially when the water is acidic. The decline of the Roman empire has been attributed to lead poisoning from the popularity of pewter dishware, containing lead, and lead-lined water conduits. Increased water acidity may have increased lead's toxicity to the Romans as it threatens our own populations exposed to acid rain. The shift of mineral absorption of crops exposed to acid rain is one of the many imponderables of our food supply - a variable which can quickly shift the metabolic norms of whole populations.

Mercury poisoning is best known as **Minimata disease** from one of the worst examples of industrial pollution of a local environment and food supply. The Chisso Co., makers of polyvinyl chlorides, dumped organic mercury compounds into Minimata Bay over many years. They have since paid $775 million in damages and spent another $407 million on filling in the bay to create a land-fill park; apparently you cannot clean up mercury pollution, you can only bury it. Mercury damages the nervous system and people who ingested large amounts of mercury-contaminated fish were blinded, paralysed and children were born retarded; at least a 1000 people died of the disease. The Japanese experience with mercury poisoning was a horrifying example for the rest of the world, but similar atrocities continue to occur in many industrialized countries.

Mercury levels in free-swimming ocean fish do not appear to be a problem. Bottom-feeding fish near sources of industrial mercury pollution are the high-risk food sources. Mercury is available in most people's mouths as dental amalgams; a small amount of mercury trickles into our body everyday and battery action in the mouth induces an odd electrolytic food chemistry. This is just another chemical pollution problem to add to our very long list of problems. **Dental amalgams** contribute only minute concentrations of mercury and are therefore not our most urgent problem. Do not have all your amalgams replaced until you have solved other, bigger problems first, especially food problems; but do ask for non-mercury fillings if new ones must be placed. A smoker, for example, asked our advice about mercury poisoning after watching a "60-minutes" documentary; the reply is that smoking has to go first; it is probably 10,000 more toxic than the amalgams. A careful, conscientious patient, who has solved food and environmental problems in large measure, but remains ill, may consider complete amalgam repalcement as a further problem-solving option.

Radioactive Isotopes

The Chernobyl incident demonstrates the early inclusion of isotopes into the food chain, with increased radiation levels found almost immediately in leafy greens growing in contaminated fields, and in cows' milk. Rain becomes radioactive. Cisterns collecting rain for drinking water are immediately suspect. Soils contaminated by radioactive fallout produce crops with increased radioactivity for years to come. Animals grazing on contaminated fields will concentrate isotopes, like **strontium-90,** in their tissues, and will pass the isotopes on to the carnivore who eats them. **Plutonium,** with a half-life of 24,000 years, is the most dangerous isotope produced in nuclear reactors.

Radioactive iodine, I-131, competes with dietary supplies of normal iodine, and may be concentrated and stored in the thyroid gland. I-131 has a short half-life of 8 days, and poses only an immediate danger to those directly exposed to radioactive fallout. Concentration and storage of the isotope in the thyroid increases the risk of cell mutation, and the subsequent emergence of cancer. Immediate impairment of thyroid function may also occur. Supplements of iodine reduce the opportunity for the radioactive isotope to be taken up. Doses as high as 100 mg of potassium iodide for 7-10 days have been recommended for those directly exposed to radioactive fallout. This is a toxic dose of iodide under normal circumstances, and should not be taken unless there is real danger. The principle of nutrient supplementation to compete with uptake of radioactive isotopes is usually not considered as an indication for nutrient supplementation, and maybe an important consideration for all of us. Strontium-90 has accumulated in the food chain from weapons testing, and is concentrated in animal and fish bones. The slow accumulation of this isotope, with a half-life of 20 years, can be expected to increase the mutation rate in bone and bone marrow, increasing the incidence of bone cancer and leukemia. Calcium supplements may compete with strontium-90 and reduce its storage. **Radioactive calcium-45** is also produced by fission; with a half-life of 164 days, it is a shorter term concern, but is another condition for full calcium supplementation in populations exposed to radioactive contamination. **Cesium-137,** with a half-life of 33 years, is also a concern, and is distributed throughout the body, taking the place of potassium. **Radioactive carbon,** with a half life of 5700 years, is distributed throughout the living world, and offers no opportunity for competitive defense.

Antioxidants, offer meagre protection against radioactive damage. The principle mechanism of cellular damage is ionization, the production of charged free radicals which behave abnormally in molecular transactions. The effects of ionization are most pronounced when the delicate mechanisms of DNA replication and repair are damaged. The result is cellular dysfunction, and mutation of the genetic program. A complete antioxidant formula offers meager protection and might include vitamin C 1000-5000 gm, vitamin E 400-1200 IU, selenium 200 ug, cystine 250mg and vitamin B6 50-200 mg per day. The following minerals should be supplemented, at least to RDA - calcium 800-1000 mg, magnesium 300-400 mg, zinc 10-30 mg, chromium 200 mcg, molybdenum 100 mcg, and iodine 100- 200 mcg per day. The dose of iodine should be calculated to body size and need, since overdose is toxic. Pregnant women may require carefully calculated increased iodine. We are assuming that the sources of mineral supplements are relatively uncontaminated with radioactive isotopes. Calcium obtained from animal bones or oyster shells will contain environmental contaminants, including isotopes, but calcium obtained from limestone (dolomite) will not be contaminated by recent radioactive fallout.

Policies for Food Selection

The **avoidance of most food additives** is a good idea. The avoidance of only specific additives, like food dyes, sulphites, and salicylates, has advocated by some authors. This avoidance turns into a game, which requires the player to carry rather long lists of foods and food ingredients to stores, where elaborate list-reading and screening procedures are carried out. The Core Program policy is less entertaining, but more practical.

You are advised to avoid manufactured, boxed, bottled, packaged, preserved, and processed foods. Packaged and processed meats are given an "X" rating. If this rule is followed, most additives are gone, and the sugar, fat and salt load is dramatically reduced.

Shopping strategy is simple; avoid the middle aisles in supermarkets. Most stores place vegetables, fruits around the perimeter of the store, and these are the foods we want the most. Frozen vegetables, fruits, poultry and fish are also desirable. You are allowed one or two dashes into the middle aisles for toilet paper and soap.

You **seldom read labels** because you seldom buy labelled food. Some canned foods such as peaches and pears have the least chemical contaminants and are preferred over fresh fruit, unless the fruit is organically grown, transported and sold without chemical spays

Frozen foods tend to be of high quality and can be ecologically sound. Frozen food values are well-preserved, spoilage is reduced, and year-round availability is assured. Improved refrigeration technology, more efficient and without Freon, will make frozen food options even more attractive.

The problem of **contaminants** can be **reduced** by two simple kitchen procedures, **washing and peeling.** All fruit and vegetables should be thoroughly washed with clean, hot water; scrubbed, when feasible; then double-rinsed, first in hot then cold water. If the food has a skin, peel it and throw away the peel. If someone admonishes you, saying that you are throwing away precious nutrients, tell them that it is okay; you are happy to throw out the nutrients with the waxes, dyes, fungicides, pesticides, insect eggs, fungi, radioactive isotopes, bacteria, and viruses.

Bacterial contamination of poultry, other meat, and fish is a concern. Food poisoning is usually caused by bacteria from 3 groups; **salmonella, campylobacter and E.coli.** the These bacteria actively infect after an incubation period of 1-3 days with acute diarrhea with abdominal pain and fever as the chief symptoms. This acute gastroenteritis may alter the immune reactivity of the GIT surface leaving new food allergy in its wake. Many patients report an acute "food poisoning" episode at the onset of a long bout of digestive symptoms, often with typical food allergy downstream (fatigue, aching, headache, difficulty concentrating, memory loss.) Other bacteria incubate in improperly stored food and produce toxins in the food before it is eaten.

Staphylococci contaminate the food from the skin or secretions of food handlers and produce a potent toxin which triggers explosive vomiting, crampy pain and diarrhea; these bacteria especially like cream puffs stored at room temperature.

Botulism is a life-threatening food poisoning produced by a potent toxin usually found in home-canned foods; the botulinus bacteria are found widely in soils and easily contaminate canned fruit and vegetables. The toxin is destroyed by heat so that often mother is the victim, sampling pickled beets out of the bottle, for example, before cooking them for her family. Botulinus spores are found in honey and may incubate in the intestines of infants, less than one year old; older GITs usually can destroy the spores before they can do anything harmful.

The list of all possible food-borne infections is very long. The following food-selection and kitchen strategies are always indicated:

Limited use of poultry meat is recommended, with skinned, defatted breast meat as the preferred portion. With all animal products, **avoid cooking the bones** and never use organ meat.

Proper handling of food can reduce the risk of bacterial food poisoning. Adequate cooking destroys the bacteria.

Proper refrigeration retards the growth of bacteria. Bacteria grow best at room temperature; therefore raw foods should be kept refrigerated (or frozen) until used.

Wash hands well before and after handling meat, poultry and fish.

Keep raw flesh away from other food and especially away from cooked food, ready to serve.

Clean kitchen counters and utensils. To kill bacteria you must remove all food residues, wash surfaces with hot, soapy water, and disinfect with chlorine bleach. Many people with allergic disease will want to avoid the chlorine, but thorough washing with hot water and detergents will suffice.

Cook fish, poultry and meat well (to an internal temperature of 180 degrees F.). Ensure that hot foods are hot and cold foods are cold, when served.

[1]Gilchrist A. Foodborne disease & food safety. Monroe, WI: Am Med Ass'n, 1981.

[2]Freydberg N, Gortner WA. The food additives book. New York: Bantam Books, 1982.

[3]Tannenbaum SR. N-nitroso compounds: a perspective on human exposure. Lancet 1983;629-632

[4]Steinman D. Diet for a Poisoned Planet. Harmony Books. NY 1990.

[5]Gunderson, Ellis. FDA Total Diet Study;(1982-1986) Dietary Intakes of of Pesticides, Selected Elements, and Other Chemicals. Ass'n of Official Anal;ytic Chemists. Arlington Via 1988

[6]Anon. Bad apples. Consumer Reports May 1989; 288-292.

Chapter 11 The Core Program

Phase 1 Clearing

The basic idea behind the Core Program is simple. If you suffer from food allergy or other food-related problems, it makes sense to stop the input of all food problems, and allow enough time to clear existing problems. This **"food holiday"** can be achieved in three ways: No food, ENFood, or Safe food. In other words, you can stop food problems by not eating; you can replace food with an elemental nutrient formula (ENFoods), specially designed to avoid food-related problems; or you can start with a simple list of basic foods that tend to be well-tolerated, and eliminate everything else.

Clearing refers to the improvement and eventual disappearance of physical symptoms and emotional-behavioral disturbances. The time required for clearing is dependent on many factors and may vary from 5 days to several weeks. On average, we expect significant **improvement to occur within the first 10 days.** We consider three clearing options:

Option One	**No Food (Fasting)**
Option Two	**ENFood (Nutrient Formula)**
Option Three	**Safe food (Clearing Diet)**

Option 1: No food or fasting is an ancient healing method, and often a spontaneous choice of patients with food allergy who say: "I fell much better when I don't eat." Ironically, in our affluent, over-indulged and overweight society, fears of anorexia and starvation dominate nutritional thinking. If you are reasonable, familiar with fasting methods, and well-supported at home there is nothing to fear and you may consider this option. Generally we advise patients to choose option 2 and/or 3 as their clearing method.

Option 2: Replace food with ENFood is the most efficient, high-tech, clearing method. You stop eating all food and supply nutrients in their pure form, as a rationally-designed, Elemental Nutrient Formula (ENF). This strategy requires the most dedication to change, since you forfeit all eating gratification and the transitional stages, discussed in previous chapters, tend to occur rapidly and intensely. The advantages include rapid withdrawal, complete interruption of negative eating habits, and a definitive clearing experience; the more serious the beginning illness, the more attractive the ENF option.

Option 3   Start with a clearing diet. You begin by eating only the most basic, well-tolerated foods, using simple cooking techniques. The Phase 1 food list is now called the "Clearing Diet" since so many patients have cleared their chronic symptoms with this deceptively simple approach. Phase 1 foods are the first foods we now introduce to infants as they begin eating solids. We tell patients; "You are now an infant starting all over again; treat yourself with the same care a doting mother devotes to her first child!" A review of the three clearing options with detailed instructions for the clearing diet follows.

Clearing Option 1: No Food = Fasting

Fasting is an ancient method of healing. The experience of fasting has much to teach us. The thought of not eating strikes most people as a most radical method of clearing and is generally not appropriate or desirable. Even if you do not intend to fast, it is useful to understand the function of fasting, and some of the problems. We always tell patients with food allergy that if in the worst case, all the problems return and you are sick, confused, desperate; don't jump of the bridge! Simply stop eating and wait for the illness and despair to subside.

Fasting means not eating food, but drinking generous amounts of water. Supplements of water-soluble vitamins and some minerals may be desirable, but all supplements must be free of allergenic substances. Fasting allows you to experience hunger, purely and simply. You go through significant emotional changes. For some, fasting is a spiritual exercise which brings you back in touch with yourself, restoring a sense of well-being and gratitude for being alive. Fasting may restore a sense of self-control, a very real and valuable asset, as you continue the transformation series. During a fast, many metabolic adjustments occur and may not smooth out right away. It is unfortunate that the first two to three days of a fast may be disturbed, but, by day 5, most people experience significant clearing of their symptoms. Not everyone should fast, and certainly not anyone who is anorexic, ill, underweight, injured, or engaged in hard work or vigorous physical exertion.

Clearing Option 2 High Tech Nutrient Formulas

A modern alternative to fasting is to take a food holiday, but supply essential nutrients in their pure, elemental form. **Biochemical theory** teaches that 40 or so simple molecules are need to run the human body. An **ENF is a nutrient mixture with all essential nutrients** in their pure form, in amounts generally known to be desirable, with few or no other ingredients. Several different ENF's have been reported in the medical literature, with a range of nutrient contents. Several studies have demonstrated normal functioning with health benefits for volunteers living on ENF for weeks at a time. NASA sponsored ENF development to define the minimum weight and volume requirement for human food. Elemental mixtures represent the ultimate reduction of food and have been referred to as "Space Diets".

A number of researchers have demonstrated the **healing capability of ENF formulas,** replacing food with an ENF for periods of days to weeks with important benefits. If the potential for dramatic, safe, rapid recovery from many illnesses with ENF therapy were announced for the first time today, there should be front page headlines and universal rejoicing. An ENF does not cure all ills, but could compete successfully with a host of prescription drugs which never resolve the underlying problem, but merely suppress symptoms. Many people get better when they stop ingest food problems and live on pure, crystalline nutrients for 7-10 days. The **ENF orders chaos,** provides rational body input and minimizes the risk of disease-causing food problems. The disease clears itself when the problematic body-input stops.

The ENF-induced clear-state may be thought of as the **normal baseline** for each person. This normal baseline not only establishes a physical-metabolic norm but also a mental-psychological norm. Many people in the clear state report remarkable **clarity of mind;** good feelings return with improved mood stability, increased pleasure and interest, and improved concentration and memory. The mind-clearing effect of an ENF is one the most exciting insights into the nature of mental experience. Any person with well-developed self-awareness and an interest in exploring the possibility of improved clarity of consciousness should do the ENF clearing experiment.

ENF's have been used in **hospitals** to manage serious digestive diseases or to provide adequate nourishment when eating food is undesirable or impossible. Several ENF formulas have been used in medical applications for several years. The formula, **Vivonex,** renamed, **Tolerex,** was most often used in hospitals by tube feeding. It had desirable properties to treat food-related illness, especially food allergy, and provided us with our first clinical ENF tool. Tolerex, however, was not well-received by patients for many reasons. The first problem with Tolerex was an unpleasant odor and taste which deterred about half the people who tasted it from continuing through a complete clearing period. Some people vomited after taking the first dose and refused more. Tolerex was also expensive and hard to get. We often had to coax and cajole patients to use Tolerex because we knew the benefits of a nutritionally-supported food holiday. Despite the obvious problems with Tolerex, the formula consistently produced "miracle cures" for us, and a devoted group of patients became loyal users of the formula which gave them the relief from chronic diseases that no other method had provided.

There were **no substitutes for a true ENF** that were better tasting. All food preparations which contain large molecules, especially proteins (and hydrolysed proteins), are avoided because they retain some allergenic effects. Hydrolysed proteins tend to have unpleasant tastes and odors. Liquid diets for weight loss, protein powders, soya protein or vegetable protein powders, and nutritional supplements (instant breakfasts, Sustacal and Ensure) remain allergenic and otherwise contain problems that we wish to avoid. Products containing herbs, "natural foods or plant materials" contain even more allergenic materials and are not acceptable. ENF's have to be manufactured from **high quality nutrient materials** which are more expensive than food-extract products like skim milk, soya protein or powdered egg white. An ENF will always be more expensive than protein powders or liquid diets.

A variety of ENF's had been designed and tested by various research and commercial groups over the past 3 decades. Nutritional theory was well tested in animal diets that were chemically defined for research purposes and we reviewed the composition of all commonly used formulas. The nutrient content of the various formulas varied a great deal; there was no concensus about the best formula. Nutrient analysis of theoretically optimal Core Program Diets also gave us clues about the proper nutrient content of a new ENF.

The development of different ENFs for different applications became a highly desirable research and technical challenge. The logic was compelling. If food problems were even remotely suspected, **a trial of clearing on an ENF, would confirm or deny food involvement in 10-14 days**. If ENF clearing proved successful, the Core Program food reintroduction could become a standard method of redefining a safe diet. Many illnesses would not require further medical intervention, as long as the patient complied with his or her new safe diet! The potential benefits for long-suffering patients are obvious and the savings in health care dollars could be enormous!

We were, therefore, encouraged to develop a series of new ENF formulations, beginning with a formula suitable for the clearing program. The criteria for the new formulations included strict hypoallergenicity, affordability, nutritional adequacy and, most of all, palatability. We knew that Tolerex had a limited application because of very low acceptability ratings from even patients who needed it the most. The new formula had to taste much better, and had to function as well. The new formulas are referred to as "ENFood" [1]

ENFood: 7 Day Clearing Program: Example Instructions:

ENFood 1 is an elemental nutrient formula that comes in a powder form to be mixed with water. It contains carbohydrate, amino acids, fatty acids, and all the vitamins, and minerals needed to maintain your health. Because the formula is nutritionally complete, there is no need to take extra vitamin or mineral supplements. ENFood 1 is designed as a clearing formula and supplies all vitamins and minerals at or above recommended daily allowances with a daily intake of 1000 KCal, your minimum daily intake; supplied by approximately 290 grams of the formula. The assumption is that you may have been depleted of some essential nutrients, and part of the recovery process is replenishing all your nutrient stores, especially trace elements. You should drink ENFood every 3-4 hours. An adequate daily intake would be 1400 Kcal, equivalent to about 1600 Kcal of food. Weight loss usually occurs at 1000 KCal per day if you remain physically active. Increased intake of the formula is desirable to sustain vigorous physical activity or to increase weight.

ENFood 1 can be used to **"washout" or clear** problems before starting the Core Program food reintroductions. Because ENFood 1 is hypoallergenic and nutritionally complete, it will provide complete nutrition for the 7-10 days during which you are not eating or drinking any other food, except for water. If symptoms are due to foods you have been eating, there is a good chance that your symptoms will be reduced or will disappear completely by the 10th day on ENFood 1. Intial weight loss if usually caused by the excretion of excess body water; this diuresis can account for a 3 -8 pound weight loss in the fist week and is associated with increased urine output. Once you have achieved your dry weight, further weight loss is slow and gradual.

It is sometimes desirable to continue ENFood 1 for longer than 10 days if clearing is incomplete; or, in the best case, if the ENFood-state is attractive enough to postpone food introduction for a further "food holiday". Patients with inflammatory bowel disease or other serious illnesses may want to continue ENFood for several weeks; physician supervision is always advised.

You may want to start ENFood 1 several days before you begin relying on it to clear your symptoms. This **introductory period** allows you to get used to the taste and function of ENFood 1. Often patients who start their clearing phase abruptly on an ENF will experience acute withdrawal symptoms and blame their distress on the ENF formula. If you use ENFood, as breakfast, for example, for at least a week before relying on it completely, you will tend to feel better, and later, you will not blame symptoms related to withdrawal on ENFood.

Withdrawal disturbances can produce headaches, fatigue, irritability and many other symptoms, lasting several days. Intense cravings are often part of the withdrawal experience. You may miss eating solid foods while taking ENFood, but you will not feel especially hungry after the initial food cravings subside. Some people report intense irritability, often with anger and denial during the first 5 days of withdrawal and then clear with renewed optimism by the end of the first week. Often the second day is the worst with clearing well-underway by day 4 or 5. You may take several more days to really feel well again. Be patient. If you understand the origin of these transient emotions, it is much easier to cope.

After you clear on ENFood, start Phase 1 foods. During food reintroduction, you can use ENFood as nutritional support, reducing the amount of ENFood as your food intake increases. We often suggest continuing ENFood as breakfast and snack food, during the first 2-3 weeks of food reintroduction.

Option 3: Clearing Diet

We can begin the clearing process by retreating to a simple list of well-tolerated, basic foods. Many people do well simply by clearing their kitchens of old food, stocking up on rice, vegetables, poultry and beginning day 1 with determination to get better. The choice of foods and their order of introduction is determined by an analysis of the experiences of patients who improved with diet revision. The best-tolerated, "safest" foods are eaten during the clearing week, establishing a basic "Core Diet" of staple foods around which you will build suitable menus. Most of the foods on the Core Program may be purchased at any regular food store. Phase 1 Special foods include rice products, vitamin and mineral supplements. The amount of food you eat is determined by your appetite.

Food List for	Phase 1	Clearing Diet
Rice, converted	Rice flour	Rice cakes
Rice cereal	Broccoli	Peaches
Carrots	Peas	Pears
Yams	Green beans	Turkey
Zucchini	Squash	Chicken
Linseed oil	Safflower Oil	Sunflower Oil
Olive oil	Pepper	Salt
Rosemary	Thyme	Oregano
Basil	Parsley	Vitamins & Minerals

Any food or beverage not listed here should be avoided

Fast Track

For routine diet reconstruction with mild or no illness, you may follow a quick food reintroduction sequence outlined below; 12 foods are eaten during the first 10 days; one to two new foods per day are then added over the next 20 days. Slower food introduction is necessary when you are more seriously ill or hypersensitive with food allergies. There are twelve common staple foods, with vegetable oils and flavoring herbs, available during the clearing phase of the Core Diet which should last at least ten days. These foods are identified as "Phase 1 Foods" and are important for long-term eating success. A more detailed profile of these basic foods is presented in *Core Program Cooking*.

The food list is limited in the first 10 days and no distinction is made between breakfast, lunch, and dinner. The food program resembles infant feeding. You cook and eat the same healthy foods 3 or 4 times per day. The choice of which Phase 1 foods are included in a given meal is up to you. You may avoid a food you already known to be troublesome. For most people, the major change is to eat more cooked vegetables for breakfast, lunch and dinner! If you have experienced compulsive eating patterns, withdrawal tends to be difficult and the program may falter temporarily as you yield to cravings, temptations, or withdrawal effects. Be patient, and persevere. Cravings fade away, normal hunger returns, and basic foods become more appealing.

We often introduce foods in the following sequence:

Day 1 rice, chicken, pears, carrots, peas, water
Day 2 rice, turkey, peaches, yams, green beans, water
Day 3 rice, chicken, peaches, carrots, broccoli, water
Day 4 rice, turkey, pears, yams, peas, water
Day 5 rice, chicken, pears, green beans, yams, water
Day 6 rice, turkey, peaches, carrots, green beans, water
Day 7 rice, chicken, pears, zucchini, peas, water
Day 8 rice, turkey, squash, peas, zucchini, peaches, water
Day 9 rice, chicken, green beans, yams, carrots, pears, water
Day 10 rice, turkey, squash, peas, broccoli, peaches, water

You can alter the menus of Phase 1 foods,
but stay with these food choices.

Vegetarian Options

If you prefer to avoid poultry (and other meat options), you can substitute another vegetable for the poultry option, combining rice with peas or green beans for each meal to improve the intake of essential amino acids; also add an extra 1-2 teaspoons of vegetable oil. You may also add a small amount (1-2 ounces) of tofu to increase protein intake. Tofu is soya protein and is not always well-tolerated. Double-check your tofu tolerance if you choose this option. You may also supplement phase 1 foods with ENFood, the nutrient formula which replaces protein with free amino acids and boosts intake of all other essential nutrients.

Slow Track: Phase 1

If you need or want to be **more careful and precise,** then slow the pace of food introduction. If you have been seriously ill or find you are highly sensitive to foods, then introduce one food at a time and pace the rate of food introduction to your level of tolerance. We may, for example, introduce **one food at a time, every 3 to 7 days to hypersensitive patients,** especially after a serious or prolonged illness. The same food lists are used to direct food choices. Day 1 becomes week 1 and so on.

ENFood 1 should be added to supply part of daily nutritional needs; thus permitting slow careful food introduction. We might decide, for example, to supply 1000 KCal per day as ENFood and begin with 500 KCal portions of first foods, slowly establishing tolerance.

Occasionally, we encounter **hypersensitive patients** who tolerate only a few foods from the Phase 1 list and a smaller number from the Phase 2 list for several weeks to months. If we encounter extreme high sensitivity, we accept a small number of safe foods and continue to supply additional nutrients with an ENF. Again, we compare the needs of a sick patient with the needs of an infant; nutritional support with a safe formula and slow, careful food reintroduction should establish a safe diet within a few months!

Professional supervision is advised if you have low food tolerance. A computed nutrient intake, weekly weights, and blood monitoring tracks nutritional status, if there is any doubt about adequacy of nutrient intake. Tolerance to other foods eventually returns, permitting further food introductions. There is no reason to hurry food introductions if basic foods, plus ENFood, and, perhaps, other nutrient supplements are providing adequate nutrition.

The **timing of food reintroduction** is based on how you feel. Often we do better if we introduce foods slowly, being sure than no adverse reactions occur to one food before adding another. Rice is usually the first food chosen, and may be presented as normally cooked rice, rice Pablum, rice flakes (cooked cereal) or boiled rice pureed in the blender. Carrots, squash, and yams are often the next foods you should try. Phase 1 foods can be subdivided into 4 groups, in order of priority of introduction. Establish Group A food first and then proceed through Group B and so on.

> *Group A:* Rice, chicken, carrots, peaches
> *Group B:* Peas, yams, squash, pears
> *Group C:* Green beans, turkey, broccoli, zucchini
> *Group D:* Salt, oil, pepper, flavoring herbs

Food Preparation Phase 1

Phase 1 foods are prepared simply with vegetable oils and basic condiments. Avoid any food that you know you are allergic to. Stop any food that seems to trigger adverse reactions. At the same time, try to eat sufficient amounts of rice and vegetables. Consult the companion volume, *Core Program Cooking* for more complete cooking instructions and recipes.

Vegetables: are the most important, most desirable foods. The vegetables must be well cooked during the first week of the diet. Steam-cook, bake, or microwave them. They may then be mashed or pureed (in a blender) to promote easy digestion. Soups made from pureed vegetables are also a good choice for easy digestibility.

Rice: This is the first and most desirable staple food. Eat 2-4 cups of cooked rice per day to provide your caloric base, the basic "fuel" for the day. Rice cakes and puffed rice cereal may be introduced in the first week. Rice cakes are substitutes for bread, crackers, and snack foods. Puffed rice, Rice Chex, or cooked rice cereal (rice flakes) are breakfast options.

Chicken and turkey, preferably breast meat, without the skin are the first meat choices. Serving poultry breast meat, well-cooked, without fat, in small amounts reduces the problems we experience with these foods. When cooking poultry, trim, drain and discard fat. Serve small portions (less than 3 oz.) initially. Vegetable foods are more important. Avoid using poultry bones in soup bases, since the bones tend to concentrate toxic material in the birds' food supply, especially tetracycline, and lead. It is best to bake, poach, or microwave poultry; avoid frying.

The poultry options can be omitted if you want to develop a vegetarian menu.

Fruit: Two fruits are selected during week 1: canned peaches and pears. Cooked, home-canned, or commercially canned fruits (without sugar syrup) are acceptable. Choose a brand without preservative, sugar, or artificial coloring or flavoring. You may use peach or pear jam or jelly without food coloring or preservatives.

Vegetable Oils: Safflower oil is our first choice; sunflower oil is an alternative and olive, oil may be used in moderation (3-6 tspn/day total). To obtain a spectrum of different fatty acids combine 3 teaspoons of safflower oil with 1 teaspoons of olive oil as your daily fat allowance. An optional oil is 1-2 tspn flax oil added to the basic mix to provide more linolenic acid. Cold-processed, organic oils, packaged in black or opaque bottles to avoid light-driven oxidation are desirable. Spend more money to achieve a higher quality oil and use less. A blended oil to balance fatty acid intake is available as a Core Program supplement. Avoid margarines. Flavor oil with a little salt and permitted seasonings. Supplemental marine lipids (EPA), borage or primrose oil (GLA) are other optional, accessory oils.

Seasonings: Pepper, and light garden herbs; rosemary, thyme, oregano, basil, parsley can be used for flavoring. It is often best not to use seasonings in the first week of clearing, then introduce one at a time, so that you notice any new symptoms they may provoke. Moderate salt intake is usually permissible. Pepper may not be tolerated.

Beverages: Water is the beverage of choice. Drink a generous amount of water; 4 to 6 glasses per day. If you doubt the quality of your water, consider buying bottled or distilled water or use a water-filter. Carbonated (no sodium) water is allowed without restriction. Soda waters (contain sodium) are allowed only in limited amounts; 12 oz/day. Peaches and pears may be quickly converted to a fruit puree in a blender and added to carbonated water, if desired, to make a homemade carbonated drink. We avoid other packaged juices during the first 4 weeks of the Core Program.

Avoid all other foods and beverages, especially hot spices, garlic, cinnamon, nutmeg, onions, coffee, teas (also excluding herbal varieties) hot chocolate, chocolate, chewing gum, chips, pop, candies, and all snack foods.

Caution: Problems During Phase 1

While we encourage a **positive, optimistic approach** to changes, it would be unrealistic not to anticipate some problems. If you have read Section 1, you will anticipate some of the typical difficulties of diet revision. Hopefully you will have recognized a description of your own predicament and have appreciated the description of the emotional-psychological responses to change in the previous chapter.

The following cautions are always attached to **clinical instructions** given to patients undergoing treatment for food-related illnesses. These warnings summarize the difficulties you might encounter. You may be lucky and sail through diet revision with ease and benefit quickly from your efforts.

Withdrawal from problematic foods often increases symptoms and distress for several days. If clearing is completely successful, you experience symptom remission and have a renewed sense of well-being. In the worst case, withdrawal may be severe. Coffee and tea withdrawal, for example, regularly results in headache and fatigue. Withdrawal **headaches** can be blocked with preventive ASA (Aspirin) tablets, taken at 600 mg twice daily for the first 3 days; only if you tolerate ASA. Acetaminophen (tylenol) can be taken to relieve the headache.

Symptoms of the preexisting illness **may flare** suddenly and intensely before subsiding. You may not sleep well. You may not have regular bowel movements. Some patients are alarmed at how ill they become when withdrawing from ordinary foods. Withdrawal symptoms include: whole-body tremors, chills, crampy abdominal pain, nausea, vomiting, muscle aching and cramps, agitation, fatigue, restless insomnia, and headache. Many patients report a severe, often aching-burning **pain** in the lower back, sacrum, extending down the back of the legs in the pattern of sciatica. Often **depression** with tears, self-doubt, irritability and anger dominate the withdrawal period for 3 or 4 days. If withdrawal is slow and gradual, the symptoms may not be so acute, but disturbances may not clear. Slow withdrawal is a limbo state, often without positive benefits, and may deter many people from continuing diet revision.

The **expected duration** of withdrawal effects is **5 days**; although more serious illnesses may take longer to remit. You might find it best to plan a 5-7 day retreat with no responsibilities and especially no social activities during the initial clearing period. You will have cravings for old favorite foods and may feel angry watching others eat familiar foods. You will tend to be compulsive if you eat wrong foods. **Avoid temptations**. You may not want to eat at all, and vegetable foods may have little or no appeal. Patience is required initially. As the disturbance subsides, you feel more hungry and a bowl of rice with carrots tastes very good. Review the discussion of emotional changes in the previous chapters, and renew your commitment to getting better.

Weight loss may occur. Dramatic weight loss in the order of 3-10 pounds in the first week is mostly water loss; a positive sign that food allergic responses have stopped. Water excretion (**diuresis**) means increased urine flow. You should notice increasingly frequent urination, high urine volumes and weight loss. Real weight loss, in the order of 1-2 pounds per week, may occur in the next 2-3 weeks. Weight stabilization occurs after several weeks on the Core Program. Further weight loss, if desirable, is achieved by aerobic exercise. If weight loss is not desirable, the use of ENFood to supply extra calories and micronutrients is recommended. A dose of 300 to 1000 KCal/day in addition to reasonable portions of phase 1 foods should prevent significant weight loss.

Sensitivity to allergenic foods may increase in the first week and continue for several weeks to months; it feels as if a previously suppressed "alarm system" is reactivated. As you get better, your body responds more quickly and dramatically to food allergens. Therefore, it is important that you are careful about making exceptions to the Core Program, especially in the first six weeks. Your increased sensitivity and new awareness of events in your body will help you track abnormal events. You will be much more aware of recurrent disturbances from reactive foods.

Nutrient deficiency may occur with the unsupervised use of the Core Program. Short term food restriction tends to be associated with dramatic improvements in health status, not deterioration, unless you have suffered malabsorption or malnutrition prior to starting diet revision. ENFood has a complete set of nutrients and can act as a supplementary source of nutrients if your food choices remain limited for more than one week. Supplementary vitamins and minerals are desirable features of your long-term maintainence diet.

Resistance to diet change comes from all directions. You are undertaking major changes in your food selection and cooking habits. The cooperation of family and friends is essential. Families who support one member by making whole-family core diet meals often produce unexpected benefits for other family members. Explain the Core Program quickly and simply to family and friends to avoid conflict, embarrassment, and the inevitable "good advice". Linda Gomez contributed to our understanding of the emotional adjustments to the Core Program She wrote insightfully about her own experiences dealing with food allergy and migraine headaches:

> *"As well meaning as they may be, family and friends can pose a frustrating problem. Initially, when you are "clearing" and have quite a few restrictions, They want to feed you. "A little bit won't make a difference" is said with caring in mind, but beware, the body doesn't forget anything. One must be persistent in one's explanations and assure them that they are really helping you to get better by not offering any tempting food. Later The same people may become your policemen when you are thinking of cheating. Once they actually see results, they monitor every morsel of food that enters your mouth."*

Do not panic or despair when problems recur. Remember the problem-solving rule: when symptoms recur, *a food or drink did it until proven otherwise!*

Vitamin-Mineral Supplements

The following table suggests a supplementation level for vitamins and minerals. These supplements are an "insurance policy" against possible nutrient deficiencies. If you follow the Core Program instructions carefully, and have a reasonable tolerance for a variety of foods, excellent nutrition is readily achieved. Occasionally, problems arise with supplements, especially allergic reactions to products and side effects of wrong doses of specific nutrients. Some vitamins, even in pure form (niacin, vitamin A, pyridoxine or folic acid, for example), may not be well-tolerated if the dose is too high. An acceptable supplement must be "hypoallergenic"; without alfalfa, yeast, corn, wheat, soy, color, flavors, binders, preservatives, or animal glandular products. **Avoid herbal mixtures.** It is usually **not helpful** to take acidophilus, lactobacilli, digestive enzymes, bile salts, caprylic acid, garlic tablets, or other concoctions sold to improve digestion or immune function. If you are concerned about weight loss, you may require macronutrient supplementation with an elemental formula (ENFood), to provide a percentage of your daily nutrition. You should not use protein powders of any description, milk-based formulas (Ensure, Sustacal), or other formulas sold for weight loss purposes since these formulas may be allergenic. **Suggested CP Vitamin & Mineral Supplement Levels**

Minerals	*Level*		*Vitamins*	*Level*	
Calcium	500 mg		Vitamin A	4000	IU
Potassium	500 mg		Beta-Carotene	5000	IU
Magnesium	350 mg		Vitamin D	200	IU
Zinc	15 mg		Vitamin C	500	mg
Iodine	50 mcg		Vitamin E	200	IU
Iron	10 mg		Thiamine	50	mg
Manganese	2.0 mg		Riboflavin	10	mg
Boron	1.0 mg		Niacinamide	100	mg
Vanadium	25 mcg		Pyridoxine	50	mg
Chromium	50 mcg		Biotin	500	mcg
Selenium	200 mcg		Pantothenate	500	mg
Molybdenum	150 mcg		Folic acid	400	mcg
			Vitamin B12	100	mcg

*mcg means Micro-gram or millionth of a gram; 1000 mcg = 1.0 mg

Laxatives

Constipation may be occur in the first weeks of the Core Diet plan, but is eventually corrected by increasing vegetable fiber intake. The best laxative to use temporarily is a bulk laxative. We prefer the plant fiber, **Psyllium Mucilloid** (Metamucil or Prodiem; choose unflavored varieties) at 1 teaspoon 2-3 times/day. This fiber is a natural gluten-free derivative of the husk of the grain Plantago ovata. The fiber absorbs water and increases the bulk of stools. The fiber absorbs bowel irritants as it normalizes colonic action. Fibre improves both constipation and diarrhea. Occasionally, psyllium mucilloid will cause abdominal bloating and must be discontinued. One caution: allergic reactions to psyllium have been reported in nurses who dispense the powder frequently (and are sensitized by inhalation), and severe anaphylactic reactions have been reported. Ground flax seed is an alternative fibre laxative. Do not expect a bulk laxative to produce the immediate action of irritant laxatives. Irritant laxatives, including cascara, senna, and castor oil, are best avoided, but if constipation remains a problem after day 10 on the Core Program a small dose of senna can be added to the psyllium for 7-10 days and then withdrawn. Increased vegetable fibre in your newly emergent core diet should solve the problem of constipation. If constipation remains a problem beyond 3 weeks, be sure to consult your physician. Avoid other herbal laxatives of any description. Herbal laxatives are mostly irritants; all plants contain potential allergens and toxins and may cause symptoms. Enemas are not recommend.

Problem-Solving

Everyone is different; our goal is to custom-fit a safe, healthy diet plan to your needs. The common beginning of this dietary program may not fit your needs exactly, but it offers a good start toward solving your health problems. You will be your own problem-solver; keep a **Daily Food Intake and Symptom Journal (FISJ)** as you follow the diet revision plan. Describe each disturbance as you experience it. Include time of onset, duration, and severity. This information will help you solve any problems which may arise. The food-symptom journal also helps you to learn more about self-monitoring and self-management. Linda Gomez offered the following suggestions:

> *"The food-symptom diary is one of the most important things when beginning the search to find problem areas. It is definitely like the work of a detective, constantly searching for clues and suspecting everything. With this idea in mind, the job becomes exciting. Write everything down; not only what is ingested during a twenty-four hour period, but also the eating times, amount of sleep obtained, environment, medications taken, and disposition. One must expand on all of the above. For example: How was your sleep? Was it disturbed and restless or pleasant? Did you wake up feeling worn-out? Did you get enough sleep? How about your moods? Are you generally irritable, or just when you have a headache? Do certain foods make you jumpy or overly tired?*

Each of the categories must include very explicit information in order to track down the culprit foods. This may seem a tedious task but it helps to keep the diary with you at all times and write things down as soon as you eat or experience them. Once the habit is begun, it becomes second nature. Also, realize that being meticulous is to your advantage and may identify problem areas sooner. Sometimes (when I was first working through my problems) I wouldn't include something which I considered trivial and ended up suffering for it later. Nothing is too trivial. I neglected to write down that I had a little lemon juice and cinnamon with my hot water and suffered for weeks. Better to get a little callous on your finger than a headache. "

Daily Check List

You may find it useful to list your most important symptoms and rate your symptoms as part of a daily check list. The **0 to 3 scale** has been most useful; 0= no problem; 1= minor discomfort; 2= medium; 3= major or disabling symptom. A chart for the first 10 days is a useful scoring tool; you rate your most important symptoms each day. For example, this record shows an increase in symptoms scores during withdrawal, with most disturbances settling within the first week. This method of recording becomes increasingly useful as you follow your progress during food reintroductions in phase 2 and beyond.

Day	1	2	2	4	5	6	7	8	9	1
Headache	2	2	3	2	1	0	0	0	0	
Sore throat	1	3	2	1	0	0	0	0	0	0
Fatigue	3	3	3	2	2	2	2	1	1	0
Irritability	1	2	2	2	1	1	1	0	0	0
Bloating	3	3	3	2	2	2	2	2	1	0
Back Pain	1	2	2	2	1	0	0	0	0	0

Symptoms During the First week are caused by:

Your primary symptoms should diminish or disappear during the first 10 days unless you are unlucky enough to have problems with the initial foods. It takes a number of weeks to fully reconstruct your food intake with balanced, proper nutrition. You may be genuinely distressed during the first week and you may not be able to assess your improvement until the second week. In the best case, improvement is obvious by Day 4 and food reintroductions cause little difficulty. Symptoms during the first 4 days are usually due to withdrawal effects which can be severe, and reduced caloric intake. It is important to eat sufficient amounts of vegetable foods or supplement your food with ENFood to avoid caloric deprivation, and acidosis, especially as the worst withdrawal effects are subsiding. With reduced carbohydrate intake, fat is used as a fuel with the production of acidic by-products; "acidosis"; the symptoms include   nausea, weakness, fatigue, irritability, and headache. Increased intake of vegetable carbohydrate prevents acidosis. Fortunately, most patients report a dramatic increase in their appetite by the end of the first week and the higher caloric vegetables (rice, yams, sweet potato, squashes, peas and carrots) become attractive and satisfying foods.

Symptoms during Phase 1 **of diet revision** **may be due to:**	* **withdrawal effects** * **metabolic disturbances** * **reduced caloric intake** * **allergy to Phase 1 foods** * **cheating** * **other problems**

Linda Gomez comments:

> *" Food withdrawal is rather unpleasant, but should only last four or five days. It is difficult to accept that one can have an addiction to food, as was my case, but one soon realizes it does exist. It is quite normal to experience nausea, cravings, and general malaise, but one must keep in mind that this state is temporary. It is very important to stick to the diet, as this is probably the most crucial time. It may be necessary to live from day to day at this time rather than thinking of long-term results.*

> *I had been told I would go through a withdrawal syndrome, but I really didn't believe it. I saw drugs, alcohol and smoking as addictive habits, but certainly not food. I had been told that withdrawal would last for four or five days. I was not addicted to food. I would not experience withdrawal. For five days, I felt worse than I had ever felt. "There I was craving these foods, feeling absolutely awful - but after I came out of withdrawal, even though I was still getting headaches, I had a wild sense of energy. My concentration was amazing and I*

could tell that, even though there obviously was still some problem because I was still getting the headaches; could something be done about my headaches?

"Once through withdrawal, one experiences a new feeling of well-being, the body being clear of all its toxins. As mentioned previously, the increase in energy, concentration, and better moods are an encouraging factor. I did not clear entirely on the clearing Diet and resorted to an elemental nutrient formula (Tolerex). Once one has been on the formula for a few days and "clears" of headaches, the feeling is wonderful with high energy and high concentration with no headaches was something I had not experienced in a long time. While still on the ENF formula, I began adding simple foods to my diet. It was like feeding a baby, first adding rice and then one by one, vegetables, fruit, chicken, fish as the list grew."

If Symptoms Persist

If symptoms are not improved by Day 11, then stop to solve remaining problems before progressing to new food additions. Four problem-solving options are available:

1. Continue eating Phase 1 foods if you are starting to improve but not all your symptoms have abated. It may take longer to complete the clearing process. The duration of clearing can be approximately equated to the duration of your previous illness or food-related problems. Some patients remain on phase 1 foods for several weeks before they feel fully recovered. If you feel somewhat better, it may only take a few more days to clear. Try to boost vegetable intake to supply adequate daily calories and reduce the amount of poultry if you have been eating meat. Add vitamin and mineral supplements. If this strategy seems to work, then start Phase 2 food introductions. If no further improvement occurs, move to the second option.

2. Review and revise Phase 1 food list. You may notice a food problem during the first week, but withdrawal symptoms and general confusion during such an abrupt change often obscures the origins of Week 1 symptoms. If you suspect any food, then remove it from the list and continue with the remainder for several more days. Also review problems you may have in your ambient environment.

3. Divide Phase 1 foods into four groups: If you cannot identify the offending food(s) in phase 1, remove group A and D foods and continue eating the Group B & C food - vegetables, turkey, and pears for 4 or more days. Reintroduce rice and chicken to reassess their effect on you.

Stop	Group A: Rice, chicken, peaches
	Group D: Salt, oil, flavoring herbs
Continue	Group B: Peas, yams, squash, pears
	Group C: Green beans, carrots, turkey, broccoli, zucchini

4. Return to Clearing Option 2, an ENF: If all the above the food revisions are unsuccessful, retreat to an elemental nutrient formula (ENFood) until your symptoms have cleared. This may take several days. You then begin slower food reintroduction with single foods, continuing to provide baseline nutrition with ENFood. You are at an early infant stage with respect to food tolerance and will need to simulate early infant feeding to define a perfectly safe Core Diet. You wean yourself from the formula slowly as you develop tolerance for solid foods. Give each new food at least 3 days to reveal any problems before accepting it as a safe food in your new Core Diet. Some of our more sensitive patients take several weeks to develop a comfortable Phase 1 diet; their experience closely parallels the timing of infant food introduction. Perseverance furthers one!

---

[1]ENFood is a registered trade mark of EnVironMed Research Inc. 3661 W. 4th Ave. Vancouver, BC V6R 1P2 (604) 731-9168..

Core Program Phase 1 foods

Rice, converted	Carrots	Rice cakes	Rosemary
Rice cereal	Broccoli	Peaches	Basil
Rice flour	Peas	Pears	Thyme
Yams	Olive oil	Turkey	Parsley
Zucchini	Linseed oil	Chicken	Oregano
Squash	Safflower oil	Pepper	Vitamins
Green beans	Sunflower oil	Salt	Minerals

Now Add Phase 2 Foods

Celery	Cauliflower	Applesauce	Watermelon
Lettuce	Asparagus	Honeydew	Cantaloupe
Turnip	Cucumber	Plums	Apples
Spinach	Onions	Strawberries	Raspberries
Brus. Sprouts	Bok Choy	Blueberries	Avocado
Mushrooms	Chives	Nori	Water chessnuts
Mung B. Sprouts	Sue Choy	Kelp	Bamboo Shoots

Rice noodles	Basmati rice	Sole	Lamb
Arrowoot flour	Rice bread	Cod, Snapper	Beef
Brown rice	Rice pancakes	Halibut	Tuna
Tapioca Starch			

Chapter 12   The Core Program

Phase 2: Food Reintroduction

If you are doing well at the end of Phase 1, you can assume that food-related disturbances have subsided and you are tolerating Phase 1 foods. These foods are kept as staple foods, and you slowly reintroduce other foods. **A slow, progressive reintroduction of single foods** allows you to evaluate their effects and make decisions about their acceptability. The idea is to test individual foods or simple combinations, keeping track of your symptoms and mental-emotional changes as you proceed. This is a **self-diagnostic method** which requires **daily decisions** about food choices and the pace of food reintroduction. Again, you choose a fast-track if you are well, and expect few food reactions; or the slow track if you remain symptomatic or prove to be hypersensitive as you try food reintroduction. Your determination to define permanent changes to your diet for lasting health benefits will be challenged during the next 3 weeks.

Our programming strategy is in the form: If condition X then do Y.

The following *if... then* loops gives you an idea of how to proceed.

> *If you are free of symptoms, then it is reasonable to add foods progressively, at the rate of one or two new foods per day.*

> *If problems recur, then slow the pace of food reintroduction one new food every 2-5 days.*

> *If you already know you are allergic to a food then avoid testing this food item; simply add it to your list of "unsafe" foods.*

> *If you eat non-allowed foods, then go back to Phase 1 foods or ENFood to clear recurring symptoms.*

If you doubt the necessity or wisdom of diet change; then have good conversations with yourself make a list of the reasons you are seeking change. Post the list in your kitchen. Review and reaffirm your motives for diet revision.

If your goal is to reduce illness, end your suffering, and to feel and function as well as you can, then be prepared to invest a good deal of time and energy in seeking a solution.

If you are simply restructuring your diet then renew your relationship with basic foods.

If you are missing old recipes and menus than then cultivate an awareness of individual foods, simplicity of preparation, and appreciation of the intrinsic taste of foods.

Phase 2: Food Re-introduction Plan

The most important goal at this stage of diet revision is to develop safe, acceptable meals with a high vegetable content. Continue to eat safe foods from Phase 1 and add the new foods listed, beginning with Phase 2 vegetables. Try to **combine rice and 3 or more vegetables per meal**.

If a food reaction occurs after a meal with new food combinations, then the meal components need to be reviewed, singly, at another time. If you feel unwell for any reason, postpone further food reintroductions until symptoms clear. Simply delay going on to the next day's new food choice until you feel better.

Continue to keep a **daily food-symptom journal** reveal any remaining problems and continue adjusting the new food choices to remove problems. You will need to reorganize meal planning and food selection. Ask for help from other family members, friends or relatives.

The food choices remain basic, familiar foods with good nutritive value and generally high tolerance. The choices include **vegetable, fruit, rice products, fish and meat options.** The vegetable options continue to have the highest priority.

Try different varieties of rice, especially brown and basmati, and rice products, including different kinds of rice cereal, rice noodles, rice paper and rice flour. You may want to experiment with rice flour and/or tapioca (arrowroot) flour to thicken sauces, make gravy and do simple baking. White fish options are introduced, if desired, with the caution that some people develop vigorous allergic reactions to fish. Fish quality is an issue and you may want to do some local market research. Wait to reintroduce red meat to the end of Phase 2 and, even if you seem to tolerate meat, keep the portions small (3 oz.) and meat meals infrequent (twice a week). Hopefully you can enjoy more fruit choices; after you have established tolerance to a fruit, include jams and jellies made with that fruit; try make your own fruit juices.

Fast Track Food Example

If we assume that the first 10 days of Phase 1 have gone smoothly, we continue to add one or two foods per day to finish the second week. Continue to serve foods from Phase 1, choosing rice (if tolerated) and 3-4 vegetables per meal.

Phase 2	Fast Track Food	Choices	
Day 11	*applesauce, sole*	Day 21	*beef*
Day 12	*lettuce, cucumber*	Day 22	*raspberries*
Day 13	*celery*	Day 23	*mushrooms, chives*
Day 14	*halibut or cod*	Day 24	*plums*
Day 15	*melon*	Day 25	*lamb*
Day 16	*bok choy*	Day 26	*pineapple*
Day 17	*avocado*	Day 27	*tuna fish*
Day 18	*rice bread; pancakes*	Day 28	*onions*
Day 19	*raw apples*	Day 29	*brown rice*
Day 20	*asparagus*	Day 30	*strawberries*

Slow-Track, Phase 2

If you encounter symptom recurrence during the earlier stages of Phase 2, or you know your food tolerance is low, proceed more slowly with food reintroduction. If a new food seems well-tolerated, allow at least 2 days to detect delayed responses, before introducing another. If there is any doubt about the food, allow, 3 or more days to notice delayed-onset symptoms.

Wait at least 3 days for symptoms to clear from a reactive food,
before introducing new foods.

Follow a food order similar to the fast-track list. In creating a balanced new diet, we are most interested in introducing a variety of vegetables, and then fruit choices. You might want to add cooked celery to your vegetable mixes first; and then try simple salad ingredients; lettuce first, and cucumber; then add other cooked vegetables such as turnip or brussel sprouts. You may want to try applesauce and then add honeydew melon or cantaloupe next. A fish option is desirable to break the monotony of poultry eating; try fillet of sole or other white fish next. Avocado is included as a fruit, although its nutritive properties resemble a vegetable. Avocado make a good spread for rice cakes and it can, of course, be included in salads. Locate and try a rice bread (as toast) during the 3rd week, and also try different kinds of rice. Wait at least until week 4 before you try beef, lamb, onions or garlic.

You might plan to introduce a new food every three days and then need to slow down after any reactive experience with one of the foods. In the following example, food reintroduction was slowed to every 2-3 days; the pace varies:

Phase 2	Slow Track		
Day 11	cooked celery	Day 25	rice bread
Day 13	lettuce	Day 28	tuna
Day 15	applesauce	Day 30	Bok Choy
Day 18	sole	Day 32	brussel sprouts
Day 21	cucumber	Day 34	beef
Day 22	turnip	Day 37	basmati rice
Day 23	honey dew	Day 40	rasberries

Meal-Planning

Daily meal plans are based on selecting 3-4 cooked vegetables, rice, 2-3 raw vegetables as salad or finger food, selected fruits, and poultry or fish (see end of the chapter for further meal suggestions). These foods are combined to make a variety of meals. Provide nourishing meals for breakfast and lunch by using "dinner" menus earlier in the day; vegetable soup, cooked rice cereals, or leftover dinner with chicken or fish, vegetables, and fruit are all good breakfast choices. Consult the companion volume *"Core Diet Cooking"* for specific meal planning ideas and recipes. Continue the Daily Food-Intake-Symptom Record as an aid to self-monitoring and problem-solving.

You now have enough food variety to cook meals with more attention to tasty mixtures and pleasing appearance. **Vegetable mixtures** can be colorfully arranged. The juices of vegetables cooked, together with simple spices, are delicious, mixed with rice. Asian cooking styles, blending small amounts of many different vegetables together, into tasty mixtures, eaten with rice, is suitable at this stage. Several varieties of commercial **rice bread** are available. The ingredients vary widely and the recipes change often. Rice breads requires evaluation. In general, avoid those containing potato starch, as well as any other untested ingredients If you have no problems with cooked vegetables (eg. carrots, celery, zucchini, cabbage) you may try them, one at a time, as raw snack and salad foods. A homemade oil, vinegar and water dressing, using safe herbs, is attempted next. Carrots and celery are good snacks if they are tolerated. Some vegetables are better cooked, especially broccoli, cauliflower, squash, sweet potatoes, and yams. You should distribute the food groups in approximately the proportions listed below:

FOOD GROUPS	PORTIONS
Rice, Rice Products	*2-3/day*
Vegetables Cooked	*4-6/day*
Vegetables Uncooked	*3-4/day*
Fruit	*2/day*
Meat, Poultry, Fish, Tofu	*1-2/day*
Vegetable Oil	*3-6 tsp/day*
Water	*1-1.5 liter/day*

An adequate diet plan consists of 3 to 4 balanced meals per day. The actual amount of food eaten should be determined by your appetite, which, we hope, will work in a more balanced and physiological manner. It is important for you to eat properly-prepared, well-balanced meals early in your activity day.

Three 2/3's rules help to distribute foods on your Core Diet:

Vegetable foods, including rice, rice products, and other grain alternatives, should account for two thirds (2/3) of your daily calories. **Cook 2/3's of your vegetable foods** and eat the rest as fresh, raw salad or snack vegetables. If you have persisting digestive difficulties, you may not tolerate raw vegetables. About 2/3 of daily calories should be eaten by late afternoon or within 8 hours of waking. **Eat 2/3's of your daily calories before 5 PM** or during the first 8 hours of your waking day.

Suggestions for Meal Plans

The best **breakfast** meals involve "real food" in the morning. The 2/3 rule suggests more of our principle cooked meals should be eaten earlier in the day. The best breakfast is a properly cooked meal. Think of poached rainbow trout, wild rice, carrots, and a sprig of parsley. A bowl of cooked rice with 2-3 vegetables (eg. carrots, peas, green beans) is a perfect breakfast. Rice can be fried (ie. warmed with vegetable oil, peas, cubed carrots, and perhaps fruit pieces in a frying pan to make a delicious breakfast; a little salt and pepper may be the only flavor required.

Eating only fruit in the morning may work well for some people and not for others. Fruit is not nutritionally complete, and its high sugar content will often induce sugar cravings. Fruit juices are traditional breakfast foods, but are not always suitable for people with food allergies. Citrus juices and apple juice have not been well-tolerated, in our experience. You can take any fruit that has proven to be "safe" and create homemade juices, using a blender or juicer. Homemade vegetable juices are highly desirable. Raw-food fans would suggest eating only fresh raw juiced vegetables; however, for many this would produce digestive symptoms and increased allergenic effects. To avoid these effects, you can make juices from cooked vegetables. Cooked vegetables may be pureed in an ordinary blender; add water to achieve the right consistency.

Cereal breakfasts include puffed rice, Rice Chexs, Rice Flakes, Rice Krispies, millet-rice flakes, or hot rice cereals, moistened with fruit and fruit juice or water instead of milk. Breakfast can be leftovers from the previous evening's dinner, perhaps mixed with fruit and warmed in the microwave. Why not have soup, salad, or stew in the morning? All over the world, for centuries, a single food pot would contain a soup-stew made of all available foods, simmering and available for every meal.

Lunch should be based, if; possible, on **dinner menus; a full-course cooked meal** is preferred. You may require a portable lunch. A Core Diet soup, a salad, and rice cakes can easily prepared at home and taken in a warm food thermos. Lunch away from home may be cold chicken/turkey, salad, carrot sticks, rice cakes with a spread or jam, fruit, or any other relatively non-perishable food. Use a cooked-food thermos and take rice and vegetables, hot soup, stew, or poultry or fish casserole.

Dinner at home is generally the least difficult meal to create. A basic meal plan would begin with the choice of:

>*A rice portion.*
>*Cooked vegetables; choose a mixture of 3 or 4.*
>*Salad vegetables; choose a mixture of 2 or 3.*
>*A poultry, fish, or meat portion.*
>*Fruit.*

Vegetables can be chosen for their complementary nutritive properties. Mix vegetables of different botanical families in tasty combinations. You can think of vegetables as color coded. For example, choose four cooked vegetables using the following criteria:

>**One yellow-orange vegetable***; these tend to have a higher caloric value and are more filling; yams, sweet potatoes, winter squash, carrots, and turnips.* **One legume***: begin with cooked peas and green beans.***One brassica** *vegetable - broccoli, cauliflower or brussel sprouts.***One green vegetable***; spinach, asparagus, bok choy.*

Phase 2 Problem-Solving

As you proceed, new foods are associated with an increased incidence of symptom recurrence. Protect yourself. **Be alert to the return of any symptoms.** After you introduce a new food you will be waiting for an adverse reaction to appear. It is fine art to relax and let nature take its course; don't over-emphasis small transient discomforts, but don't ignore a significant warning symptom. You will find immediate reactions (within 3 hours) easy to identify, but delayed problems will not be so obvious. The morning is a good time to do a whole-body check and decide if you are having delayed symptoms from yesterday's food.

Remember that important changes are not straight-forward and your responses to change are not necessarily rational. Many forces will act to distract you from the business of getting better. Unstable moods and emotions associated with social experiences will interfere with your rational plan to rescue yourself from old destructive patterns. The **emotional responses** to change tend to peak during phase 2. Paradoxically, the more you improve, the more intense the emotional responses are. Review the description of the **stages of transformation** in the previous chapter when you experience difficulties. Maintaining control should involve daily negotiations with yourself. Linda Gomez comments:

> *"The old story of Wimpy in the Popeye cartoons comes to mind with Wimpy saying "I'll pay you Tuesday for a Hamburger today." Sometimes when one is faced with a particularly favorite food, there occurs a type of "wheeling and dealing" so commonly used by car salesmen. Unfortunately, the body does not go for "bargains" or "deals." There is no late payment accepted for total compliance at another time. It is an "all or nothing" contract, with the body calling all the shots."*

You will learn to monitor your progress better if you continue to keep a daily food-symptom journal. It may be useful to rate your energy level, mood, and score your symptom levels as suggested in phase 1 instructions. A simple record might be two columns in a convenient notebook with food intake written on the left and a description of how you are doing on the right. For example:

Food Intake	Symptoms
AM; vegetable soup with rice peaches, water	nose congestion =1; headache=0
Noon; Rice, turkey, carrots, peas, squash, cantaloupe, hot water	fine all AM; a little gassy after lunch
Dinner; Rice, broccoli, yams, sole, pears, rice cakes, peach jam	good day so far; energy 2/3; headache=0

And so-on through the day, each day. A brief description of how you are each day will help you to remember the details of your experiment when you return to your notes at the end of the week, and at the end of the phase to reconsider the meaning of all you have experienced. Try to be a good **scientist, making daily observations,** reasonable hypotheses, and keeping your head, in spite of the chaos and confusion which surrounds you.You might add a symptom **flow chart** to your note book to keep track of your progress over a period of 2-3 weeks. The record allows you to enter a short-form notation of the foods introduced and a symptom level for each of your major disturbances.

Invent your own **symptom list.** Use the 0 to 3 scale; none, little, medium, a lot. Some of our patients have monitored 12 or more parameters every day over a period of many months. Some skeptics might accuse them of being overly concerned with their symptoms, but we think it is good home science, and we have learned a great deal from these records.

Example of a food-introduction/symptom flow chart from day 10 to 18:

Day #	10	11	12	13	14	15	16	17	18
New Food	*Ap S*	*Lett*	*Cuc*	*Blue*	*Cod*	*Cod*	----	-----	-----
Bloating	1	0	0	0	1	2	2	1	0
Diarrhea	0	0	0	1 **	2 **	3	2	1	1
Headache	1	1	0	0	0	0	3	2	1
Aching	1	1	0	0	0	1	2	2	2
Edema	0	0	0	0	1	1	2	2	1

This symptom chart shows recurrent symptoms which start with loose bowel movements on day 13 and progresses to a maximum symptom level on days 15&16; subsiding by day 18. A migraine type headache didn't occur until the third day of this disturbance. The food intake record showed blueberries on day 13, 14 and cod introduced on day 14 and again on day 15. Both foods were suspects. The patient returned to phase 1 foods and symptoms cleared again over the next 3 days. Blueberries and cod are entered into a list of suspect foods to be tried later (wait at least 4 weeks) if desired. If adverse reactions occur, then decide what food is most likely responsible for the problem and drop it from the food list. Often you will not be certain, but our goal is to develop a perfectly safe therapeutic diet and, therefore, doubtful foods are not permitted at this time.

If you have recurrent symptoms on the fast track, **slow down!** Stop for a few days until your symptoms clear then slow the pace of food introductions to one new food every 3 days. Two foods in the above example remained suspects for several weeks; you accept the uncertainty simply because your policy is only to accept foods that feel perfectly OK; doubt is resolved by taken the simplest, safest course of action.

Later introduction of blueberries revealed a similar delayed type response and cod was exonerated - it could have been the other way around. The clue was that a loose bowel movement occurred on the evening of the first blueberry day but this was not conclusive right away; too much fruit of any kind can induce gas and loose stools without being allergenic, and without progressing. You could not tell that their was a significant, expanding problem until the third day after blueberries were introduced. Your experience with these foods may be quite different You may have to return to an earlier phase to clear recurrent symptoms. It is often desirable to eat very simply for several weeks, pausing at an early stage of phase 2 to adjust to new food selection and preparation habits and to reset your awareness of a new, better level of feeling and function. **Patience** at this stage of diet revision pays off later with sustainable good health. It is desirable that you do not "skip ahead", trying phase 3 foods before they are listed, nor should you consume foods or beverages not listed. Also, keep in mind that food mixtures act differently from food eaten in isolation.

The most important problem-solving rules are as follows:

> *If symptoms persist or recur; then* **retreat** *to an earlier phase of your Core Diet menus. If you cleared during Phase 1, you can always reestablish clearing by going back to Phase 1 for 3-7 days. Remember that* **no simple test can predict** *complex responses to foods; foods must evaluated by real-time, real-food, whole-system observation. Remember also that* **allergic effects are not consistent.** *Do not expect to observe the same reaction each and every time the food is eaten.*

Alter food Timing, Portions, Frequency

Some foods can only be eaten comfortably in smaller amounts, less frequently. Here are some examples of the most consistent **dose-frequency** reporting during phase 2:

> **"I can only eat food A every 4 days. If I eat it everyday I start to feel sick again. * "I can eat food A as long as I limit the portion size to about 3 ounces, and I don't eat it everyday. * "I introduced beef on day 18 and I found I was OK until 5 days later when my joints began to ache again and I felt tired and generally awful. * "I ate it everyday for the first week then I began to notice mouth tingling and bloating each time I ate, so I stopped by day 20 and started feeling better."*

Rotation diets have been advocated for many years as a solution to food allergy problems. Rotation meant that each food is eaten at intervals; every 4 days, for example. Even allergenic foods were allowed. Rotation was based on an old idea that you would be sensitized to foods you ate it all the time. We now know that the opposite is true; we develop tolerance to foods eaten all the time. Rotation diets may have partial benefit because they reduce the total dose of reactive foods over time, but many foods will not be acceptable even with a low dose and frequency.

Sensitization to foods is easy and probably occurs with the first few exposures to a food. We are born sensitized to foods our mothers ate!

What determines our reactivity is a **complex interactions** among tolerance-inducing and reactive mechanisms. We know this is a variable balance, at best. If charted, the net reactive level would look like a **stock market graph** with daily fluctuations, overall trends and occasional crashes.

We know from careful observation of many patients over time that food allergic symptoms were related to the **amount and frequency** of food eaten, as well as the timing and circumstances of the meals. The Core Program is based on an awareness of the **complex interactions** which govern food hypersensitivity and tolerance. There are many variables to consider

To make problem-solving simple we constantly apply our rule *<a food did it until proven otherwise>* and add a dose-frequency factor *< because I ate too much, too often>*. Too **much fruit,** for example, often causes sugar cravings, rashes, itches, intestinal gas or diarrhea, and increased frequency of urination.

Solution: identify and withdraw offending fruit (eg. apples, apple juice); reduce the amount of fruit eaten - 2 portions/day or less is appropriate. Fruit also triggers cravings for more fruit or other sweet foods and may block your appetite for vegetable foods which tend to be safer and more nourishing. Reducing fruit intake to two portions per day and changing the fruit choice each day may resolve the problem; for example:

Mon	Tues	Wed	Thurs	Fri	Sat	Sun
peach	pear	apple	melon	plum	berries	pear

A similar **alternation of poultry, fish and meat choices** may be required. Even if beef is tolerated, limit beef intake to a maximum of 2 days per week and keep the portion size to about 4 oz. maximum. Similarly, chicken should not be eaten all the time nor in large amounts; a maximum of 3 days/week would be suitable.

Mon	Tues	Wed	Thurs	Fri	Sat	Sun
chicken	fish	turkey	beef	fish	chicken	beef

Exceptions to the Core Program

If you eat foods not on the list, simply record the experience in your daily record. It is important to understand the reasons for your "cheating" on the Core Diet. Do not feel guilty! Eating wrong food is inevitable. Everyone, young and old, makes exceptions, sometimes frequently. Food selection discipline is one of the high arts of human endeavor. A professional woman, offered the following report of relapsing after a "treat":

"I was doing so well and had reached day 25 feeling much better than I had in years. I couldn't eat peas because of bloating and fatigue, avoided the beef, but otherwise ate all phase 1 and 2 foods without incident. It was the holiday weekend and I was asked out for "coffee" by a close friend. I decided that I was doing so well I would treat myself to a cup of coffee and a cinnamon bun. The bun tasted good; it had gobs of cinnamon and butter stuffing . The coffee tasted oddly bitter, but familiar, and reassuring.

"My pleasure didn't last very long; within 15 minutes I had terrible heartburn; I was yawning, then sneezing and my eyes began to burn. I couldn't follow what my date was saying and I began to resent him – I don't know why. .. 30 minutes later I was feeling so awful, I tried to explain what was happening to my date, but he looked skeptical and started to argue that coffee and a cinnamon bun shouldn't bother me, so I excused myself and went home.

" I was feeling so tired and weak that I went to bed. The heartburn got worse and I bloated; a headache – the kind where someone is jabbing knives into your temples – started about an hour later. It took me two days to recover, and I went back to phase 1 foods gladly. I probably won't do that again for a long time."

As long as you can return to Core Diet foods, all deviations from your safe food list serve as random experiments and can teach you more about the way your body responds to foods. Sometimes, the response is so severe we vow never to allow it to happen again; at other times, there is little problem and we feel more confident about exceptions or treats.

If a major slip from the Core Diet results in a burst of disturbance lasting several days, **retreat to Phase 1** and await symptom-clearing before you proceed to other food introductions. Linda Gomez comments:

> *"The final stage of acceptance may take some people a long time to achieve and others a short time. Once acceptance is achieved, the person can really start working with what they can eat instead of living in the past. Acceptance brings about a new, healthier lifestyle, a whole new outlook on life."*

> *" Acceptance is a stage of new beginnings, with a lot of energy and a new, positive sense. Adapting to a new lifestyle may be like a game, with little twists, modifications to recipes and new ways to deal with old problems. When one finally does accept their food sensitivities, they can clean out the fridge and the cupboards with a clear conscience. Some may remain in Acceptance permanently, while others may have momentary lapses to Denial and eat some problem foods. "It only takes a few days of being ill to bring back all the memories of the times when feeling good was just a dream.*

Phase 3 Foods

Celery	Lima beans	Vanilla	Carob
Leeks	Peanuts	Ketsup	Sesame
Daikon	Apricots	Vinegar	Currie
Radish	Cranberries	Sugar	Garlic
Lotus Roots	Nectarines	Honey	Ginger
Yellow wax beans	Mango	Wasabi	Marjoram
Azuki Beans	Grapes	Miso	Mustard
White beans	Blackberries	Tofu	Tofu products
Chickpeas	Papaya	Tofu ice cream	Soy infant formula
Kidney beans	Lemon-lime	Soya beans	Soy Milk
Lentils	Buckwheat	Soya flour	Soy sauce
Split peas	Millet		

Phase 4 Foods

Cabbage	Cornstarch	Orange	Lobster
Tomatoes	Corn	Currants	Trout
Artichokes	Pumpkin	Pineapple	Salmon
Kale	Chard	Prunes	Shrimp
Parsnip	Potatoes	Cherries	Crab
Kohlrabi	Garlic	Abalone	
Beets	Mint	Prawns	

Chapter 13   Core Program Phases 3 to 5

Phase 3: Stabilization, Flavors, Legumes

Phase 3 consists of securing the gains you have made thus far, **problem-solving**, and then proceeding with further food reintroductions. The idea is to stabilize in a new, healthier mode, before making food selection more complex. We usually pause to solve any remaining problems and write standard meal plans for the week. The foods that you now tolerate well are the staple foods which will continue to serve you well.   A growing friendship with these foods is the basis of your long-term success.

The separation of Phase 3 from Phase 2 may seem arbitrary. During medically supervised diet revision, the beginning of Phase 3 corresponds to a problem-solving visit to the physician. The visit agenda includes reviewing progress to date with a look at the daily food-symptom journal to interpret and suggest solutions for any remaining problems. Usually, you are starting the second month of the Core Program. In the best case, you have followed the program successfully and may just need encouragement to continue.

You may be "bored" with the same foods all the time. Our patients will offer ambivalent remarks such as: "I'm fine as long as a I stay on the Core Diet, but it's boring, and I can't go out for dinner! What can I add that is more flavorful and entertaining?"

Boredom has important advantages and we welcome this report at the end of Phase 2. Boredom means that you have settled into a new stable pattern with limited but healthy food selection. Patients who are cheating, eating in restaurants, and "falling off the wagon", may not be bored but they are getting sick again.

Relapses are common in the second month and therefore devote time and attention to securing the new pattern, making small adjustments and additions to regular meals. Emotional changes, in terms of the 4 stages of grief are resolving. You should be through anger, denial, and still negotiating with your body for the "best deal" in food choices.

The stage of acceptance is just around the corner. Random experiments, eating off your Core Diet w,ill give you a better definition of the limits of your tolerance. You need to better define the **safe eating zone** and recognize when you have gone beyond safe eating. The safe zone may be very tight and only a few foods may feel perfectly OK; if you are lucky, the safe zone is rather permissive and you may find that you can add quickly to your Phase 1 and 2 foods with no problem. Let your body be the judge. Pay attention to the feedback signals! Chaos wants to take over again.

Keep the kitchen stocked with Core Program foods; maintain order with a daily food-symptom record, meal-plans, shopping lists, reminders to yourself of your best intentions to a achieve lasting, healthy, safe diet.

Symptom recurrence is common as you try new foods or stray from your Core Diet. Hopefully, your distress will be minimal and infrequent. Our most important problem-solving rule is: **a food did it until proven otherwise.**

You will likely discover that symptom responses are variable. Some foods will prove perfectly safe and acceptable every day in any amount. Other foods will bother you if eaten too much, or too often, or too fast, or in combination with certain other foods. review the problem-solving strategies, described in Phase 2. Remember that your body works in a complex manner, and it remains your task to stay tuned-in to how you feel so that your decisions about food choices will produce good results.

Continue your policy of protecting yourself from wrong foods and adverse environments. Remember that irritability, sleep disturbances and/or depressed feelings signal recurrent food reaction until proven otherwise. Give yourself non-food rewards for good compliance with the Core Program rules. Maintain a regular meal schedule. Become more involved in play, sports, and other physical activities.

Phase 3   Food Reintroductions

The next goal is to make more interesting meals and you begin another round of food reintroductions. You add more flavorings, more substitutes for missing cereal grains, and seek more opportunities to try different recipes, perhaps from Chinese or Japanese cuisines. You seek to develop variety in basic meal-plans. The next food list includes herbs, spices, sauces, fruits, soya, products and legumes; all these choices help us to slowly improve flavor and menu variety .

Write out a **standard meal plan** for the week. This your emerging Core Diet which will work best if you diversify your menus and distribute the safe foods on your food list. List the safe foods you have established and select the prerequisite number of foods from each food group. Assign these foods to the meals you are planning.

The goal of your menu-planning is to balance food intake between stability of nutrient and energy supply, and taste diversity. You may eat staple foods every day if they are well-tolerated. You will do best if your follow standard menu plan for the week and add single food items, flavors and sauces to basic meals. The idea, of course, is that a stable, safe meal plan acts as a baseline of normal function so that you can assess the results of adding foods.

Add **new flavors** to meals that have worked well before, so that you can decide if the flavorings have any adverse effects. Add one at a time, alternating a flavoring addition with a new food introduction. Try **fruit juices** with the awareness that we experience more symptoms with commercially-packed fruit juices than with the fruit itself. You will always do best to make your own juice at home from fruit which you enjoy and have eaten without adverse effects. Carbonated fruit drinks are more common on the market now and are good choices.

We are interested in **Asian recipes** at this stage and highly recommend **Wok cooking**. Vegetables suitable for stir-fried meals include bok choy, sue choy, mung bean sprouts, lotus root, bamboo shouts, and mushrooms. Seeds can also be added to cooked meals and salads. Roasted sesame seeds are used for flavoring. Sunflower and pumpkin seeds can be cooked with rice to add flavor and texture. We often observe adverse effects when these seeds are eaten in quantity as snack foods or as "butters" and do not recommend this use. **Millet** is the second grain to be introduced in the Core Program, and if you are unfamiliar, you will need some recipes to help you prepare Millet into tasty dishes. **Buckwheat** is another grain-like food to try, especially in pancake recipes and as a cooked breakfast option.

Legumes are nutritionally desirable, especially lentils and beans, but also can be tricky foods to prepare, and complicated in terms of adverse reactions. Legumes have moderate allergenic potential and contribute to excess gas and other digestive problems. Dried beans need careful cooking. Avoid eating several legumes at once (eg. peas, lentils, soy milk, tofu).

Peanuts are also favored as snack food, but have many problems, including the potential to trigger anaphylactic reactions. Peanut butter may be introduced first as a spread on rice cakes or rice bread. Compulsive eating of peanut butter is common and must be avoided. If peanut butter seems okay, limit the daily dose to 2 ounces at the most; dish out the daily amount into a serving dish or plastic container and keep the main supply out of reach.

We also try **soy products** which have great appeal as substitutes for dairy products and meats in vegetarian, Chinese, and Japanese cooking. **Tofu** is refined soy protein, a good food to begin evaluating adverse responses to soy. This is a nourishing, highly versatile food which can be a real asset if you tolerate it. Tofu is utilized as a base for making many food products that substitute for dairy and egg, including ice cream, chip dips, and mayonnaise. Clever cooks turn tofu into many meat-like dishes for vegetarian diets. Soya milk may also be tried. Infant **soy milk formulas** (Soyalac, Isomil, Nursoy, ProSobee) are complete foods, useful in cooking and occasionally as a nutritional supplement for adults who need to gain weight. You can use the canned infant formulas, as if they were condensed milk, on cereals and in baking. Try rice pudding using, for example, rice, vanilla, soy milk, and raisins (leave the cinnamon and nutmeg out).

Miso is another soya product to try; it is the base for the delicious Japanese consume. Miso is a fermentation product of soya as is soya sauce and tamari. Try wheat free soya sauce, and even if you tolerate it, use the sauce sparingly and not every day. Soya flour is also a baking option. Soy protein, unfortunately, is allergenic and produces adverse reactions in up to 30% of our patients. You may have to ration the amount of soy products in your diet to stay below a safe dose-frequency threshold. Often, only limited amounts of soy protein are well-tolerated.

Phase 4 Further Food Reintroductions

Again, the transition between Phase 3 and 4 may seem arbitrary. Our intention is to continue reintroducing foods if everything is going well. Usually, Phase 4 begins informally after the interesting food choices in Phase 3 have been successfully incorporated into your core diet.

Phase 4 foods are separated for a reason - these foods are to be considered optional extras and not staple foods. For example, the nightshade vegetables, potatoes, tomatoes, and peppers have be a source of trouble in too many patients to be considered staple foods, but if your tolerance permits, enjoy a serving of these vegetables once or twice a week. If you have arthritis it is unwise to these foods except as occasional "treats". The citrus fruits and bananas are similarly rationed, even if you seem to tolerate them well. Other fruits may be more suitable for regular eating. The seafood options, including shellfish and crustaceans, may contribute to interesting variations in your basic recipes but generally should not be eaten too frequently. Immediate hypersensitivity type of allergy to shrimp, crab, lobster and prawns is well-recognized.

Remember that foods are added now with the same care and concern that we exercised when first introducing foods into your Core Diet. You must be convinced that the new food is well tolerated before you keep it in your diet. If symptoms recur, wait longer before attempting new food introductions.

> *If you continue to have recurrent symptoms for any reason, postpone this phase of food reintroductions until symptoms clear. Retreat to a safer eating position, rather than making things more complicated.*

More vegetable and fruit choices are always desirable. New fruit options are often appreciated. Introduce one new fruit per week during Phase 4; for more of a treat use jams, jellies, fruit salads or desserts. We continue to observe a variety of problems when patients eat too much fruit. Continue to limit daily intake to about two portions. Be cautious about fruit juices as well. You must be convinced that the fruit and/or juice is well tolerated before you keep it in your regular, safe food list. For baking, cereal grain alternates and substitute flours are introduced. The exclusion of wheat, rye, oats, and barley remains a firm policy of Phase 4.

Meal Planning

Recall our basic meal planning outline: You should continue to distribute the foods available on your safe food list in approximately the proportions listed below:

FOOD GROUPS	PORTIONS per Day
Rice, Rice Products	2- 3
Vegetables Cooked	4- 6
Vegetables Uncooked	3- 4
Fruit	1- 2
Meat, Poultry, Fish, Tofu	1- 2
Vegetable Oil	1-3

Combine cooked vegetables in groups of 4 or more; choosing among:

yellow, orange, red	yams, sweet potatoes, winter squashes, carrots, and turnips, parsnips, beets.
legumes	peas, green and yellow beans, dried beans, lentils, and split peas
cabbage group	broccoli, cauliflower, cabbage, cabbage brussel sprouts.
green vegetables	bok choy, sue choy,spinach, asparagus, beet greens.
nightshades	potatoes, tomatoes, peppers
flavoring vegetables	onions, garlic, celery, parsley, chives

Phase 5   Maintenance of Your Core Diet

The Core Program is a sequenced program of change, designed to reveal and then correct food-related health problems. The changes that you make by thoughtful, conscientious self-management are not temporary adjustments that you abandon once you are well. Maintaining an asymptomatic, healthy state requires a continuing, determined effort to monitor yourself and to regulate your food supply. Phase 5 may again seem to be arbitrary. The beginning of phase 5 corresponds to a follow-up visit to a Program supervisior to discuss the final touches to your core diet, and to plan the longer term strategy. Any remaining problems with food choices, compliance and nutritional status are resolved. Meal plans should be well-organized and routine. Appropriate cooking skills should also be second-nature. Most the social problems of diet change should be resolved. You are settling into the long-term plan.

Our basic maintenance strategy is to follow the custom-fitted Core Diet, that you have created, as closely as possible, allowing treats and exceptions of convenience or necessity if adverse effects are not too serious. Continue to think of your Core Diet as a safe eating zone. If you wander beyond the limits of this safe zone you may enjoy some food experiences and you may suffer ill-effects. The adaptive trick is to return as soon as possible to the safe zone, your Core Diet, if old symptoms recur or new symptoms emerge. Always invoke the rule *<a food did it until proven otherwise>*.

You need to be good at self-monitoring and develop a flexible, adaptive approach to feeding yourself. Often dietary advice implies that living is uneventful and easy, with few distractions from the business of looking after our needs. This illusion of an orderly, rational existence is misleading at best, and at worst, inspires real guilt and despair in those who believe others have an easier time of it. Since the Core Program is an exercise in problem-solving, careful and systematic observation tends to reveal patterns of dysfunction and disease which otherwise remain mysteriously troublesome.

The task is to continue problem-solving because **everything changes**. Reject the idea that you are "on a diet" and accept the idea that your are "in an adaptive, healthy state". One of our patients remarked after a few months that friends were still expressing sympathy that she was on "such a restrictive diet". She replied: "not restrictive - selective, and don't feel sorry for me; I am perfectly happy to feel as well as I do."

We observe a range of coping skills and styles over the long-term. The most successful people are positive about change, open to new experiences, and good at self-monitoring. They are adaptable and develop new food-shopping patterns, cooking techniques, and develop an interesting cuisine, even if their food list is limited. Successful people tend to treat themselves to safer food indulgences and backtrack quickly if they get symptoms; they may go to a Japanese restaurant for Sushi, and miso soup for example, instead of insisting on pizza and beer.

The people who resist change in the beginning, forced by their disease to consider change, but feeling deprived, continue to cheat, eating foods that make them ill, as if they were rebelling against an unseen parent. Either they stay in the anger and denial stages of change or fall back easily. Many eventually realize that the first person they cheat is themselves and advance to the negotiation stage, perhaps seeking a compromise solution; a relatively safe Core Diet most of the time, but exceptions based on convenience, pleasure, and social pressures. If you wander too far away from safe Core Diet foods, you need to retreat to Phase 1, clear, and restore a sense of well-being with renewed control over food choices.

The long-term Core Program **food-selection policy** is based on the goals outlined in chapter one. These are sincere, serious goals that require our dedicated effort to permanently change our habits. Our experience to date suggests that people who stay on their own version of the Core Diet do best over the long term. They do best in all departments; general health, work performance, mental-health, growth, body-shape and size, athletics, and self-esteem.

Problem-Solving

There are **many variables** which decide how you react to food. All you can count on is change. We all change continuously, food changes, the planet changes. Your food selection will change, if you are doing a good job of adjusting to your changing needs and tolerances. Recall that increased sensitivity is expected during the first few months on the Core Program. **Hypersensitivity** tends to stabilize after a few weeks and slowly decreases. Increasing tolerance for more foods is experienced by many patients during the first year. Increasing tolerance means that more foods can be safely eaten; more treats and exceptions can be enjoyed. However, long term success depends on your ability to monitor your mental and physical status and your willingness to adjust your food intake, if problems recur.

We are aware of **cyclic changes** in food tolerance. Short daily cycles interact with lunar and seasonal cycles. Short daily rhythms effect us. Many people report little food tolerance first thing in the morning, and more in the evening. Others report decreased symptoms if they exercise right after eating.

Women regularly report increased sensitivity **premenstrually** and we can explain some premenstrual symptoms as increased allergic reactivity. Many people find that they tolerate more foods in the summer, or when they are happy, relaxed, and well rested. Conversely, some report that their food tolerance drops severely in the winter, or if they are tired, angry, or infected with a virus. The following excerpt from a daily journal, kept by a professional woman, reveals typical difficulties. This description reminds us of the many levels through which we conduct our existence. It also reminds us that we are in continuous, **complex interaction with our environment,** and when circumstances around us change, so do we.

"...Not a very good month or five weeks - seemed to deteriorate just before getting my period and never recovered. I have had sore throats, off and on, aching in calf muscles, dry lips and headaches. I was under a great deal of pressure at work before I left on vacation...to Jamaica. I was okay there for a few days, I had a small glass of rum punch and after that never felt the same. Slept a lot in Jamaica - could not stay awake very late. Played tennis five evenings in a row for one hour each time. Did not seem to affect me."Food was difficult there in the hotel as it was geared to American diets - bought fruit for our room (bananas, tangerines, papaya, mango), and had rice cakes along with me - ate out as much as possible for Jamaican food - was okay with pumpkin soup, red bean soup, codfish and akee, cho-cho, rice and peas (red beans), curried goat, yams. In the hotel, through hunger I ended up eating bread once a day for several days in a row (bun or hamburger bun), had chicken salad with mayonnaise two or three times - no strong reactions at the time. The menu offered almost nothing that was okay for me except gazpacho soup.

"The dry, swollen lips started mid-week and I felt tired and irritable despite the sun and relaxation. Once I got home, I had a lot of trouble adjusting to the time change, and found myself wanting to go to sleep early in the evening (but I did not), and then waking up at 3:30 or 4:00 a.m. for well over a week. It seems that almost every time I eat I get some reaction - sore throat, sometimes dry lips, but my temperature has finally come down from 98.6 or 98.8 (high for me) to 97.4 (normal for me). I have a very stiff neck and headachy feeling just before my period "

Advance and Retreat

She had remained hypersensitive for many years and found that she had to follow a precise diet to remain well. When her body received the wrong input, a delayed illness pattern emerged that tended to persevere for a week or longer. Her recovery program usually involved returning to **Phase 1** for several days, often on an elemental formula. Our food supply is **constantly changing.** Environmental variables throw many unknown complications in our direction. The best method of dealing with variations in food tolerance and variations in the food supply is a common-sense, problem-solving strategy: Advance and Retreat.

Advance with increased food choices when you are feeling perfectly well. **Retreat** to a safer food list when symptoms return to recover and rest. Cravings and compulsive eating are often triggered by wrong foods, and may lead you back to a prolonged session with recurrent illness. The most successful self-managers learn to retreat promptly to a simpler, safer eating program and wait until the disturbance clears.

The most efficient technique of **Retreat-Recover** is to return to **Phase1** clearing. Choose either Phase 1 foods and/or ENFood until recurrent symptoms clear. We have found that minor symptom recurrences will clear by skipping a meal and having ENFood instead. Moderate symptom recurrences require ENFood or the clearing diet for 3 days at least. Major recurrent illness will require more than a week of clearing. Once you are clear of symptoms again, advance to your complete Core Diet food list, and promise yourself better compliance in the future.

The most radical feature of Core Program food selection is the exclusion of milk products, eggs, wheat, oats, rye, and barley. Coffee, tea, chocolate, and alcoholic beverages are also gone. The less radical but equally important exclusion of popular drinks, packaged, canned, and bottled foods continues to be a problem to many people. There is always a strong pull back to old food habits and the more typical eating patterns of the community. We continue to be bombarded by food advertising. Recent TV advertisements show self-indulgent actors complaining that life is not worth living if they cannot have their favorite mayonnaise or dessert. Your adult personality is intelligent enough to resist this child-level persuasion. But, the child-side of your personality will buy the message without hestitation.

Social pressures, old habits, and recursive loops triggered by reactive foods will all draw you back to problem foods. You may be less tempted at home, but struggle to stay on track in restaurants, fast food outlets, parties, and other social events. You are battling a culture which conspires against healthier, self-responsible eating habits. You may be battling cravings and compulsive behavior which return as you react to foods, eaten as occasional treats, or as inadvertant exceptions when you eat-out. Advance and retreat. Do not give up!

Policy Re: Dairy Products

Well-funded advertising insist that you drink milk, but we do very well without it. Milk products are likely to trigger recurrent problems and we are reluctant to suggest reintroducing milk. You should assume that milk allergy is a life-long possibility. You might find that small amounts of dairy foods as treat, an ice cream cone on a hot Sunday afternoon, for example, may be pleasurable and tolerated. Often, small amounts of milk creep back into a Core Diet through baking, restaurant foods, and treats.

Small amounts may be well-tolerated with minimal symptoms such as nasal stuffiness, or increased throat mucus. Many increase their intake of dairy products, only to realize, weeks or months later, that their general status has deteriorated with increased digestive symptoms, "colds", fatigue, depression, aching and other symptoms. Some people remain hypersensitive to milk and even small amounts will trigger diarrhea, congestion, coughing, asthma, or headaches. If even small doses of dairy products are not well-tolerated then find substitutes: dairy-like products include Rice Dream, a variety of soya or tofu products including tofu "ice creams", and Dole Whip.

Eggs are similar to milk. **Egg white** is the prototype of allergenic proteins and will often trigger recurrent symptoms. Egg yolks are less allergenic but contain cholesterol. The use of occasional egg yolks in baking may be acceptable, but returning to regular egg meals is unwise.

Policy Re: Beverages

Coffee, teas, herbal teas, coffee-substitutes and chocolate drinks remain unwelcome on the Core Diet. Tasty, safe, non-toxic hot beverages include safe-fruit drinks, your own soups and consumes, and delicious hot water, perhaps with honey or a touch of fruit. When you do consume coffee, tea, and other beverages note the adverse effects. Once you are off these beverages for a while their negative effects tend to be very obvious. Avoid falling back into regular use patterns since you will renew the addictive cycle and face withdrawal again (many do this repeatedly over several months or years before they are finally convinced abstainers, the author included).

Alcoholic beverages also remain unwelcome for best functioning, although some people tolerate small portions of white wine, cider, or sake. Spitzers and coolers may also be enjoyed occasionally by some successful Core Dieters. If you drink compulsively or get any symptoms from the alcoholic beverages, you would, of course, continue to abstain completely.

Policy Re: Convenience Foods

Keep the number of processed packaged foods to a minimum and introduce each new product as a separate new food. Be sure that you are OK before you include any product in your safe food list. If symptoms recur, automatically exclude all manufactured food products as part of your retreat and recover strategy. There are unexpected problems even with products prepared from apparently "safe foods".

Packaged fruit juices have been a special source of disappointment. Dried fruits also may bring unpleasant surprises. Of course, we look for products that have no chemicals added, but even this precaution is no guarantee that all will be well.

Eating Out and Traveling

Traveling and eating out are the most hazardous activities for Core Dieters. You must be firm in your resolve to protect yourself. Your task is to approximate proper food selection when ordering food in restaurants or accepting meals invitations. sometimes it is difficult to make the distinction between the immediate but brief pleasure of a food in the mouth, and the hours of suffering that may follow the ingestion of an allergenic food. Some people are good at saying "no". Others court temptation.

When you travel, take your own food whenever possible. Carrots, celery, rice cakes, and fruit are portable foods. ENFood is a safe, convenient travel food; mix with water to make a quick, complete meal.

Be selective when you eat out. The cheaper, fast-food restaurants have rigid, mass-produced food choices with many chemical additives and synthetic materials. Avoid these food outlets. Choose restaurants which allow you to select individual food items. Simple written directions given to the waiter or waitress help get your message to the chef.

The following example is a restaurant note by a patient; it was simply typewritten and photocopied on pocket-sized cards to hand out. Cooperation with this written request was good.

I am on a hypoallergenic diet. I am unable to eat milk,
dairy products, eggs, and wheat (flour).

Please:

Prepare vegetables steam-cooked without sauces.

Bake or microwave meat, fish and poultry
without breading or sauces.

Avoid using sulphates on fresh vegetables and MSG
or tenderizers in soups or on food.

Thank you for your consideration.

If we become more specific and discriminating in choosing restaurant foods, it will eventually influence restaurant practices and make it easier for everyone with food intolerances to receive the appropriate consideration. Success in redeeming oneself and pursuing a healthier life-pattern is the first step toward healing a sick and troubled earth. As you improve your well-being, direct some of your time and energy to improve the conditions around you.

Cereal Grain Reintroduction

What if we reintroduce wheat products, some bread or pasta, for example? Some people, especially after 2-3 months, tolerate small to moderate amounts of cereal-grain foods. Others get recurrent symptoms, food cravings, mood and behavior changes and must withdraw all grain-foods again to remain normal. If you are doing well after 2-3 months, consider introducing one grain portion 3 days a week. You might choose a pasta portion or 2 slices of french bread or a breaded coating on poultry or fish to begin your wheat evaluation. If after 3 or 4 weeks you are convinced that there are no recurrent symptoms, especially digestive symptoms, fatigue, irritability, thinking or mood disorder, then introduce a wheat portion 3 days a week as a regular feature of your expanded Core Diet.

No attempt is made to reintroduce wheat, oats, barley, rye as daily foods if your initial problem list included:

Chron's Disease	Celiac Disease
Dermatitis Herpetiformis	Ulcerative colitis
Other diarrhea	Arthritis
Depression	Schizophrenia

If the wheat portion is well tolerated 3 days a week for three weeks, introduce one portion per day. Continue to emphasize Core Diet foods with rice and rice products (if tolerated) a staple foods. Increase wheat and related grain (oats, rye, barley) foods to a maximum of 2 portions/day after 6 weeks if you remain symptom-free. Decrease or discontinue all cereal grains, if symptoms recur, especially bloating, aching, fatigue, or if your mood deteriorates; wait another three months before repeating the experiment. You can assume if symptoms recur with wheat challenge that you will have a long-term limit on the amount of cereal grains in your Core Diet.

SECTION 3

Further Discussion of Nutrition, Food Allergy and Tests

AA Amino Acid

Allergy: immune-mediated dysfunction and disease.

Antigen: any substance which stimulates an immune response, usually proteins.

Antibody: proteins made by immune cells to identify antigen.

BIN Blood Immune Network, the blood and bone marrow compartment of the 'immune system".

CFP the ratio of carbohydrate, fat and protein in a food or diet.

CHO carbohydrate, the sugar, starch, and fibre components of food.

CCHO complex carbohydrates - starches and fibers.

Complement is a series of blood proteins that chain-react to produce explosive allergic reactions.

ENFood is brand name for Core Program elemental nutrient formulas, a series of different nutrient mixtures, designed to replace food in part or totally during DRT.

FA Fatty Acid

FAC Food allergy complex: incorporates all the pathological mechanisms for food-immune system interactions, and all the diseases that result from these abnormal interactions.

GIT Gastrointestinal tract

IMD Immune Mediated Disease: a new, more comprehensive term for "allergy". There are at least 4 major mechanisms of immune injury (see Types below). Combinations of these mechanisms make IMD exceedingly complex .

Type 1 or IMD1: immediate hypersensitivity = typical allergy.

Type II or IMD2: cytotoxic of cell damaging hypersensitivity; for example, hemolytic anemia

Type III or IMD3 : circulating immune complexes, associated with more serious and prolonged illnesses often leading to or associated with IMD4.

Type IV or IMD4: cell-mediated hypersensitivity = inflammation and damage in target organs.

IMAD Immune mediated Affective Disorder: the mood and arousal disturbances that accompany immune-mediated diseases.

IME Inappropriate Molecular Entry: the concept that food molecules may enter the bloodstream before they are completely digested; the common basis of food allergy. IME leads to IMD.

IN Immune Networks: an updated systems description of the "immune system"; three immune compartments have their own acronyms - BIN, TIN, LIN.

LIN Lymphatic Immune Network: the lymphatic compartment of the "immune system".

MALT Mucosa Associated Lymphatic Tissue

PUFA Polyunsaturated Fatty Acid

TIN Tissue Immune Network: involves cells living in or migrating through or invading (damaging) tissue spaces.

Chapter 14 Core Program Nutrition

This chapter is a brief review of nutrition, refreshed with 1990's systems theory. **Nutritional Programming** (NP) is a new approach to medical therapy that utilizes insights into nutritional biochemistry. References to "NP" in this chapter indicate nutritional programming concepts. The Core Program can be thought of as a Nutritional Program, designed to resolve food-related illnesses, improve nutritional status, and prevent endemic disease in the longer term.

We recognize two kinds of foods: **Primary and Derivative**. Primary foods are in their close-to-natural state, and come directly from the farm or the sea. Both fresh or frozen plant or animal tissues can be considered primary foods, as long as they are not processed in any way. The optimal food is unsprayed, garden-fresh produce from rich healthy organic soils, free of acid rain, radioactive isotopes, and other forms of air pollution. All foods which are preserved, processed, manufactured, cooked, baked, smoked, packaged, or bottled are derivatives. Derivative foods, of course, have increased burdens of non-nutrient chemicals, additives and contaminants.

Macronutrients are the heavy materials in food, consisting of sugars, fatty acids, and amino acids. These molecules must be supplied in sufficient quantity to fuel the body and to replace structural material lost through secretion, excretion, or injury. Minerals required in gram quantities (calcium, magnesium, sodium, and potassium) may also be considered macronutrients.

Micronutrients are vitamins and minerals, required in smaller amounts, mostly as co-factors or catalysts to enzymes. Enzymes are responsible for the millions of different molecular transactions which sustain our life. Many enzymes must have one or two vitamins and at least one critical mineral to function. The basic equation of life chemistry has the following form:

Nutrients----> Enzyme + Vitamin + Mineral----> Cell Product

To make the neurotransmitter, serotonin, the amino acid, tryptophan , derived from food is transported to the brain. At the appropriate place inside a brain cell, two enzymes and vitamin B_6, transform tryptophan to serotonin. Serotonin is then transferred to the sending end of the neuron (the terminal bouton of the axon), where it is used as a molecular messenger to carry information across the synapse to the receiving neuron.

The serotonin synthesis equation is:

STEP 1. Tryptophan----> 5-Hydroxytryptophan

STEP 2. 5-Hydroxytryptophan (5HT)----> Serotonin

via enzyme 5HT-Decarboxylase

A-2: Prenutrients

The size and identity of food molecules are important to us when we consider the problem of food allergy. For example, proteins should not be considered "nutrients". Proteins are large molecules containing hundreds of amino acids. Cells do not utilize protein to make protein. Food protein is digested in GIT into amino acids which are transported across the GIT wall and transported via the blood, first to the liver and later to all body cells. The amino acids are then assembled in intracellular factories, ribosomes, to make new proteins. It is therefore wrong to say that "we need protein in our diets". We need essential amino acids in our diets. The meaning of a protein molecule in ingested food is totally different from the meaning of the amino acids which make it up, just as these words have meaning which their letters alone do not imply.

The construction of large molecules in the leaves of plants by **photosynthesis** and the breaking down of the same large molecules by animals is the basis of life on earth. The sun energizes the whole cycle and our metabolic energy is indirectly an expression of the sun's energy. One can make an excellent case for staying close to the sun in choosing proper foods. Staying close to the sun means eating plant tissues. This is also thought of as the "top" of the food chain, the most biologically efficient location for a food consumer.

The idea that we should eat food combinations that result in a defined proportion of Carbohydrate, Fat, and Protein is basic to nutritional thinking. Standard recommendations have suggested the proportions:

Carbohydrate	53 %
Fat	35 %
Protein	12 %

The main area of dispute in this recommendation is the proportion of fat and carbohydrate. Increased concern about the role of dietary fat, especially animal fat, in arterial disease and cancer has prompted suggestions that the fat proportion be decreased and complex carbohydrate increased. The **Core Program** favors increased vegetable content and tends toward the following proportion goals:

Carbohydrate	74 %
Fat	14 %
Protein	12 %

The short-form notation for **CFP proportions is C74:F14:P12.**

The idea of macronutrient proportion is linked to food group choices. Standard nutritional advice encourages us to choose foods from **four food groups:**

Four Food Groups	**Daily Servings**
Grains	3
Dairy	2
Vegetables and Fruit	2
Meats	2

Proportion rules and daily servings make diet design a relatively simple undertaking. Dieticians have used these rules in recommending "normal diets". Medically altered diets have tended to follow the same basic rules, simply altering proportions. Diverse weight reduction diets have altered the rules in every conceivable way, without any scheme demonstrating weight-reduction superiority. Several major problems arise when the four food group scheme is used rigidly for meal planning and recommending diets. Many people suffer from food allergy and other adverse reactions to food and must not eat one or more of the four food groups. Others have religious, cultural, moral, esthetic, and economic reasons for not eating from one or other of the food groups. There is a general trend away from killing and eating animals, for example. Abstinence from meat may reflect a combination of moral, esthetic and ecological motives.

Milk and wheat disease are common health problems and abstinence from these foods makes four-food-group meal planning obsolete. The Core Program is designed to replace the four food group method of meal-planning. From an NP vantage point, food-proportion rules are programming precepts. The four food group rules are too general to be all that useful. Similarly CFP proportions are too general to construct diets that address individual needs. What about the different kinds of fats, carbohydrates, and proteins in different foods? What about the distinction between saturated fat, found in animal foods, and polyunsaturated fats, found in vegetable oils? What about different fatty acids and their cis or trans formations? What is the difference between sugar carbohydrate and complex vegetable carbohydrate or the different metabolic effects of sucrose, glucose, and fructose?

Carbohydrates

Carbohydrates (CHO) are sugar-base molecules of great diversity. Complex carbohydrates (CCHO), like starch, are found in plant foods everywhere. Starch is a polymer or long string of sugar molecules, just as a protein is a long string of amino acids. Starch-containing plants are the universal staple foods. The success of the Core Program depends on increasing vegetable carbohydrates to about 2/3 of daily caloric requirements. Rice, millet, potato, and maize have long been the major carbohydrate-supplying food plants, and, more recently, the cereal grains and their flours have dominated as staples, especially in the industrial nations.

Currently rice, wheat, and maize or corn are the world's most important staple foods. Vegetables are a major source of complex carbohydrates. In the US, about 15% of agricultural production is devoted to vegetable cultivation. High-starch vegetables tend to be roots or tubers like potatoes, yams, turnips, winter squash, carrots, and beets. Yams and sweet potatoes are important, high-caloric root vegetables. The green leafy vegetables are more chemically diverse and interesting foods, supplying less digestable carbohydrate, but more vitamins, minerals, and non-digestible fiber. The seeds of 30 or so common legume species are important vegetables, since they are cheap, available and high in protein and fatty acids. Soybeans are perhaps the most important legume, supplying carbohydrate as well as oil and protein. Beans, peas, lentils, and peanuts are the other common legumes.

Sugar

Sugar is a maligned, and misunderstood food component. The principal sugars are glucose and fructose. These are the simplest CHO molecules, known by their single ring structure as monosaccharides. **Glucose** is the **fuel** of all living things, supplying energy to all living cells, plant and animal. The creation of glucose begins in plants with the magic of photosynthesis. The sun's photons are the original energy source used by the chloroplasts of leaves to drive carbon, hydrogen, and oxygen atoms together to form glucose. Plants then use the newly synthesized glucose to fuel all their other synthetic processes, constructing tissues so that animals have food to eat. **Fructose** is the first cousin of glucose and occurs in fruit and corn syrup .

Sucrose is the sugar that is commonly called "sugar", often with negative connotations. Sucrose is the dominant sugar in most of our sweeteners, and appears in refined form as white table sugar. Brown sugars and molasses are cruder sugar products which contain the same sucrose in the presence of many other substances not yet removed. The preference for brown sugars, syrups, molasses, and honey, in place of refined white sugar is not based on any important biological information. White table sugar has the advantage of containing less extraneous molecules and contaminants. **Honey** is preferable only by taste and implication (visions of bees, flowers, summer days) and contains the same sugars, glucose and fructose. Honey also contains bees' wings, legs, poop, pollens, and other assorted hive contaminants, and may offer some allergic reactions to sensitive individuals. Honey also carries the spores of the botulinus bacteria, and should not be fed to infants, since the spores can germinate in their intestine producing the deadly botulinus toxin. I personally prefer honey by taste, implication, and a lingering identification with Winnie the Pooh.

Large carbohydrate molecules form the structure of plants, and to a lesser extent, animals. A carbohydrate polymer, or **polysaccharide**, is a string of sugar molecules linked together. The cell walls of plants are constructed of elaborate polysaccharides made from 12 basic sugars. **Cellulose** is the main structural carbohydrate, and is a polymer of glucose units, linked together to form a tough fiber. We lack digestive enzymes to break down cellulose, and miss some of the nutritive value of plants. Vegetarian ruminants utilize special stomachs which host bacterial populations that break down cellulose. **Starch** is the most obvious and most valuable polysaccharide. The starch molecule is tree-like, with branches of varying length. Starch digestion begins in the mouth with salivary amylase, and continues in the small intestine with pancreatic amylase. Short chains of glucoses are referred to as alpha-dextrin, maltotriose (3GL), and maltose (2GL). Glucoamylase breaks these short chains down to individual glucose molecules which are absorbed. Starch is our best fuel, supplying sustained-release glucose. There are several different types of **carbohydrate polymers** in fruit and vegetables that we are unable to digest. This material passes through the GIT as bulk **fiber**, undergoing modification and digestion by colon microorganisms. Several fibers have benevolent roles. The benefit seems to be the absorption or neutralization of the irritation or toxicity of other foods. Carbohydrate fiber contributes to the well-hydrated bulk of soft, easily-passed stools. Increased dietary fiber over a lifetime is associated with decreased incidence of bowel cancer and cardiovascular disease.

Proteins and Amino Acids

Food supplies the building materials to permit continuous cellular renewal and growth. Protein forms a major part of our **structure**. Most of our body protein is **recycled** and we do well by ingesting very little protein. About 3% of the total body protein is recycled every day (approximately 200 grams). In a healthy adult, net protein loss in a day may be as low as 2 grams. Dietary requirements for protein increase with activity, growth, and protein losses, especially following injury or during illness. The average American diet supplies 11-14% of total calories as protein, or 25-100 gms/day. Protein digestion and absorption are generally efficient. A minimum average protein intake is approximately **25 grams.** Since all amino acids contain a nitrogen atom (N), protein balance is synonymous with nitrogen balance. When nitrogen intake exceeds nitrogen loss, there is net protein synthesis. **Anabolism**, or tissue construction, prevails. When nitrogen losses exceed intake, protein tissue is being broken down and **catabolism** prevails. Loss of protein-tissues occurs with malnutrition, following surgery, injury, and chronic illness. Adequate intake of energy molecules, both carbohydrate and fats, is said to "spare protein", permitting a small protein intake to maintain positive nitrogen balance. In metabolic studies, the total amount of nitrogen intake is compared with the total excretion of nitrogen to assess protein balance. Excess amino acids may be converted to fuel.

When amino acids are "burned" as a fuel, **ammonia (NH_3]** is the waste product. Ammonia must be carried to the liver, converted to urea and excreted by the kidneys. One of the penalties of amino acid excess is ammonia excess, a potential cause of body malfunction following a high protein meal. The blood measurement of urea nitrogen (BUN) shows the balance between urea production by the liver and excretion by the kidneys. The BUN rises in kidney failure and serves as a measure of ammonia or nitrogen. In liver disease, reduced ability to synthesize urea leads to ammonia accumulation. Ammonia is neurotoxic and contributes to the syndrome of brain dysfunction in liver failure, hepatic encephalopathy.

Patients with reduced kidney or liver function are required to restrict protein, since their ability to handle the nitrogen waste of oxidized amino acids is limited. Fluctuating levels of ammonia influences brain cell function, and should be considered whenever brain function is abnormal. Some children are born with metabolic abnormalities in the handling of amino acids and ammonia. They often present with malfunctioning brains.

Essential Amino Acids (AAs)

Amino acids (AAs) are the alphabet characters of body proteins. Proteins are chains of amino acids linked together like beads on a necklace. The individual amino acids fall into two groups: the essential AAs, which must be ingested, and the non-essential AAs, which can be synthesized in the body and need not appear in the food. Nine amino acids are considered essential, while another 11 AAs can be synthesized from the essential amino acids. There are other amino acids which appear in nature and are not included in protein structure. These odd amino acids appear especially in plants, where they may have roles as insect deterrents. Non-nutrient amino acids can be toxic. Other non-nutrient amino acids, usually synthesized within may be useful as accessory nutrient;s taurine and carnitine are prime candidates.

Fat and Cholesterol

Dietary fats are a heterogeneous mixture consisting of about 93% triglycerides, 6% phospholipids and lesser amounts of sphingomyelins, glycolipids, cholesterol, and phytosterols. Fat is usually fully digested, with less than 5% remaining unabsorbed and excreted in the feces. If fat digestion is impaired by pancreatic enzyme deficiency, an oily diarrhea results, with foamy, floating stools (steatorrhea). Ingested fat mostly consists of triglycerides. The molecule, glycerol, acts like a rack to which three **fatty acids** (FA) attach. There are many different fatty acids, and their individual metabolic effects are not well-known. FA are chains of **carbon molecules** with the form -C-C-C-. If carbon atoms are joined by two of their available four bonds -C=C=C- the FA is described as "**polyunsaturated**" (PUFA). A single bond -C-C-C- is "saturated".

The double bond facilitates molecular re-arrangement in the body, and everyone has been told that -C=C=C- is better than -C-C-C-. There is, however, evidence that increased total fat is harmful, regardless of the bonding arrangements. Increased incidence of skin, breast, and colon cancer may be correlated with increased intake of PUFA. The exact nature of each fatty acid may be more of a specific determinant than its general biochemical properties. Vegetable oils, liquid at room temperature, tend to be unsaturated, and animal fats, solid at room temperature tend to be saturated. Margarines are made from vegetable oils by saturating the carbon bonds chemically, and this procedure robs the oil of its metabolic advantages. Another variable of fatty acid structure is that the double bonds may have one of two forms; **cis** and **trans**. Only the **cis** form functions normally in us and is the natural form. The processing of vegetable oils to produce margarine and other cooking fats increases the **trans** forms of the same fatty acids, an undesirable result. The altered fatty acids produced by margarine hydrogenation are potentially harmful, and probably should be avoided. One of the least desirable foods in a store is cheap margarine. Most margarines contain milk proteins (as whey) and are not suitable on the Core Program.

The disadvantage of unsaturated carbon bonds is that they are easily oxidized, and oxidized FA tend to be toxic. If vegetable oils are cooked at high temperature in the frying pan or deep fryer, oxidation occurs rapidly. This is the argument against fried foods. Slow fat oxidation underlies rancidity of fat. Most oils are preserved with anti-oxidants to prevent rancidity, and this appears to be a good idea. Fresh vegetable oils (PUFA) are desirable; if no preservatives are added, the oils should be stored under refrigeration. Light exposure increases fat oxidation, and can be reduced by brown or black bottles and dark-room storage. Careful manufacturers may supply sensitive oils in hydrogen-packed, black, sealed bottles and instruct you to store opened bottles in the fridge.

The only fat components that are truly essential are the fatty acids, **linoleic acid** and alpha-linoleic acid. Arachidonic acid is sometimes considered essential, but may be produced inside cells by the conversion of linoleic acid. Animal fats have been associated with several major diseases; atherosclerosis, which leads to heart attacks and strokes; cancers of the colon and breast; and obesity. Fat is energy dense, supplying **9 Kcal/gram.** Dietary fat surplus is stored as body fat, and high fat intakes are associated with obesity, except in Eskimos who continue to follow traditional patterns of sustained hard work in extreme cold weather. Current recommendations for fat intake are shrinking progressively from 35% of total calories to 20%. Typical American diets contain as much as 42% fat, an extravagant surplus. Our needs are supplied by 15-25 grams of fat per day, 1-2% of total calories for adults and 3% for infants. Fat intakes close to minimal need may be desirable, especially for those at risk of fat-related disease. The goal for a Core Diet level of fat intake is 14 % of daily calories, with 60-70% as polyunsaturated vegetable oil. **Safflower or sunflower** oils are chosen because of a high content of linoleic acid.

Cholesterol & Atherosclerosis

Cholesterol is a normal, useful body substance, from which we manufacture essential things, like steroid hormones. Blood (serum) cholesterol remains a chief predictor of coronary heart disease, and current recommendations set target goals of less than 200 mg% for blood levels. So-called "normal levels" range from 180-300 mg%, depending on age and sex. As discussed in chapter 2, atherosclerosis is most associated with increased blood levels of **low density lipoprotein (LDL).**

Circulating **LDL is a spherical packet** containing 1500 molecules of cholesterol attached to fatty acids and surrounded by an envelope of phospholipid. A single protein, attached to the LDL sphere like a handle, allows it to bind to **receptors (LDLR)** on the surfaces of cells. The protein handle, **apolipoprotein,** is essential for LDL clearing, and deficiencies in it lead to another type of "fat transport disorder". Circulating LDL is removed when the apolipoprotein binds to LDLR on cells, who then swallow it, and metabolically process its contents. Liver cells remove half the circulating LDL. A typical LDL sphere lasts 2-3 days in the blood stream. If LDL clearing is impaired, fat accumulates in the blood, making it thick and viscous like gravy. If a blood sample is allowed to sit for several hours, the cells drop to the bottom of the tube, and the normally clear, straw-colored serum stays on top. The serum with increased LDL looks milky and opaque, with fat droplets.

Some of the LDL in the blood stream makes its way into the **arterial wall** where it tends to lodge as an extracellular deposit. The arterial wall seems incapable of breaking down the LDL derived fat, and a progressive tumor develops in the arterial wall, growing outward to obstruct the flow of blood. Fat tends to accumulate in the arterial surface where blood flow is turbulent. Arteries branch like trees, and the first turbulent areas to develop fatty plaque are the points of bifurcation of the blood vessels. Once a fatty plaque pushes into the lumen of the artery, more turbulence develops, which promotes more fatty deposition.

Obviously, any deficiency of, or defect in, LDLR will reduce the ability of clearing blood LDL. Paradoxically, dietary fat reduces LDLR activity, so that the more you eat fat, the less you are able to clear LDL from your blood stream. A genetic disorder, familial hypercholesterolemia, arises when the LDLR is defective, and blood LDL cannot be cleared; accelerated atherosclerosis leads to heart attacks by the age of two years! One child with this disorder was given a transplanted liver which cleared the drastic hypercholesterolemia, as the lipoprotein receptors in the new liver began to function.

Another form of transport cholesterol, **high density lipoprotein, HDL,** is "good cholesterol". The ratio of HDL to LDL should be as high as possible. The Core Program is designed to lower fat and cholesterol intake. Sunflower and safflower oils are chosen because of their high intake of the essential fatty acid, linoleic acid; Olive oil has a high level of oleic acid. Both linoleic and oleic acid appear to lower levels of LDL and should have a protective effect against atherosclerosis.

Many articles have been written to recommend fish intake to prevent heart disease. Epidemiological evidence suggests that fish eaters suffer less cardiovascular disease. **Eicosapentenoic acid (EPA)** is given the major credit for this protective effect. EPA influences many aspects of our biochemistry, especially inflammatory mediator synthesis and fat metabolism. This is an omega-3 FA, mostly found in fish, especially salmon, and herring. A recent study of patients with elevated cholesterol and triglycerides showed 12% reduction in cholesterol, a 40% reduction of triglycerides, with a 5% rise in HDL on 20 capsules of MaxEPA per day. MaxEPA is a commercial preparation of marine lipids containing 180 mg of EPA, and 120 mg of docosahexaenoic acid (DHA) per capsule. Such a high dose may not be required for a long-term protective effect, since in epidemiological studies, the ingestion of fish a few days per week seems to protect against heart attacks. Salmon oil is high in EPA .

EPA looks useful in several directions, beyond the prevention of heart attacks and strokes. Pain-relieving, anti-inflammatory action has been demonstrated in arthritis, and migraine headaches. A recent study has shown that EPA is incorporated into immune cell membranes where it alters the immune-reacting behavior of the cells. EPA enriched cells release less leukotriene B4 which acts to recruit more cells to a site of inflammation. Less leukotriene B4 means less inflammation. EPA may be acting as a competitive inhibitor of arachidonic acid at 5-lipoxygenase sites. EPA at a dose of 10 1.0 gm capsules/day improved patients with atopic dermatitis or eczema. Eczematous skin has elevated levels of LB4. EPA may be desirable in patients with Multiple Sclerosis, which involves immune-mediated ("allergic") destruction of myelin. Myelin is a composite of fat molecules, with EPA acting as a structural component. The idea of using nutrients as biological response mediators is appealing.

Gamma-linoleic acid (GLA), is another fatty acid that has been marketed as a nutritional supplement. GLA is an omega-6 FA, derived from the oil of the evening primrose (Effamol) and from borage. GLA is a first cousin of LA, of course, and is usually synthesized in cells from LA. Three grams per day of primrose oil, containing both linoleic acid and GLA can reduce LDL cholesterol significantly, and may lower blood pressure. GLA has been used to treat women with premenstrual syndrome, and 3 gm/day can reduce breast pain, tenderness and nodularity in the fibrocystic breast syndrome. **Methylxanthines** in tea, coffee, chocolate and coke aggravate fibrocystic disease and should be removed from the diet of any woman with this disorder.

Alcohol ingestion reduces the production of GLA by blocking the liver enzyme, delta-6 desaturase. Supplements of GLA may helpful in the treatment of recovering alcoholics. GLA also helps atopic children with eczema, and may be a good adjunct to the hypoallergenic diets, which cure these children of their disease. GLA may also be added to the hypoallergenic diets used to treat both children and adults with affective disorders, especially moody, hyperactive children. [1]

Nutrient Intake Goals

The destination of all nutrients is the intracellular assembly lines which require all raw materials to be present simultaneously. Naive statements, like "Vitamin A is good for your vision", should be reserved for preschool nutritional instruction. This is like recommending "rubber" to Ford Motor Company as "good for their production line". It is much more satisfying to think of the trillions of biosynthetic events per hour which keep you going and to develop a good feeling for the molecular flow supplying raw material and catalytic substances to this busy living machinery. The NP idea is to establish a range of nutrient intakes as a guideline for adjusting food selection and designing supplement programs. The baseline values are the **Recommended Daily Allowances (RDA)**. The RDA is an evolving committee-style guesstimate of adequate nutrient intake. The data supporting the committee decisions has been the best available, but is not yet adequate for definitive nutrient recommendations.[2] The RDA committee[3] prefaced their recommendations:

> "RDA are recommendations for the average daily amounts of nutrients that population groups should consume over a period of time. RDA should not be confused with requirements for specific individuals. Differences in the nutrient requirements of individuals are ordinarily unknown...the RDA values are recommendations established for healthy populations. Special needs for nutrients arising from such problems as premature birth, inherited metabolic disorders, infections, chronic disease, and the use of medications require special dietary and therapeutic measures. These conditions are not covered by RDA."

Well-formulated diets with total calories in excess of 3000 Kcal per day tend to supply all Vitamins and minerals at RDA levels and higher. As the total caloric intake drops, nutrient deficiencies begin to appear, although the overall effect of the food choices may be quite positive. One of the dogmas of standard dietetics is that all nutrients should be obtained from food. The recommendation to increase food intake sufficient to achieve RDA levels of nutrients may be counter-productive. The prescription of a reasonable nutrient supplement permits food selection, free of this nutrient-deficiency concern. Proper supplementation is a safe, cost-effective, intelligent way to assure optimal nutrient intake without compromising safe food choices.

Dieticians follow the four food-group rules and the RDA guidebook in recommending diets. Clients are advised to eat food from the traditional four food groups to achieve nutrient concentrations up to the RDA levels. The RDA nutrient values are based on a low-end estimate, the amount of the nutrient which prevents deficiency disease. RDA has some allowances for error and individual variation, but perhaps misses the advantages available by increasing intake of selected nutrients. If, for example, you were convinced that the data at hand suggested that 20 mg of Vitamin C per day would prevent scurvy, you would recommend that everyone ingest at least 40 mg per day to be on the safe side. Later, you may learn that Vitamin C is destroyed by storage and cooking, and that food estimates of Vitamin C content may mislead your trusting clients. You raise the RDA to account for food variation to 60 mg per day. Then you realize that various factors, such as smoking and drugs, interfere with the metabolism of Vitamin C and you adjust upwards to 100-200 mg/day for individuals at risk. Then Linus Pauling suggests important benefits from much higher doses, 1000-5000 mg per day. You are skeptical, but eventually test the idea with disappointing, but not entirely negative, results. Norman Cousins cures himself with high doses of intravenous Vitamin C and funny videos and becomes a professor at UCLA. Others advocate new reasons for higher doses, like the antioxidant effect of Vitamin C or the stomach cancer protective effect. Still others boldly treat cancer or AIDS patients with huge intravenous doses of Vitamin C, up to 100,000 mg per day! Now we are far from the RDA and are only reassured by the realization that even huge doses of Vitamin C are well tolerated. The range of actual "recommended" use of Vitamin C is 60-100,000 mg/day! Whose advice are you going to follow?

One of the most persuasive arguments for the use of extra Vitamin C over a lifetime is its ability to scavenge **free oxygen radicals.** Cellular combustion can be compared to a stove, which needs adequate protection to do its job without burning the house down. As we burn fuel in our cells, some oxygen atoms are given an extra electron and become the radical, O_2^-. Oxygen will also combine with hydrogen in the free hydroxyl radical -OH or in the highly reactive hydrogen peroxide molecule, H_2O_2. If O_2^- floats free of the energy engines, it may interact vigorously with other molecules. Cell membranes are vulnerable to O_2^- injury; damaged membranes disturb the function of the entire cell. Extra O_2^- reacting with DNA can make the code sticky and can cause mistakes in code reading or replication, resulting in cell mutation. The cumulative damage of trillions of random O_2^- encounters with critical molecules over many years contributes to accelerated aging and cellular dysfunction, like cancer. Cells contain oxygen detoxification enzymes: peroxidases, superoxide dismutase, and catalases. Several molecules combine harmlessly with O_2^- and are referred to as "antioxidants". Vitamin C is the cheapest, safest, and best antioxidant in town. If you can raise the amount of Vitamin C in cells, you may soak up enough O_2^- to make a long-term difference. The effect of Vitamin C is enhanced if you present two other nutrient antioxidants alongside, Vitamin E and selenium. You cannot take superoxide dismutase by mouth and expect benefit, since it will not arrive at the intracellular locations where it is needed. Intravenous injection of the enzyme may, however, be an effective treatment of inflammatory disorders.

Active Transport of Nutrients

The RDA of several nutrients may not be sufficient if the mechanism of absorption is impaired. Many nutrients are selectively and carefully carried across the GIT wall by enzyme systems. This active transport is the input regulator to body space. Vitamin B_{12}, for example, requires a transport molecule, called intrinsic factor, before it can be actively transported across the small bowel wall. If you lack intrinsic factor, even large amounts of Vitamin B_{12} in your diet will not help you avoid pernicious anemia, the overt B_{12} deficiency disease. Without intrinsic factor, Vitamin B_{12} shots are needed to get the Vitamin inside. Sodium, potassium, iron, and calcium are all actively transported minerals. Amino acids and fatty acids are also actively transported.

An important principle of NP is that **each person has an individual best-fit.** The Core Program relies on a well-tested, thoughtful approach to diet re-design. Once an adequate intake of vegetable foods, rice, poultry, and fish is established, adequate, if not superior, nutrition is available. The intake goal is to achieve nutrient levels within an **optimal range.** In conventional dietetic theory all nutrients are best delivered in food. In practice, it is seldom possible to balance all nutrient levels within the optimal range by manipulating food choices alone. The optimal range for each nutrient is a best-guess estimate. An optimal range allows enough room to accommodate the biochemical variability of individuals and the upper values permit "therapeutic" levels of the nutrients without risking toxicity. To resolve food-related disease, it is often best to offer nutrients in their pure and elemental form. Indeed, from the NP point of view, accurate body programming is most readily achieved by crystalline-pure nutrients, not food. An elemental nutrient formula (ENF), custom-formulated, will be the optimal nutrition of the future for many people.

---

[1] Horrobin D F. Clinical Uses of Fatty Acids. 1982.Eden Press Inc.

[2]Hegsted DM. Jour Nutrition 1986;116:478–481.

[3]Food and Nutrition Board, National Research Council. Recommended dietary allowances. 9th edition. Washington, DC: National Academy of Sciences, 1980

Chapter 15 Food Allergy and Immunology

In Section 1, a wide array of disturbances was attributed to food allergy and the mechanisms of food allergy were introduced. In this chapter we will further develop the idea of food allergy. Our initial assumption is that many patterns of illness can be explained if we recognize that ingested foods interact complexly with the body and can trigger a variety of immune responses in any part of the body. The word **allergy** refers to any immune-mediated disease. We recognize at least **four different mechanisms** that produce immune injury. Combinations of these defense-injury sequences increase the variety and complexity of allergic reactions.

Some physicians limit their definition of allergy to a subset of immune-mediated disease - the immediate or Type 1 reactions. The word **hypersensitivity** has been used in the past to describe immune responses which cause symptoms and do damage. If you use **allergy** in its original sense, then all immune-mediated disease is allergy. Rheumatoid arthritis, multiple sclerosis, lupus erythematosis - all could be referred to as "allergy" since they are immune-mediated diseases. The use of the word "allergy is more than a semantic choice. The idea of allergy is useful when we enquiry into the nature and mechanism of these diseases, since allergy implies reactivity, and reactivity means there is something to react to. Usually, the cause of these terribly destructive immune-mediated diseases are listed as "autoimmune" or even idiopathic - cause unknown. If we think "autoimmune", then we stop looking for the outside cause. If we think "allergy" we continue to search for immune reaction triggers in the food, air and water. When you see antihistamine advertisements for "allergy", the reference is to hay fever and the term "allergy" is used in the narrow sense of immediate hypersensitivity. Type 1 hypersensitivity is mediated by a specific antibody type, IgE, and specific populations of immune cells, basophils and mast cells. The limitation of the term "allergy" to Type I hypersensitivity may suit a drug company's advertising strategy or a physicians' pattern of medical practice, but is a major error to confuse the narrow self-interest of the company or the physician with the disease phenomena that exist in the real world. WIRGO is quite another story.

Food allergy involves the broadest set of immune reactions. Immune responses to food materials are diverse and capable of producing many symptoms and many diseases. The idea of food allergy is to modern disease concepts as the idea of infection was to disease concepts in the 19th century.

When you do not know about food allergy you are surrounded by mysterious diseases. When we know about food allergy, a lot of common illness patterns begin to make sense.

Food allergy can be understood as a **multisystem disorder** caused by the **distribution** of "wrong-stuff" throughout the body. Immune responses to food antigens typically involve a symptom complex. The multi-symptom process begins to make sense when one considers the progression of events from GIT to blood stream to mediator release to whole-body response to long-term consequences of inflammatory tissue events, which, once set in motion, tend to persevere. **Target tissues** tend to localize or concentrate food antigens and suffer damage from the immune responses to them.

The symptoms may be limited to GIT; eg. the pain and diarrhea, associated with gastrointestinal allergy. The lungs are the major target organ in food-induced asthma, the skin in atopic dermatitis, and the joints are target organs in food allergic arthritis. Muscles and connective tissue react with pain, stiffness, and swelling which, along with fatigue, are among the most common food allergy symptoms. The brain is the target organ when fatigue and somnolence occurs and whenever disorganized, disturbed thinking, feeling, remembering and behaving occur. As we have so often repeated in this book, the psyche is completely vulnerable to the biological mechanisms involved in food allergy; mental-emotional disturbances are a consequence of food allergy, not a cause of it!

The distribution and timing of immune responses following meals may be appreciated by thinking of the flow and distribution of food materials in the body. Obviously, every cell needs nutrients delivered everyday and food is the origin of these nutrients. Wrong materials are also distributed to every cell in the body and we can expect a bewildering array of adverse effects. Since there are multiple effects following ingestion of food, no explanation of adverse reactions, based on one mechanism alone, will ever account for the multiplicity of effects reported and observed. Our best theories assume complex interactions; simultaneous immunologic, physiological and biochemical mechanisms.

We further assume that everyone has some adverse effects from eating food, especially in a modern world with new strange eating habits and many problems built into the food supply. All biology is understood as a distribution of common characteristics, so that in any population, the adverse effects from food will range from a little bit to a lot. People, who get very sick from their food supply, are hypersensitive with respect to someone who claims: "I have iron stomach... never sick a day". Hypersensitive people may react to food, air, drugs, smell, people, ideas, feelings in an exaggerated manner. Mental and emotional symptoms arise from the same biological mechanisms that produce physical symptoms. When hypersensitive people get conspicuously ill, the rest of us are soon to follow.

The idea of "boosting your the immune system" has become popular. Odd diets, herbs, gland extracts, and vitamin-mineral products are promoted to enhance your immune system". From the allergy, immune-mediated disease, point-of-view, we often want less immune response. Allergic reactions involve **increased, damaging immune responses.** If the immune system is working overtime to defend against materials arriving in the body in air, water and food, there is a penalty to pay. When patients report recurrent colds and flus or chronic fatigue, they often to refer to their "depressed immunity" but, actually, they often have food allergy or hypersensitivity. The solution is stop the intake of allergenic foods and wait for the immune activity to subside. If the allergic disease is severe we use immune-suppressant drugs especially corticosteroids (cortisone, prednisone) or drugs such as cyclosporin (often use after transplant procedures) to save patients from immune injury!

Any molecule which excites an immune response is called an **Antigen.** Antigens can be constructed of smaller molecules attached to proteins. Many drugs, food additives, and food contaminants are small molecules which enter the body through GIT and are transported in the blood, attached to carrier proteins. These improvised antigens are numerous and difficult to track.

The **timing** of allergic responses cannot be predicted accurately, but can be followed by careful recording of symptoms, emerging in response to food challenges. A burst of symptoms, emerging over hours or days, can be explained if we assume that material from food has triggered GIT responses and antigens have entered the bloodstream from GIT, triggering a variety of alarm and defense procedures

A plausible theory of food allergy must recognize that digestion in GIT determines how food will affect us. The theory must also recognize that the surface of GIT is an immune sensing device that immunizes us to materials flowing through it. If digestion and absorption of nutrients proceeds in an ideal fashion, all may be well. But if GIT reacts to food materials and malfunctions, we are in trouble. But what kind of trouble? One major concern is that GIT may be excessively permeable, and may "leak". The wrong molecules may enter internal body space, not just normal, nice nutrients.

Food allergy can be understood as a variety of consequences following this admission of "wrong stuff" into the body. We have chosen the formal term **"Inappropriate Molecular Entry"** (IME) to describe the admission of antigenic food molecules into the body. IME can initiate complicated patterns of **Immune Mediated Disease** (IMD). Immune defense plays a major role in screening the traffic of food molecules through the gastrointestinal tract (GIT) and, later, in body spaces.

Immune defense must recognize the "wrong stuff" that enters appropriately or leaks through GIT inappropriately. Immune defense, like military defense, has both a cost and a destructive aspect.

No diagnostic tests completely define the body's dysfunctional response to food. Spot sampling, so typical of clinical medicine, is seldom helpful in discovering what is wrong. Skin tests, best used to diagnose airborne allergens which cause hay fever, will not reveal the more complex forms of food allergy. A distinction between immediate, obvious allergic reactions and delayed, less obvious, chronic immune injury is useful.

Immune Networks

We refer to the "immune system" although this is not an appropriate description of WIRGO, since immune function tends to be scattered and chaotic. The immune response is distributed through several body systems and involves several **migratory populations of cells**. A more meaningful description might be **immune networks** (IN) which are collections of different, diverse, often unstable, components. INs tend to produce characteristic responses and tend to be essential for our survival. Activation of INs is not always welcome. More people are sick with and die of increased immune response than deficient immune response.

When the term **"system"** is used we may get the wrong image of a well-defined, orderly device, perhaps similar to a new car or a computer with an instruction manual. A more appropriate analogy might be bee or ant colonies; there is al lot of swarming, moving about, with different job descriptions in the hive and a **meta order** achieved by the collective behavior of many individuals. The overall activity of the hive or colony decides what the society or system looks like.

We are not quite the coherent entity that we like to think we are. We are really a community of cells in prodigious array. Some of our cells stay in place and do more or less predictable things. Immune cells tend to wander around and, like bees, forage in our various body parts looking for items of interest. They have the property of getting excited, recruiting their peers and attacking interlopers. When you try to picture immune responses think first of swarms of bees and stingers - this is the "system". The second analogy that helps visualize immune responses is that immune activity resembles the interests and organization of the military. Once engaged, chaos is more a property of these cell networks than is orderliness.

In Chapter 7, we established the relationship of immune networks and our nervous system. Recall that the **information and control** properties of the immune system are analogues of brain function, with the four major functions of sentience: **Sensing, Deciding, Acting, Remembering.** There is significant overlap of immune regulation with the **chemical senses** (taste and smell), and appetite control in the brain. Brain information processing is more detailed and complex than IN information processing by several orders of magnitude. These systems overlap at the most primitive, basic levels of body control.

Immune networks (INs) tend to tolerate antigens which appear regularly. Tolerance is most likely to occur with antigens presented orally. The eruption of symptoms of food allergy may represent the loss of tolerance, rather than new or different sensitivities. Many patients do not understand how foods eaten routinely over many years can produce disease; how can these reliable foods now make me ill? But, nothing really stays the same, especially body functions and food quality. The adaptive dysfunctional state, described in chapter 1, may permit bad habits to continue for years, but sooner or later, decompensation occurs. Loss of tolerance is one interpretation of worsening trends. Increasing sensitivity is another, complementary interpretation.

Three Immune Network Compartments

There is a mobile **blood immune network (BIN)** that originates in the bone marrow, and circulates in the blood stream. This division of the immune network has several distinct cell populations and receives a lot of attention in transplant programs. BIN is specially vulnerable to carcinogens - uncontrolled overgrowth of these cell populations is leukemia. Another division is the **lymphatic immune network** (LIN with both stationary structures like hives (nodes) and migratory populations of lymphocytes that move around looking for antigens as bees look for pollen. The thymus gland is the master controller of LIN and a large population of lymphocytes are said to be "thymus-dependent" and a re referred to as T-cells. The third immune division is the **tissue immune network (TIN),** mobile populations of cells that move through our tissues. Mast cells are important TIN cells in the allergy business.

These networks are prodigious; trillions of cells are involved; with rapid turnover; millions of antibody types are produced as defensive weapons by B-lymphocytes. Hundreds of different chemical messengers are used in communications among IN cells and between the IN and the rest of the body. Cells move from one IN compartment to another, transforming in shape and function. The most likely movement is from blood to tissue spaces; BIN becomes TIN.

Some cells identify the characteristic **molecular shape of an antigen** and respond by proliferation. A virus, for example, will have protein identifiers stuck to its capsule which mark it, much like an **ID badge.** Several cell populations will emerge when the virus is present to identify and combat it. One cell group manufactures antibody, a protein specific to one antigen. Molecules in the food supply, especially proteins, act similarly, as antigens. Food additives and contaminants may increase the probability of allergic reactions to food. Immune cells do not know the difference between viral, bacterial or food antigens. We expect, and regularly observe, similar immune reactions to both antigen sources!

Immune Networks as Defense

The principle function of INs is defense against infection and invasion of the body by foreign molecules. We can also think of INs as military organizations with many divisions and complicated strategies. Immune defense intends to stop infection and otherwise protect us from invasion by foreign substances. We think of certain immune cells as **sensors** which, like **alarms,** trigger emergency responses in the presence of antigens. Other cells are **effectors** and carry out defensive actions, once activated. Some cells are both sensors and effectors. Other cells are **modulators** and regulate the reactivity of sensor and effector cells. These cells **communicate** with each other via a set of chemical messages which are received by receptors on the cell surface. Immune cell populations are large and dispersed so that messages are of a very general nature and reach millions to billions of cells during any given event. Some messages cause cell populations to migrate, other messages trigger rapid proliferation of cells, and/or change the appearance and behavior of cells during an activation sequence.

The general impact of these chemical messages is to amplify a small triggering event into a large, prolonged response. We used to call this the "Philadelphia Effect" after Philadelphia police burned down several city blocks by using a smoke bomb to flush out some alleged terrorists from one apartment. We now call this the **"Bush Effect"** after President George Bush, who amplified a relatively minor world event into a major, international, military crisis.

If the planet is thought of as an organism, you can make interesting analogies with immune events. Awful things occur on the planet every day with prodigious loss of human life, cruelty, senseless killing, hunger, famine, poverty - a seemingly endless need for intervention and control. Tolerance, in planet terms, really means that political-military defense is restrained and often ignores atrocities, despite tremendous need. Until, one day, a critical sensor (Bush) encounters an antigen (Hussein) and triggers an immune cascade and we have Persian Gulf anaphylaxis.

Allergy attacks are similar; a person may be doing all sorts of terrible things to his body over many years until one day, apparently out-of-the-blue, he drops dead of anaphylaxis ("a heart attack"). Perhaps a spokesperson for the IN would claim: "We had to draw the line somewhere." If a reactive body (country) makes it through the initial conflagration, a chronic inflammatory state may set-in; this is the cell-mediated immune response.

Chemical communications involve immune mediators which are responsible for causing the symptoms of an allergic response. Mediators produce events such as flushing, fever, itching, swelling, pain, coughing, wheezing, vomiting and diarrhea. The effect of mediators depends on where they are released and how they are distributed. Obviously a mediator released in the blood circulates throughout the body in a matter of seconds; mediators released in tissues may remain localized. The effect of mediators released in tissues also depends on how important that tissue is and how disruptive the immune event is. A hive appearing in the skin is a minor annoyance; a similar event in the retina of the eye may result in loss of vision.

Immune events are not orderly, but probably have the chaotic appearance of guerilla warfare, more than the orderly chaos of a football game. Allergy or injury is the flip-side of defense. You cannot have defensive immunity without risking injury from it. Within the TIN are populations of cells which lurk under every body surface exposed to the environment: skin, respiratory tract, gastrointestinal tract, and genitourinary tract. **Surface defense** features the Type I or immediate hypersensitivity response. This is a property of mast cells, often using IgE antibodies as sensors. Immune cells are also distributed in LIN, in the organs of the lymphatic system, which includes lymph nodes, tonsils, liver, and spleen. The immune network in the bloodstream, BIN, is highly reactive and occasionally mounts life-threatening anaphylaxis reactions and may involve other dangerous features, such as cell destruction and/or clotting. Blood defense is designed to counter life-threats such as infection and injury. Immune cells and molecular weapons are delivered by the blood to any tissue that is threatened. Special relationships between BIN cells and the cells lining the surface of blood vessels give BIN cells access to any tissue space.

Of all the organs of the body, the brain offers the least access to itself. The **blood brain barrier** is a property of the blood vessel linings in the brain that control the molecular and cellular input to the brain. The brain has a limited TIN; if frequent immune skirmishes occurred in the brain as they do, for example in the skin, none of us would remain mentally intact. **Multiple Sclerosis** is a terrible disease that results from **lymphocytes** attacking the **myelin** insulation in the nervous system circuits; this probability involves cell populations which move from LIN to BIN to TIN. We think food allergy could cause Multiple Sclerosis if lymphocytes, sensitized to food antigens and activated in GIT, moved through the blood and gain access to brain through a defective blood brain barrier. These food-activated lymphocytes would recognize a component of myelin as their own antigen and attack. The food antigen may coincidentally resemble myelin antigen, a case of molecular mimicry. Or the food antigen may be myelin basic protein or similar molecule that you ate; the myelin in meat resembles your own myelin. Whenever myelin is stripped from nerve circuits, information flow is interrupted; numbness, paralysis, loss of vision are typical consequences.

Lymphocytic attacks on myelin occur sporadically and major events tend to be infrequent; this is an **avalanche effect** - a number conditions must be aligned before the damage occurs. In tracking the progress of immune events in M.S. it is therefore important to pay attention to minor symptoms which are occurring more often than major events. If minor symptoms increase (like warnings of a major earthquake), precautions can increase, including food control and immune-suppression treatment with, for example, prednisone. As soon as an acute attack begins, we suggest going on an ENF and taking a large dose of prednisone in an effort to get the immune attack to stop. If you wait too many hours the damage is done and now it will take months to repair.

The **surface of blood vessel walls interacts** in dramatic ways with immune cells. If blood vessels are thought of as controlled access highways, and immune cells as emergency vehicles, then immune defence procedures must involve opening vessel walls to immune cell traffic. A common IN event is the flow of fluid and cells into tissue spaces; the swelling aspect of inflammatory reactions. Blood vessel wall events may injure the blood vessel and trigger clotting. Platelets in the blood are responsible for initiating clotting and may be activated by immune mediators especially platelet activating factor, known to play an important role in asthma. Activated platelets quickly manufacture a prostaglandin, thromboxane, a potent constrictor of blood vessels which can trigger the clotting mechanism. ASA (aspirin) is effective in blocking thromboxane production even at a low dose of one tablet a day, and has been recommended in the prevention of heart attacks and stroke. The possible significance of food allergic events inside blood vessels has already been mentioned.

The IN cells who produce antibodies are called **B-lymphocytes** in BIN and **plasma cells** when the move into tissues. Antibodies are proteins which identify antigens, specific foreign molecules or cell-surface markers. Other immune cells directly attack foreign cells or infecting organisms, removing them from the body space. Improperly labelled cells, as in tissue transplanted into a body, will be rejected and destroyed. Transplant surgery is made possible by matching donor and recipient as closely as possible for the same cell labels, known as **histocompatibility antigens.**

Imagine (but do not do) an experiment: make a small incision in the skin of your arm and place a few fibers of meat (eg.scraping from the surface of a steak) in the incision; tape the incision closed and cover with a protective dressing; observe at daily intervals. The meat fibers include muscle cell components from an animal whose tissue is foreign to yours. Many of these cell components will act as antigens. Immune cells will swarm around the foreign cells and, within 48 hours, local inflammation will set in. The small wound will swell and fester. The typical signs of inflammation, redness, swelling, pain, heat will persist for many days, leaving a scarred lump behind as a permanent reminder of the event. This experiment would illustrate the transplant rejection reaction. Similar zones of inflammation can be set up in your tissues by meat-fiber antigens arriving via an internal route. Food allergy can trigger events in target organs that resemble transplant rejection!

LIN or the "Lymphatic System"

LIN tissues have always been called the **Lymphatic System.** Everyone has had the experience of lymph nodes swelling during the course of a viral or bacterial infection. **Tonsils** are part of the lymphatic defense system and are naturally enlarged, particularly in children who are often busy fighting threatened infections, making new antibodies, and accumulating resistance or immunity. **Lymph** is a watery fluid that washes through all our tissues, passes through **lymph node** filters, and eventually returns to the blood stream. Lymph is' therefore' a second fluid circulation through the body; lymphocytes wander through the lymph spaces in the body, rest and proliferate in lymph nodes. One of the typical signs of food allergy is enlarged tonsils and swollen lymph nodes in the neck. If you have an infected finger and observe a red streak going up your arm, you are seeing a lymph channel, marked by the release of inflammatory mediators. The streak reminds us that pathogenic bacteria can also travel along lymph channels and spread rapidly; if immune defense does not stop them, then it is usually a choice between antibiotics and death.

Humoral Immunity: Antibodies and Mediators

The immune system has a cell-defense strategy and a molecular weapon system. **Antibodies are proteins** made to fit specific molecular shapes, or antigens. We can think of an antibody as a **connector** which links a foreign antigen with cells that deal with alien substances. One end of the antibody connects with the foreign antigens. The other end connects with immune cells which then specifically deal with that antigen. Other sites on the antibody can trigger a molecular weapon system, called complement. **Complement** is actually a series of proteins that change rapidly in a chain reaction, once triggered.

Complement products have numerous, powerful body actions, including cell damage. Some very nasty food and drug allergic reactions occur by antigen-antibody combinations triggering the complement cascade. Complement can be triggered directly by drugs, bacteria, and food materials.

Anaphylaxis, the dramatic, life-threatening, allergic reaction, is mediated in part by complement products. We think that complement activation is a major player in food allergy; the worst afflicted patients are probably "chewing-up complement" every day. Some would argue that direct complement activation is not "true allergy" and use ridiculous terms such as "pseudo-allergy". Our patients who are told they have "pseudoallergy", leave to the "pseudodoctor" who generally is no help at all and find a real doctor who can help them avoid the complement explosion.

The Cells of Immune Networks

Immune cell populations are diverse. BIN cells are collectively referred to as white blood cells. **White blood cells** (WBC) are routinely counted and recognized on stained blood smears, one the most common medical lab tests done all over the world. The different WBC groups include lymphocytes, neutrophils, eosinophils, basophils, and monocytes. These cells are made in the **bone marrow** and the **lymphatic tissues** (lymph nodes, thymus, spleen, and gut-associated lymphatic tissue). A diverse population of very important cells present antigens to other immune cells, initiating immune responses. These **antigen-presenting** cells are found, found for example, on the surface of blood vessel, especially in the liver and spleen, acting as monitors and filters of the blood stream. In tissues these cells are called **macrophages**.

Lymphocytes are the cells which recognize antigens presented by macrophages, proliferate after contact with antigens, attack antigen-labelled cells, and manufacture antibodies. These cells belong to many different functional groups which interact in a complex way, resembling a large policing organization. Some **T-Lymphocytes** (Killer cells or K-cells) act directly to attack cells, identified by specific antigen, and are responsible for cell-mediated delayed immune-injury. Some T-lymphocytes act as controllers of the antibody-producing cells, the **B-Lymphocytes**. Controller T-cells fall into groups which remember how to respond (Memory cells) and other groups which enhance immune response (Helper cells). B-lymphocytes are transformed to make antibodies to specific antigens. B-lymphocytes are activated by helper T-lymphocytes via chemical mediators, the interleukins.

Tolerance to food is achieved by some pattern of signals which turn off responses to regularly appearing antigens. Immunologists have postulated an opposing group of suppressor T-cells which would control and perhaps stop immune responses; we still do not know if these cells really exist. We do know that the system works by delicate checks and balances, and is prone to error. People with high levels of food reactivity probably have defective tolerance mechanisms or super-effective activation responses.

Most immune cells live and die in a resting state. **Activation** of cells can be specific, by antigens which alert only cells armed with specific antibody; or, activation can be non-specific with whole populations of cells turned-on by a super-antigen or overabundance of cell-stimulating mediators, like **interleukin 2**.Patients often report a sudden **onset of hypersensitivity** after an acute illness or injury; this always suggests non-specific activation of immune cells. The non-specific stimulus might be a bacterial or viral infection, a drug-induced allergic event, childbirth, surgery, or exposure to an environmental toxin.

Non-specific hypersensitivity is often expressed as food allergy with very limited food tolerance, even complete loss of tolerance to foods. Many patients in this predicament report reactions to numerous foods and airborne antigens and often need radical changes in diet, and environment to get better. The hypersensitivity might last a few weeks to several years. Often diet revision, air quality control and immune-suppressant drugs are all needed to control runaway hypersensitivity. Prednisone, cimetadine, sodium cromoglycate and ketotifen are sometimes useful drugs to reduce this hypersensitivity.

Different Patterns of Allergy

The clinical practice of "Allergy" as a specialty has tended to restrict the definition of allergy to one specific pattern of immune reactivity, described as **"Atopy"** by Coca and Cooke in 1925.[1] The term "atopy" simply meant **"strange disease"**. Allergists noticed connections among the "'strange diseases" including hay fever (seasonal allergic rhinitis and conjunctivitis), asthma, eczema, and urticaria (hives) in the atopic group. The original definition of the term "atopy" could still apply to the ever expanding list of immune-mediated and ill-defined "strange diseases" which plague us at the end of this century of extravagant biological misadventures.

Study of atopic hypersensitivity revealed a common immune mechanism which further confirmed the allegiance of many allergists to atopy, with the exclusion of other allergic diseases from their field of interest. It was found that a single antibody species, IgE or "reaginic antibody", was responsible for at least some atopic problems. Immediate and obvious allergic reactions occur an allergen meets a reactive cell populations under the surface of the skin, respiratory, gastrointestinal and genitourinary tracts. For example, an inhaled allergen (antigen), grass pollen, meets antibody-coated mast cells waiting in the mucosal surface of the nose, and a typical hay fever attack with sneezing, itching, and nose congestion results. A similar reaction in the throat produces soreness, mucus flow, swelling, and difficulty in swallowing and breathing (pharyngitis, laryngitis). The same reaction in the lungs produces cough, mucus obstruction to airflow, and asthmatic wheezing (bronchitis, asthmatic bronchitis).

Type 1 Allergy and Mast Cells

The mast cell is an immune cell filled with powerful mediators which are released if an antigen reacts with IgE antibodies coating the cell's surface. When the mast cell is triggered, it releases packets of chemical mediators which cause the allergic symptoms. The inherited tendency to make excessive amounts of IgE antibody is one the characteristics of atopic individuals. A convenient correlation between nose-reactive IgE and skin-reactive IgE was discovered. By introducing tiny amounts of suspected antigens into the skin, a local wheal and flare reaction, like a mosquito bite, is produced, if reactive IgE is present on skin mast cells. The association of hay fever, asthma, and skin tests with allergy practice was further confirmed by the relative success of "allergy shots". These shots came to characterize the allergist's office, and other aspects of allergy practice often were neglected.

Allergy shots, or desensitization, are immunological treatments or "Immunotherapy". The immune response to any reactive substance can be modified by giving repeated challenges of the reactive substances. Allergy shots for hay fever start with a serum containing the antigens which caused positive skin responses. The antigens are then administered in increasing concentrations by regular injections under the skin. It remains unclear how the shots work. One response to the injected antigen is the production of a second antibody population of the IgG class. These IgG antibodies are thought to compete with IgE antibodies, "blocking" the allergic response. It is also possible that the antigen injections stimulate suppressor T-cells or inhibit helper T-cells and reduce production of IgE.

Allergy shots have limited therapeutic application. The hay fever sufferer and some asthmatics with specific inhalant reactions to grass pollens do well with desensitization.[2] Immunotherapy also protects patients who have had anaphylactic reactions to bee and wasp stings. Patients with complex reactivity, food reactions, and drug reactions do not do well with allergy shots, and the shots are not usually recommended. There are dangers with allergy shots, including life-threatening anaphylaxis, delayed immune responses associated with generalized symptoms, and, rarely, a grave illness like polyarteritis nodosa. Indeed, the delayed reactions to allergy shots are typical of the immune-mediated disease process which is characteristic of food allergy. **It is our policy to avoid allergy shots in patients who have food allergy and other forms of delayed immune responses.**

Neutralization is another immunotherapy technique of repeated injection of antigen at different concentrations. The idea is that if one concentration of antigen will trigger a reaction, another weaker injection will "neutralize" it. While this mysterious method refers to a well-known immunological idea that immune cells do respond differently to different concentrations of antigens. These dose-response characteristic of immune cells have been observed in laboratory experiments with cell cultures responding to one antigen at a time. It is unlikely that neutralization method has a practical application. We consume kilogram quantities of food materials daily with thousands of potential antigens coursing through our body; INs are responding, often in a chaotic manner to numerous events. Even if single-antigen neutralization worked in controlled circumstances, (and many allergists doubt that it does work) there is too much (chaos) happening in our food-consuming lives for this technique to offer practical relief to suffering patients.

The reason for the definition of "allergy" to shrink toward a narrowly-defined clinical practice probably was the skin test. If anything distinguished an allergist from his /her colleagues, it was the passion for skin tests. By a practical evolution of allergy practice, those clinical problems which were diagnosable by skin reactions became the special property of allergists. Allergy therapy became synonymous with the desensitization (immunotherapy) injections.

Immediate-Reacting Food Allergens

For some time, it has been appreciated that food allergy operates in a more complex and mysterious way than inhaled allergy. Although skin tests were used to test for food sensitivity, many allergists also prescribed various kinds of allergy diets on clinical grounds with satisfactory results. Allergists generally appreciated that allergy shots containing food antigens were not helpful. Nevertheless, the IgE model was the easiest route to follow in the study of food allergy. This model encourages us to search for specific food allergens and to trace the occurrence of similar allergic substances in related foods. An allergic reaction to peanuts, for example, suggests that the peanut protein sensitizer may appear in related legumes like peas or soybeans. This "cross-reactivity" has been noted for several food groups. The study of food antigens or allergens has focused on the special antigens which produce immediate allergic reactions. A profile of antigenic proteins suggests that

glycoproteins of a certain size and weight are common allergens. These proteins can be isolated from foods and are used to skin test sensitive individuals. Specific protein antigens have been characterized from a variety of foods, particularly cow's milk, eggs, soybeans, peanuts, fish, crustaceans, wheat, oats, corn, rice, citrus, and some other foods. Laboratory studies of the interaction of these specific proteins and antibodies present in the blood of sensitive individuals have confirmed the immediate hypersensitivity model of allergy as a reaction between specific proteins and specific IgE antibodies. This model of allergy is immensely satisfying to researchers, because of its simplicity and the ease of testing for sensitization; but, it selects only a special population of people with type 1, IgE-mediated allergy. While this is an important reaction pattern, some physicians have claimed it is the only valid form of allergic reactions to food. Their opinion is no longer acceptable.

Delayed Patterns of Food Allergy: IMED

The **Food Allergy Model** attempts to explain many well-known diseases and ill-defined illness. Beyond Type 1 or Immediate Hypersensitivity, there are numerous possibilities for immune injury. We often refer to the other, more complicated problems as "Delayed Pattern Food Allergy", following the lead of Dr. William Knicker[3], Dr. J. Brostoff[4], and others. At the risk of repeating the most important concepts, let us review the basis for delayed pattern food allergy.

Several mechanisms of immune injury, described in immunology literature as Types II, III, and IV immune hypersensitivity mechanisms are responsible for the more varied and complex forms of food allergy. The essential concept of food allergy is that we are immunized to food molecules by GIT and then develop immune-mediated or allergic disease after entry of food antigens into the body by GIT error and/or inappropriate selection of food. Now we realize that GIT errors mingle with all body responses to food ingestion every day. Drs. Coombs and McLaughlin summarized the problem simply in a 1984 discussion of food allergens:[5]

> *"Food proteins in the gastrointestinal tract and their absorption into the body as antigenic molecules have immunologic significance both in (i) initiating an allergic state and (ii) in the subsequent challenge(s) where, by a variety of mechanisms, they may cause some form of 'food-allergic disease'."*

Immune responses to food must be one of the most common abnormal consequences of eating. GIT permeability to molecules, other than nutrients, is a key determinant of what happens to us after eating or drinking food materials. Antibody synthesis occurs at all body surfaces, when antigen is presented. GIT is the obvious choice for major antigen sensing and encoding, since it contains the largest surface area and largest amount of mucosal lymphoid tissue of any body surface. Antigen is selectively sampled from the soupy contents of the GIT by "M cells" in specialized areas of GIT which probably recognize most food antigens. Therefore, we are routinely sensitized to many, if not most, of the foods we ingest.

A local GIT surface reaction to food antigens may release mast cell mediators and produce a local inflammatory swelling which in turn increases GIT permeability and permits increased entry of undigested large molecules. Unfortunately, many people ignore or suppress GIT symptoms and continue ingesting injurious substances. The most obvious form of food allergy is this contact sensitivity of the GIT. The principle symptoms of GIT surface reactivity are sore throat, heartburn, abdominal pain, nausea, vomiting, diarrhea, rectal itching-burning, and distended-tender hemorrhoids. All of these symptoms disappear when the allergenic foods are eliminated. The more complex food allergy problems occur **beyond the GIT**, but depend on GIT surveillance of food. GIT immune sensors transmit food reaction information to the entire body. We then become reactive to food antigens in all our tissues! Surveillance information from GIT is distributed throughout the body by **wandering lymphocytes.** These cells sensitize the whole body in a discontinuous distribution. B cells (IgA precursor cells) migrate from GIT via the draining lymph nodes, and are subsequently found in the spleen. Cells originating in GIT have a tendency to return to GIT, but some find their way throughout the lymphatic system.

Mast cells living in skin and connective tissue are also sensitized by food-inspired antibodies of the IgE and IgG classes. These "swat teams" can then react to circulating food antigens anywhere in the body. If you are immunized against an antigen presented to GIT you can expect a response to the same antigen in any tissue. This localized distribution in different tissues of sensing, reacting immune cells is one of the reasons for the topologically distributed reactions to circulating antigens.

Increased GIT Permeability

Many factors allow allergens access to the body by interfering with GIT-surface defenses. Deficiency in the surface IgA antibody defense typically leads to delayed forms of food allergy, triggered by IMED. Without adequate IgA, large molecules are routinely absorbed through the GIT wall. We know a little about dietary factors which increase GIT permeability. Alcoholic beverages are perhaps the most important agents of increased GIT permeability. Any bacterial or viral infection which induces inflammation in the wall of GIT may increase GIT permeability. Reduced blood flow to the GIT (ischemia) increases GIT permeability and may be associated with abdominal injury, surgery, or arterial narrowing from atherosclerosis. Water retention and swelling of the GIT wall (edema) may increase GIT permeability. During the premenstrual week, many women show increased food allergic effects as they experience generalized edema. Anti-inflammatory drugs, used to treat pain and arthritis, increase GIT permeability and may perpetuate the diseases they are used to treat. Cancer chemotherapy and radiation therapy damage the GIT and increase GIT permeability. Agent X, any molecular stressor or toxic food element, may also be involved.

Deficiency of the antibody, IgA, promotes food allergy. This antibody is secreted on the surface of intestinal cells. The role of IgA is to trap undesirable molecules and block their entry into the absorbing surface of GIT. Deficiency of IgA would permit the entry of more allergenic macromolecules into body space via the bloodstream. Newborn infants are deficient in both serum and secretory IgA. IgA levels rise progressively in a normal child to an adult range over the first four years. IgA deficiency continues in some people as an isolated abnormality, perpetuating food allergy.

Immune Complexes and Complement - Type III Reactions

Von Pirquet first described **serum sickness**, the prototype of **Immune Complex disease** in 1925. Horse serum proteins were the first antigen stimulus used to produce this effect. Any food protein entering the circulation in sufficient quantity can produce symptom patterns resembling serum sickness. If antigens make it into the blood stream, they combine with circulating antibodies to produce **circulating immune complexes (CICs)**. BIN cells interact with CICs, triggering immune reactions with the release of symptom-producing mediators. Serum sickness manifests as a systemic illness, typically evolving over a 7-10 day period. Manifestations include general malaise, fever, flushing, sweating, hives, swelling, bruising, aching in joints and muscles, progressing in the worst case to inflammatory disease in target organs with protein in the urine from kidney damage.

Food-enriched blood, coming from the gastrointestinal tract, goes through the liver where most immune-complexes are removed. If circulating complexes pass the liver filter, they may cause disturbances in many organs. The other path of absorption of molecules from the GIT is through lymphatic drainage. The lymph channels flow together to form the thoracic duct, a flimsy vessel which drains its contents into the subclavian vein. This pathway may direct antigenic molecules directly to the lungs where food antigens may excite asthmatic attacks, bronchitis, or more serious and enigmatic inflammatory lung diseases. The combination of antibody with antigen in the blood stream is a **circulating immune complex (CIC)**.

CICs have the general form of:

Antigen—Antibody

CICs may simply be removed from the circulation by macrophages or they may trigger a cascade of events which lead to multiple symptoms, and possibly tissue damage:

CICs —> Mediator release —> Symptoms

Mediators + Immune cells —> Inflammation

CICs activate **complement,** a circulating system of 25 proteins which interact to produce a variety of defensive molecular weapons. CICs may not cause tissue injury unless access to tissue spaces is increased by leakiness of blood vessels, allowing influx of CICs and cells.

The complement system modulates and amplifies the biological effects of CICs. Once activated the complement cascades through a series of changes, producing powerful effects including anaphylaxis and blood cell damage. At the same time, certain complement products are essential to clear CICs. Individuals with deficiencies of complement proteins are at greater risk of developing immune-complex disease.

CICs leave capillaries to trigger inflammatory events in target tissues. A classic model of complex-induced pathology is the **Arthus reaction,** which appears 3-6 hours after antigen challenge and involves large insoluble (type 3) complexes with complement (C3b) passing through vessel walls to excite inflammatory responses in target tissues. The Arthrus reaction can be prevented by depleting C3 with Cobra venom.

Inflammation

Inflammation is the most potent effect of immune defense. Inflammation is recognized as swelling, pain, heat, and redness in the affected tissue. Inflammation is produced by immune cells within the tissue, releasing specific mediators which control local circulation and cell activities. The ancient purpose of inflammation is to war on invading microorganisms. Thus, inflammation describes a battle-ravaged tissue. **Inflammation** occurs around a skin infection like a boil, or may occur within a tendon (tendinitis), a joint (arthritis) or a vital organ. The suffix "**itis**" simply means inflammation. Many of the serious, unsolved diseases of modern civilization are expressions of chronic inflammatory processes. Medical therapy is often directed at controlling inflammation. Apparently, nature has provided a good protective strategy in the inflammatory process, but it goes too far too often. The pathologist recognizes different stages and patterns of inflammation from acute to chronic. Under the microscope, an inflamed tissue is invaded by a variety of immune cells. Many of the chronic and unsolved diseases which plague our civilization are inflammatory disorders.

Type IV Cell-Mediated Immune Response

Chronic inflammation is a product of the Type IV hypersensitivity mechanisms. Cell-mediated immunity is initiated by several cell populations, including mast cells and neutrophils, and then sustained by lymphocytes. All these cells must invade a tissue space by migrating from BIN to TIN. As a tissue space becomes inflamed, neutrophils release enzymes, and a variety of mediators such platelet activating factor, interleukinns, and leukotrienes. This early response can be triggered by immune complexes containing food antigens and/or complement products.

Lymphocytes are activated by the secretions of other cells and are selected for specific activation by cells who present antigen to them. If the antigen matches the lymphocytes antibody receptors, they respond to antigen presention by proliferation. The result is an expanding population of activated "clones" which, like good soldiers, do the job they were brought up to do. Some produce antibody, others secrete messenger molecules, others swarm in the local area, looking for antigens to attack. On any average day, we probably have billions of food-sensitized lymphocytes in antigen-specific clones, numbering in the thousands. If a lymphocytic network is activated by food antigens the pathogenic consequences depend on: the dose, frequency, and distribution of antigen; the location of lymphocytes; host factors - tolerance vs. hypersensitivity; target organ dysfunction (eg. nose vs. retina). The net effect is inflammation in target organs, associated with systemic symptoms from mediators, especially interleukins, leukotrienes, prostaglandins, and peptides.

Lymphocytes are mobile, **migratory** cells. Their traffic patterns are now being studied, and prove fascinating. A basic pattern seems to be for the various kinds of lymphocytes to become sensitized in MALT and then to wander inward to other organs of the lymphatic system. After a holiday in lymph nodes, liver, or spleen, the same lymphocytes seem to wander back to their place of origin. Sensitized lymphocytes who wander off in other directions may be distributing antigen recognition codes from one MALT defense unit to another. The traffic patterns of these nomadic cells must have a great deal to do with the success of immune defence and the tenuous balance between reactivity and tolerance. The distribution of the ability to recognize and react to foreign antigens, is one of the keys both to successful immunity and to the problems of allergy. We know too little of this traffic to easily understand the complex phenomena of immunity and allergy. **Helper cells** specific for IgA synthesis predominate in Peyer's patches, the antigen-sensing structures, distributed along the intestinal wall. Similar IgA-helper cells migrate to mesenteric lymph nodes but not to the spleen. The migration of lymphocytes, following oral administration of antigen, from Peyer's patches to mesenteric lymph nodes and spleen has been described.

The chronic inflammation in eczema (atopic dermatitis) serves as a visible example of cell-mediated inflammation. The most important experiment to perform is to stop all food intake, replace this antigenic material with an elemental nutrient formula and await spontaneous resolution of cell-mediated inflammation in the skin over the next 2-3 weeks.[6]

Symptom Timing

A simple classification of food allergy symptom patterns is based on the timing of symptoms:

> The **immediate responses** are symptoms emerging in 1-60 minutes. As the allergy process unfolds, at least two other time periods are readily recognized.

> Symptoms like headache, drowsiness, dizziness, cognitive dysfunction, and aching tend to arrive 1-8 hours after eating, and may be classed **intermediate**.

> **Delayed symptoms** emerge in 8-72 hours after eating, or may follow a dose/frequency dependent pattern , requiring several feedings over a period of days to weeks.

The onset of symptoms tends to vary with nature and amount of the food, digestion and absorption delays, and type of immune response, but other "host variables" contribute to complexity. A body reacts to an adverse stimulus, not just in one burst of activity, but with **rhythmic, oscillating disturbances.**The profile of a single pulsing response may be different from the next, similar event. Allergic reactions follow our rhythms and are not consistent over time. Patients will always complain one feeding of a food was OK but the next time was a disaster; or they will say they experienced minor symptoms with three feedings and a major response with the forth.

The failure to recognize rhythms and patterns leads to many wrong assumptions about the timing and patterning of allergic reactions. Smolensky and D'Alonzo, writing about Biological Rhythms and Medicine[7] stated:

> *"...biological processes and functions are precisely organized not only in space but also in time. Thus living organisms have both a physical and temporal anatomy. Unfortunately most physicians are only vaguely aware of chronobiology, the science concerned with biological rhythms and their mechanisms...".*

They go on to describe **biological clocks,** different cycles in us and relate their insights to diseases such as asthma which tend to occur at night, during sleep and may cycle through monthly and seasonal changes. Several immunological observations have documented rhythmic change in immune activity. For example, the secretion of the protective antibody, IgA, follows a 24 hour rhythm. The maximal secretion occurs between midnight and 8:00 a.m., and the minimum between 6:00 and 9:00 p.m. A longer seasonal cycle has been noted for the total RBC count, which peaks in December for most people. There also are rhythmic changes in immediate sensitivity, or IgE, reactivity. Skin itching peaks between 8:00 and 10:00 p.m., and again, between 6:00 and 8:00 a.m. The "itch threshold" is 100 times lower at midnight than it is at two in the afternoon. Patients who suffer hay fever are likely to be most congested when they wake up in the morning, and experience another peak in the late evening. Asthmatics' reactivity peaks around three in the morning. It is a common experience for an asthmatic to awaken with severe breathing problems. This **early-morning crisis** is associated with the lowest levels of adrenalin-like hormones in the blood.

There are clear **lunar rhythms,** more obvious in women because of the menstrual cycle marker. Allergic phenomena increase during the premenstrual week. This change is likely due to ovarian or pituitary hormones, although the exact mechanism is unknown. Often premenstrual symptoms are food allergy amplified by a hormonal response. In seeking control of severe premenstrual symptoms or PMS, women may have to be very careful with their food choices a week prior to their period, but and relax and eat more foods in the 2 or 3 weeks following their period. Migraine headaches are especially likely in the premenstrual week. Food control is, however, more difficult in the premenstrual week with most women reporting cravings and compulsive eating.

Symptom Sequences

The distribution of food antigens helps to determine symptom sequences we observe. We can imagine the path through the body of group of food allergens, let into the blood stream like burglars in a shopping mall. During initial contact with the lips and mouth, food antigens may trigger an immediate, contact reaction. This **contact response** leads to sensations on the lips, mouth, and throat which include tingling, numbness, itching, and pain. The symptoms are associated with visible changes; swelling, small ulcers, and reddening. A similar surface reaction may extend along the esophagus and into the stomach. As the path of surface reactions extend inward, the symptoms change their character. An **esophageal-stomach inflammatory response** would be felt as chest and abdominal pain, usually burning in quality. Nausea and vomiting often accompany the pain. Further along the small intestine, a similar surface reaction would be felt as crampy abdominal pain and diarrhea. If food antigens are digested they lose their immune identity and the problem stops. Individual amino acids do not trigger immune responses.

If antigens are admitted through the GIT mucosa into the circulation or lymphatics, then another series of complex contingencies will result. The antigens may be identified by circulating antibodies who attach to them, forming **circulating immune complexes**. These immune complexes pass to the liver where they may be cleared by specialized cells. Or, if the immune complexes are passed beyond the liver, they will then circulate through the lungs, back to the heart, and out to the rest of the body space. Complexes can activate the **complement cascade** anywhere in the circulation, triggering an **explosive event** with both local and general symptoms. The **liver** may occasionally react with some degree of liver inflammation or hepatitis. Transient liver swelling is felt as pain in the upper right abdomen, often under the ribs on the right side. Since the liver sits mostly within the rib cage, right-sided chest and back pain following a meal may be liver swelling.

If circulating immune complexes travel to the **lung**, breathing difficulties, asthma, and lung inflammation might ensue. An asthmatic with immediate hypersensitivity typically experiences an acute wheezing attack within 20 minutes of exposure to an airborne of allergen. This **initial attack** is followed by remission for a few hours, and then return of worsening breathing problems. The second or **late phase** is associated with swelling and edema of the tubes of the lung, a more prolonged and serious threat to breathing ability. The variable delay of absorption of food antigens and the biphasic asthma response makes for a confusing variability in symptom-sequences, following food ingestion. We, therefore, expect symptoms for at least 48 hours after food ingestion; although peak onset is usually within 12 hours.

A typical **symptom sequence** combines nose and throat congestion with generalized connective tissue inflammatory activity, felt as muscle tension, aching, and stiffness. If immune-complexes, aberrant protein or peptide molecules, complement fragments or other immune mediators penetrate the blood brain barrier, brain function may be disturbed. The **blood brain barrier** should protect us from major disruptions of our psyche, but once breached profound disturbances can be expected. We experience brain disturbances as changes in thinking, sensing, seeing, hearing, feeling, remembering, and behaving.

One of the common food allergy symptoms is **edema or increased tissue water.** Under the influence of peptide **permeability factors,** water moves from the circulation to tissue spaces in increased amounts. Tissue spaces swell with the extra water, noticed as puffiness of hands, feet, face with sudden weight gain. Extra water may move into critical organ spaces. In the brain, extra water globally interferes with brain function, manifested as fatigue, depression, and confusion. This water retention is not dependent on salt intake, and attempts to control it with salt restriction fail. When the allergenic foods are removed from the diet, water moves back into the circulation and is excreted by the kidneys. Increased urine flow is noted with sudden weight loss and improvement in brain function.

Topology of Immune-Mediated Events

Another fascinating aspect of food allergy symptoms is the **distribution of symptoms** in body space. A patient will describe a typical reactive sequence beginning, for example, with itching and burning of the feet, followed in minutes by shooting pains over the right temple, followed in 2 or 3 hours by low back pain, and itchy welts involving the skin of the neck. Another patient will describe nasal stuffiness, swelling of the neck lymph nodes, followed by right shoulder pain and dry cough. Many patients experience symptoms preferentially on one side of their body, suggesting a brain controlling effect over the expression of the allergic reaction. It is common for each person to have reactive zones on their skin surface which preferentially react with itching, flushing, hives, rashes, eczema, or psoriasis.

Internal body reactive zones also are established, according to rules which are not usually apparent. Sites of old injury are foci for recurrent inflammatory events, for example. There are general reactive zones that behave similarly in most people; the diamond shaped area, defined from the nape of the neck to points over the mid-shoulder blades to a point in the middle spinal area, is a common reactive zone. Increased muscle tension and pain in this area typically occur during a food allergic reaction. This **pain-tension** complex in the **neck-shoulder-back zone** receives a lot of attention from doctors, osteopaths, chiropractors, physiotherapists, and massage therapists who think in terms of a structural-mechanical model, often blaming poor posture, slipped vertebrae, tension, or stress for the symptoms. Mediator release in connective tissue and inflammatory reactions are a better explanation of this common symptom complex. The structural-mechanical model, popular in both physical medicine and chiropractic, forgets that the body is made of living cells, continuously metabolizing, changing their structural-mechanical properties quickly and dramatically with changes in the molecular stream which flows through them.

The paradox is that a population of antigens is distributed throughout the body in the circulation, but the perceived response to the problem is often localized. **Localization of response** can be viewed as a functional body map that tells us about the distribution of antigenic molecules, the distribution of immune-sensing cells, the distribution of modulators of the immune response, and the role of the brain both in influencing immune reactivity and in perceiving its effects. The role of **brain modulation and perception** of allergic responses is further complicated by the involvement of the brain in dysfunctional patterns. **Topological mapping** of these patterns is another area of research needed before we thoroughly understand internal body-space allergy patterns.

Food allergy is best recognized by the **confusing barrage of symptoms** which come and go in a haphazard manner. The technique of keeping a daily food-intake-symptom record may help reveal the patterns of dysfunction, although we never attempt to identify reactive foods on an uncontrolled diet; there are just too many variables. We rely on clinical skills to properly evaluate a patient's symptoms.

The physician must assess patients' symptoms as manifestations of an underlying pathophysiological process. Often the exact mechanism is not know precisely, but this limitation of knowledge should not prevent clinical diagnosis and proper treatment with diet revision. Because symptom production mechanisms are so variable and complex it is essential to simplify a sick state by controlling food intake with a clearing program and then attempt slow food-introduction. You can usually identify the entire symptom-production mechanism to single foods as they are reintroduced.

Mediators Produce Illness Patterns

Each of our chemical mediators produces its own signature of symptoms. The possible symptom complexes of mediator reactions are too numerous to catalogue here. A sketch of histamine's activity will serve to illustrate how different mediators will produce a characteristic series of symptoms. Several mediators are released routinely from the GIT as digestion proceeds, regulating GIT activity. Other GIT mediators are released in special circumstances. Many GIT messengers also travel to the brain, affecting how we think and feel. The brain effects of allergic and inflammatory mediators are not well understood, but play an important role in the production many mental and emotional disturbances.   **Symptoms**, following a food challenge, may be read as a specific physiological code. But, before we try to interpret the code, we have to realize that there are at least dozens of mediators, released in complex patterns, as allergic reactions unfold.

The best recognized mediators of symptom production are **histamine, serotonin, bradykinin, heparin, mast cell peptides, leukotrienes, and prostaglandins.** All are major players in allergy production. Prostaglandins, for example, are sythesized at the site of of reaction, are short-lived and may produce flushing, fever, pain, shortness of breath, racing heart, constricted or dilated blood vessels, diarrhea, abdominal cramps, and then vanish as mysteriously as they came. The synthesis of several prostaglandins can be blocked by acetylsalicylic acid (aspirin), and other similar anti-inflammatory drugs. Mediators act in concert and in sequences. Histamine may dilate blood vessels and act with prostaglandins, PGE_2 and PGI_2 to produce the early swelling, redness and heat of an inflammatory response. The same mediators may sensitize nerve endings to other pain-producing mediators such as bradykinin. An initial burst of mediator activity will often set a series of cell responses in motion which will amplify and prolong disturbances for days or weeks. Once inflammation is established in tissues by immune cell invasion and mediator release, recovery may take several weeks.

Almost everyone has taken an antihistamine drug to relieve cold symptoms, treat hay fever or itching, relieve nausea and vomiting, or as an aid to sleep. The popularity of antihistamines is a mute testimony to the negative effects of histamine. To get a good idea of what histamine can do, let us imagine the effects of an injection of a small amount.

Histamine Symptoms Might Include:

* **Headache** is felt as a pulsating, whole-head pain, often with a sense of great pressure or bursting within the head.
* **Fast heart**, blood pressure falls, irregular beats are common with an alarming sense of "palpitations".
* **Skin sensations** begin with a local itching or burning sensation, followed by flushing and a disagreeable heat.
* **Stomach pain** as acid secretion increases immediately; the small intestine contracts vigorously, often with unpleasant crampy pain.
* **Respiratory** – local nose effects include swelling, congestion, and sneezing. An asthmatic attack may be provoked.
* **Anxiety and agitation** with diffuse, deep, odd body sensations:"...my bones are on fire", "I feel weird all over", "...a deep pricking, crawling sensation...".

Histamine carries its message to a large number of cells by attaching to a special receptor on the cells' surfaces. There are two kinds of histamine **receptors, H1 and H2.** The H1 and H2 receptors both receive histamine as a messenger, but the meaning taken by the different receptors is different. H1 receptors tend to produce the symptoms already listed, and activate the allergic reaction. H2 receptors tend to act as negative feedback receptors and turn the allergic reaction off. H2 receptors also exclusively activate the acid-producing, parietal cells of the stomach lining.

Antihistamines are drugs which block the receptors so that the histamine messages are not received. We have drugs that selectively block both kinds of histamine receptors. The common antihistamines; Benadryl, Chlortripalon, Atarax, Seldane, Hismanal; are H1 blockers. The H1 block is useful to treat allergic reactions. They also act on brain H1 receptors causing sedation, a dangerous side-effect if you are driving, operating machinery, or otherwise need to be alert and vigilant. Antihistamine sedative effects are increased by concurrent alcoholic beverage ingestion. The powerful sedative effect of some foods like milk and wheat in susceptible people is not blocked, but enhanced by antihistamines. The new antihistamines, Seldane, Claritin and Hismanal, are less likely to cause drowsiness than the older H1 blockers. The H2 receptor blocker, cimetadine, first marketed as "Tagamet", joins Valium as one of the best-selling drugs of all time. The H2 block reduces stomach acid secretion. This acid reduction helps to prevent and to heal peptic ulcers. Cimetadine may be thought of as an allergy reaction modifier and antacid combined. A better treatment of many gastrointestinal symptoms would be appropriate diet revision.

Milk Allergy

The allergy to cow's milk is the best studied form of food allergy.[8] [9] Cow's milk contains many **proteins** which are **antigenic**. Infants and any adult with gastrointestinal tract disease may have difficulty digesting these proteins and may absorb them as antigens. **Casein is the most commonly used milk protein in the food industry; lactalbuminn, lactoglobulin, bovine albumin, and gamma globulin** are other protein groups within the milk. There are at least 30 antigenic proteins in milk. Digestion probably increases the number of possible antigens to over 100. On food labels milk protein is identified as whey, caseinates, skim milk powder, and milk solids. Digested fractions of each of the milk proteins may induce the production of IgE, IgA, and IgG antibodies and may trigger complex, variable immune responses. The digestion of any given protein will vary, and depends on multiple factors. Complete breakdown of a protein into individual amino acids will prevent an injurious immune response to a food. Incomplete digestion of a protein, leaving larger, antigenic fragments would encourage an immune response. The symptom response is variable and emerges from minutes to hours after eating foods containing milk proteins. The variability of symptom production can confuse both patients and physicians.

The incidence of cows' milk protein allergy (CMPA) has been underestimated at about 7% of infants and children. Among atopic children, the estimated incidence of milk allergy is 14-30%. We have read the opinion that milk allergy is "rare in adults"; an absurd opinion. Allergy incidence estimates are based on the narrowest definition of "allergy" and on inadequate experience treating patients with delayed forms of milk allergy. We believe the incidence of milk allergy is much higher and assert that **Milk Disease** is a major endemic health problem. The Core Program assumes that everyone is allergic to milk, until proven otherwise.

Milk allergy usually presents as part of a food allergy complex. Digestive symptoms are common; indigestion, heartburn, excessive gas, and crampy abdominal pain are common symptoms along with constipation and/or diarrhea Milk allergy may interfere with the digestion and absorption of other nutrients and sometimes presents as anemia, secondary to blood loss. Any food allergy which disturbs gastrointestinal tract function tends to multiply its effects. This is why a major comprehensive dietary change is often necessary to resolve a food-allergy.

Typical **respiratory** tract symptoms include nasal congestion, excess throat mucus, middle ear fluid, cough, bronchitis, and asthma. Loss of hearing and ringing in the ears often occurs. Recurrent ear "infections" are common in children, less common in adults. Permanent hearing loss may result from neglected food allergy. Skin eruptions vary from common eczema to measles-like rashes and hives. Flushing (red, hot) of cheeks, ears, and neck occurs in adults and children. Milk allergy commonly produces generalized aching and stiffness, with joint pain leading to frank arthritis. The unlucky patient will develop a disabling inflammatory arthritis. Again, if the correct diagnosis of food allergy is not made, these patients continue to ingest milk and other food allergens, and suffer from an unnecessary disease.

Skin tests are not helpful in making the diagnosis of food allergic arthritis.

In infants and older children, the behavioral effects include irritability, temper tantrums, hyperactivity, restless sleep, nightmares and clumsiness or incoordination. At school, these children show **attention deficits** and often have learning disabilities. Many adult patients describe a history of childhood difficulties, with recurring or persisting concentration problems, hyperactivity and/or **depression**. Childhood dysfunction may evolve into adult disabilities. Adults report chronic fatigue, mental fogginess, difficulty concentrating, recent memory drop-outs, anxiety and sleep disturbances. Sometimes dairy products (and wheat) are very sedating and trigger uncontrollable **sleepiness** after ingestion; some patients are diagnosed with **narcolepsy**. Other nervous system effects are described by patients; restless legs, itching, prickling and burning sensations deep inside arms and legs, or a generalized body discomfort and agitation which may be dramatically disturbing.

Elimination of milk and milk products is the essential treatment for anyone with milk allergy. Milk allergy is assumed on the Core Program and dairy products are excluded. Often milk-exclusion is prescribed without other diet modification. Further diet revision is necessary because food allergy is a non-specific disease, involving many different foods. Substitutes, milk for cows' milk include goat's milk and soya milk. Goat's milk may also cause allergic responses and is often expensive or difficult to obtain. Soy milk formulas (Isomil, Soyalac, Prosobee, Nursoy) are used to feed infants and can be useful in adult nutrition. Soy protein allergy is common, however, and soy milk formulas may produce as much disturbance as cow's milk formulas. The incidence of soya allergy is about one third that of cow's milk.

Cereal Grain Disease

Foods made with wheat are staples in North American and European diets. Unfortunately, wheat and its close relatives, oats, barley, and rye, have proved to be a major problem in the diets of our patients. An important feature of the Core Program is the complete exclusion of the four cereal grains. Wheat diseases have already been discussed in several chapters of Section 1. There are many possible reasons for cereal grains to become pathogenic. We do not pretend to know all the reasons for the recurring observation that wheat disease is a common problem in our modern urban patients. Craving and compulsive eating of flour-based foods is common, especially reward and dessert foods, containing wheat, sugar, milk and eggs, the 4 foods of the allergy apocalypse. Whole grains also contain phytates which bind desirable minerals, preventing their absorption. Mineral malabsorption calcium, magnesium, and zinc deficiencies may occur with diets high in whole grains. The role of glutens in depression, schizophrenia and possibly other neurological diseases has been reviewed in Section1.

Wheat proteins are collectively called "Gluten". Wheat is closely related to other cereal grains, especially rye, barley, and oats. Enthusiasm for "whole grains" to increase intake of dietary fiber, especially in the past decade, lead to increased consumption of whole cereal grains. Relatively unrefined grains, often in combination, as with granola cereals and whole wheat breads fortified with bran, coarse flours, and other additives are now eaten in large quantities. Gluten is a mixture of individual proteins classified in two groups, the Prolamines and the Glutelins. The prolamine fraction of gluten concerns us the most when grain intolerance is suspected. The prolamine, Gliadin, seems to be a problem in celiac disease; gliadin antibodies are commonly found in the immune complexes associated with this disease.[10] We eat the seeds of the grain plants. The seed has a bran casing, a starchy endosperm which contains 90% of the protein, and a small germ nucleus which is the plant embryo waiting to grow. Any flour made from the starchy endosperm contains prolamines and is potentially toxic to the grain intolerant person The different grains; each has its own prolamine:

Grain Type	Prolamine	% Total Protein
Wheat	Gliadin	69
Rye	Secalinin	30-50
Oats	Avenin	16
Barley	Hordein	46-52
Millet	Panicin	40
Corn	Zien	55
Rice	Orzenin	5
Sorgum	Kafirin	52

Celiac disease is a model of wheat allergic disease. When wheat is the principle problem food, barley, oats, and rye must be excluded as well.[11] Millet is intermediate in the list of offenders; corn and rice are usually tolerated when gluten prolamines are the chief and only food intolerance, although corn triggers food allergy for its own reasons. Triticale is a new hybrid grain with the properties of wheat and rye, and is excluded on a gluten-free diet. The identity and the amount of the prolamine decides the kind of reaction that is likely to occur. It should be noted that there is considerable variability in the prolamine content of various foods made from cereal grains, and this variability is one of the many reasons why food reactions are not consistent. Recently marketed grains, spelt and kamut, appear to be wheat relatives; we have not yet had enough experience with them to define their acceptability for gluten-free diets.

The **mechanisms** by which wheat or any other food can cause disturbances are numerous, as suggested in earlier chapters. Painful inflammatory states may be the presentation of wheat allergy. The occurrence of pain in joints, particularly the hands, with slight swelling and stiffness is the early presentation of allergic arthritis; it can occur strictly as a manifestation of gluten allergy. A wheat gluten mechanism has been studied in rheumatoid arthritis patients. The clinical observation is that wheat ingestion is followed within hours by increased joint swelling and pain.

Dr. Little and his colleagues studied the mechanism, as it developed sequentially following gluten ingestion.[12]The mechanism involves several stages:

> GIT must be permeable to antigenic proteins or peptide fragments, derived from digested gluten.
>
> The antigen appears in the blood stream and is bound by a specific antibody (probably of IgA or IgG, not IgE class), forming an antigen-antibody complex, a circulating immune complex (CIC).Immune complexes
>
> The antigen-antibody complex then activates the rest of the immune response, beginning with the release of mediators - serotonin is released from the blood platelets.
>
> Serotonin release causes "symptoms" as it circulates in the blood stream and enhances the deposition of CICs in joint tissues.
>
> Once in the joint, the immune complexes activate complement, which in turn damages cells and activates inflammation. More inflammation results in more pain, swelling, stiffness, and loss of mobility.

While this complex of events is known to occur with gluten antigens, many food allergens can trigger arthritis. Dr. Parke and colleagues concurred with this explanation of the gut-arthritis link in their report of three patients with celiac disease and rheumatoid arthritis.[13] An additional hypothesis is needed to explain the difference between common aching disorders and severe destructive arthritis. If IMED involves a defensive immune response to "foreign" antigens derived from food, but if the reactions are suppressed, the inflammatory activity goes no further than aching pain and mild disability. If immune suppressors are deficient, a more explosive and destructive defense occurs, with aggressive inflammation damaging tissues. To develop the more serious, crippling arthritic disease, the immune response also may involve the error of an attack on "Self", an autoimmune attack. This autoimmune attack represents a failure of the immune system to recognize and tolerate "Self" antigens. This error might occur if the foreign food antigen was different enough to initiate an immune response, but similar enough to a self antigen to excite an immune attack directed at one's own tissues!

[1]Coca AF, Cooke RA. On the classification of the phenomena of hypersensitiveness. J Immunol 1925;10:445.

[2]Cantani A, Buscinco E, Beninicori N. A three year controlled study in children with pollinosis treated with immunotherapy. Annals of Allergy 1984;53:79-84.

[3]Knicker W. Non-IgE Mediated and Delayed Adverse reactions to Food or dditives. Handbook on Food Allergies, Ed Breneman J.C.; Marcel Dekker Inc. N.Y. 1985.

[4]Brostoff J. Mechanisms: Food Allergy and Intolerance; Balliere Tinbdal; 1987

[5]Coombs RRA, McLaughlan P. Ann Allergy 1984;53:592.

[6]Villaveces JW, Heiner DC. Experience with an Elemental Diet. Annals of Allergy 55:783-789

[7]Smolensky M.H., D'Alonzo G.E.
 Biological Rhythms and Medicine; Am Jour Medicine 1988; 85(1B); 34-46.

[8]Gerrard JW et al. Cow's milk allergy: prevelance and manifestations in an unselected series of newborns. Acta Pediat Scand Suppl 1973;234:2.

[9]Hill DJ. Cow's milk allergy in infants: some clinical and immunological features. Annals of Allergy 1986;57:225-228.

[10]Keiffer M et al. Wheat gliadin fractions and other cereal antigens reactive with antibodies in the sera of of celiac patients. Clin Exp Immunol 1982;50:651-60.

[11]Bell L, Hoffer M. Recommendations for foods of questionable acceptance for patients with celiac disease. J Can Dietetic Ass'n 1981;42(2):143-158.

[12]Little C, Stewart AG, Fennesy MR. Platelet serotonin release in rheumatoid arthritis: a study in food intolerant patients. Lancet 1983;297-9.

[13]Parke Al et al. Celiac disease and rheumatoid arthritis. Annals of Rheum Dis 1984;43:378-380.

Core Program Master Food List			
FRUIT	RICE	FISH & MEAT	VEG. OILS
			Oils
Apples	Converted Rice	Beef	Safflower Oil
Applesauce	Basmati Rice	Chicken	Sunflower Oil
Apricots	Rice flour	Cod	Olive Oil
Avocado	Brown rice	Halibut	Flax oil
Bananas	Rice Cakes	Lamb	Marine lipids
Blackberries	Rice Noodles	Mackerel	Primrose oil
Blueberries	Rice bread	Red snapper	
Cantaloupe	Rice pancakes	Sole	
Cherries	Rice "ice cream"	Tuna	HERBS
Cranberries	Rice crackers	Turkey	
Currants			Basil
Grapes	LEGUMES & SOY PRODUCTS		Bay leaves
Honeydew,			Carob
Kiwi Fruit	Adzuki Beans	Miso	Celery
Lemon	Chickpeas	Soy infant formulas	Curry
Lime	Kidney beans	Soy Milk	Dill
Mango	Lentils	Soy sauce	Garlic
Nectarines	Lima beans	Soya beans	Ginger
Orange	Peanuts	Soya flour	Marjoram
Papaya	Split peas	Tofu	Mustard
Peaches	White beans	Tofu ice cream	Oregano
Pears	Yellow wax beans	Tofu products	Parsley
Pineapple			Pepper
Plums	FLOUR SUBSTITUTES		Rosemary
Raspberries			Sesame
Strawberries	Arrowroot	Amarinthe	Thyme
Watermelon	Buckwheat	Cornstarch	Wasabi
	Quinoa	Millet	
Lotus Root	Tapioca	Soy flour	
Bamboo shoots			
Mushrooms			
Daikon	Vitamins & Minerals		
Water chessnuts	ENFood		
Water Cress			

Chapter 16 Tests and Treatments

Confusion about the nature of food problems, diagnosis and treatment is widespread. Patients are often disappointed when they learn that even sophisticated medical laboratories and expensive imaging devices cannot pinpoint the nature and origin of their suffering. Evaluation of nutritional status is not difficult if a physician takes an adequate medical history, including a detailed diet inventory, does a physical examination and measures basic blood and urine values. A diet history and computed nutrient intake (from a 4 day food intake record you keep) will provide adequate nutritional information. A fasting blood sugar and blood lipids will provide a snapshot of your metabolism with respect to diabetes and cardiovascular disease. Normal blood counts rule out the advanced stages of most common nutrient deficiencies; iron and Vitamin B_{12}. If you go beyond basics and measure serum vitamin and mineral levels and other more elaborate tests the investigation becomes very expensive; the value of spot measurements of the blood diminishes as the costs go up.

One of the most abused tests is the **glucose tolerance test,** which we no longer do, since it does not simulate real eating conditions and does not provide useful information. If diabetes is suspected by an elevated fasting blood sugar, and /or sugar in the urine, an abbreviated glucose challenge test can be done to asses the degree of sugar intolerance. The diagnosis of hypoglycemia by challenge with high doses of sugar is usually meaningless. If low sugar levels are thought to explain symptom occurrence, blood sugar levels should be measured during a symptomatic episode; this can be down with a home-testing kit. The information supplied by a physical examination depends on the skill experience of the physician.

We have seen far too many patients who were told "nothing is wrong" when even with a casual glance, they display signs of conspicuous problems; flushing, allergic shiners, edema, skin rashes, blood vessel changes in their skin, inflammation of the nose lining, excess weight, joint swelling, and so-on. Confusion arises when there is a discrepancy between your history of illness and the results of physical examination and basic tests. You may feel quite ill but your Doctor says he or she can find nothing wrong. By now, we know that an **insightful physician** will not dismiss your complaints but may **collaborate** with you on changes in your biological circumstances; changes in your food supply, your environment, your level of physical activity, your expectations, and so-on. A clinical diagnosis of one or more of the food allergy patterns can and should be made on the basis of history and examination. A trial of diet revision, following the Core Program then acts to confirm the diagnosis. The Core Program is, above all else, a no-nonsense, practical method of dealing with the complex of food-related illnesses. We hope the Core Program will spare many people needless, prolonged, and expensive investigation and futile treatment attempts.

This chapter addresses, briefly, some of the testing and treatment issues and confusions about food allergy. Ignorance of food allergy and other food-related problems in clinical medicine and disputes within the allergy community have left many people suffering, frustrated and confused. Many patients, who are not properly diagnosed, undergo expensive prolonged investigation, treatment, and sometimes unnecessary surgery. The lack of convenient, reliable tests for food allergy is one of the reasons for diagnostic failures. The lack of well-promoted, effective drugs to correct food allergy is another major reason why this problem has received such little attention in clinical medicine. Only one pharmaceutical company, Fissons Inc., has marketed a food allergy drug, Nalcrom, and only Fissons makes any effort to alert physicians to the problems of food allergy. Without drug company interest, there is little or no medical interest.

At the same time as **medicine defaults** in the diagnosis and treatment of food-related illnesses, many non-medical practitioners have launched careers in the food and chemical "sensitivity" business, using diverse, sometimes curious and bizarre methods, and infrequently advocate fraudulent tests and treatments. Unfortunately, we have seen many examples of bizarre and expensive non-medical "treatment" of patients with food allergy. Even well-intentioned efforts to diagnose and treat allergy are often based on faulty premises and fail to deliver proper results.

Testing For Food Allergy

The desire for simple, definitive tests for food allergy is easy to understand, but difficult to fulfill. The idea of a simple office "test" for food allergy should seem unlikely if you have read and considered previous chapters in this book. The problem of food allergy is too complex and variable to ever be evaluated by a simple test. Food interacts complexly and sequentially with our body with many different consequences. It is unlikely that food allergy occurs in a consistent manner, because of all the variables discussed in previous chapters, and no single test will ever reveal the complex nature of this reactivity.

Dr. J. Gerrard, a prominent Canadian allergist summarized the problems of evaluating food allergy:[1] "... foods can cause not only classical IgE-mediated allergy but also the irritable bowel syndrome, migraine, arthritis, and disturbances of behavior. The identification or confirmation of IgE-mediated allergy is simple, for it correlates well with skin prick tests and radio-allergosorbent test results. The identification of other adverse reactions to foods is more difficult and is sometimes hampered by preconceived ideas both on the part of the patient and the physician. To throw light on this problem we have admitted patients, thought for one reason or another to be reacting adversely to foods, to a hostel unit where they have first been fasted for four days on spring or filtered water, and have then been given single foods one by one so that adverse reactions to them might be recorded by both the patient and the physician. The patients studied had for the most part a combination of symptoms which included nasal stuffiness, headaches, irritable bowel syndrome, arthralgias, eczema, and neurological problems such as depression and lassitude. 33 patients have been investigated so far. In 6, symptoms persisted unchanged, the presenting symptoms being headache in 3, neuralgia in 2, and asthma in 1; symptoms cleared completely in 12 and diminished to 50-90% of previous levels in 15. When foods were reintroduced the reactions were unexpected, both by the patient and by the attending physician, for neither knew beforehand that foods, let alone which food, were precipitating symptoms. Had the patient been aware that foods were playing a part in causing his symptoms he would have avoided them."

"Foods seem to play a part in severe chronic disorders which have no recognized aetiology. To establish the role of foods in precipitating these disorders we need hospital units where patients can be fasted and then tested individual with foods, with biochemical and immunological studies if required. Investigations such as these are inexpensive and, when foods are implicated, the treatment, food avoidance, is cheap. When food avoidance prevents headaches, the irritable bowel syndrome, arthralgias, and depression, it is more effective and less costly than traditional treatment, and the observation also throws light on the aetiology of the disorder."

What is the Value of a Test?

The following questions must be asked about every proposed test:

What is the test simulating?" Is the simulation related to eating real food in real time, by real people, exposed to many other influences? Does this test do a credible job of simulating digestion and absorption? Are the testing substances representative of foods, actually eaten? Are the results reproducible? Are the test results just spot samples or do they represent the sequential interaction of food with body systems? Does the test simulate IMED, and does it demonstrate the different responses to varying doses and fequency of food ingestion?

The only test that answers all the simulation criteria, is to actually eat the food as meals over days to weeks and observe what happens! Some **absurd notions** preoccupy some food allergy researchers. The notion that **double blind food challenge** is essential for the diagnosis and before diet revision is prescribed is among the most impractical, and sometimes refractory ideas. **Food allergy research** should include studies of people who are given concealed doses of food materials in a variety of circumstances. This is one method of isolating the mechanism of food allergy. Very limited conclusions can be drawn from these isolated experiments. We have learned a lot about possible mechanisms this way. We never learn, however, to discredit the evidence that patients bring us after their forays in the real-world.

However, the double blind fanatics suggest that it is necessary for routine patient management to hospitalize their patients and administer food extracts by capsule or stomach tube over many days to weeks observing reactions. This procedure is expensive, impractical, and usually punitive to patients who just want to get better. Medical insurers should examine these extravagant demands for " controlled food challenges". Even if we could justify the expense, inconvenience and discomfort of food challenges, would the results be meaningful when the patient left the hospital and resumed eating food everyday? Do the capsule challenges meet our criteria for simulating the natural disease mechanisms? No! More sophisticated concepts of food allergy have been presented in this book and we know about dose-frequency factors, biological rhythms, context-dependency, chaos theory and the avalanche effect. We are too smart to settle for a single, contrived experiment to tell us what is going to happen in the confusion and chaos of the real world over a longer period of time.

The Core Program is actually a diagnostic procedure and, at the same time, it is a treatment program. It is a real-world experiment. The diagnosis of food allergy is confirmed by remission of symptoms on the Core Program, and is further confirmed by return of symptoms after offending foods are again eaten. You perform your own food challenges as you reintroduce foods. The use of an elemental nutrient formula, to replace food during the clearing phase of the Core Program, is the most definitive method of assessing the role of food in producing any illness. If remission occurs on the ENF, food allergy and/or other mechanisms of food intolerance are responsible. You may not be interested in the precise mechanisms, as long as you can get better; therefore, for practical purposes, there is no better test for the presence of food problems than a trial on ENFood.

Your results of food challenge may never be precise and that is appropriate, since the mechanisms of food reactions are never precise; recall all our information which characterizes food allergy and rhythmic, periodic, variable and always changing. The hospital, double-blind food challenge assumes that you are a deluded fool and cannot make correct decisions for yourself. We reject this patronizing style of medicine. On your own, you can achieve practical, effective diet revision, learning as you go to be self-regulating and self-responsible.

Allergy Skin Tests

People expect skin tests when they see an allergist and are disappointed when told that food allergy is too complex to be diagnosed by this means alone. Skin tests are often effective in pinpointing inhalant allergens such as house dust mites and the pollen antigens which cause hay fever and seasonal asthma, but their use beyond these specific problems is doubtful. Skin tests, with protein extracts from foods, have proven to be disappointing and often misleading. The food scratch or prick test survives in office allergy practice because too few allergists have critically reviewed the reliability and predictive value of the skin test. Often studies in food allergy are limited to those patients with positive skin tests and all the interesting problems, not revealed this way, are neglected or denied.

Skin tests can reveal some of the immediate-type hypersensitivities to food materials and are always of interest, when distinctly positive. If a food extract produces a wheal response (like a mosquito bite) with itch and surrounding redness, the food should not be eaten. However, the skin test does an enormous disservice if it is used to deny food allergy. A negative skin test for food is meaningless. The entire spectrum of delayed pattern food allergy lies beyond the predictive abilities of this elementary form of immunological testing.

"Provocation" Tests

A group of environmentally aware physicians, known as **clinical ecologists**, developed "provocation tests for food sensitivity". Clinical ecologists have tended to be more interested in food allergy than their allergist colleagues. They wanted to simulate, in a convenient and quick way, the responses of a patient to eating the food. The **sublingual provocation test (SLPT)** was invented as an office procedure. Dropping the allergenic extract of food under the tongue was an obvious sort of simulation to try. The idea is that some of the food antigens would be absorbed through the mouth lining, and would interact with immune sensors and reactors in the blood. The SLPT simulation would perhaps detect the immediate type responses of circulating basophils. The problem with the SLPT is that it is completely unreliable. A patient who is already symptomatic cannot be tested meaningfully. The test responses are subjective; the absorption of the antigen under the tongue is variable and unreliable; the responses to small doses of antigen are not representative of the illness problem; one major reaction to a sublingual challenge makes the patient untestable for several days...the list goes on. The SLPT is not a good diagnostic test of food allergy.

Provocation Tests: by Injection

Provocation tests by needle injection of food proteins into the skin have also been used. The **intradermal (ID) injection** test has proven to be more effective in showing IgG4 reactivity to antigens, and will occasionally show a delayed, cell-mediated response in 24-48 hours. Again, symptoms may develop as injected antigen reacts with skin mast cells, or reaches circulating basophils and triggers an amplified, immediate alarm-response. Injected antigen can cause a dangerous anaphylactic response by complement activation and/or the mast cell-basophil mechanism.

There is no question that injected antigen can sometimes demonstrate symptom-production in the allergic patient. Indeed every allergist is concerned about triggering life-threatening anaphylactic reactions with any injection. If major symptoms do occur to one injected antigen, further testing is invalid for several days. Clinical ecologists claim to "neutralize" the reaction by injecting further doses of antigen at different concentrations, and often test many substances in one session, lasting several hours. No meaningful conclusions can be drawn from these testing marathons. The subject tends to have fluctuating, confusing sensations, and is extremely vulnerable to suggestion from the testing person. The ID provocation test is not reliable in predicting responses to foods, actually eaten, and should not be used as the basis for recommending diet revision. A small study by Jewett and associates in California[2] questioned the validity of provocation tests; 18 patients were tested by this method and they concluded that subjects hard a hard time differentiating active from inactive solutions, and the neutralizing effect was not related to the concentration of the active ingredients.

The authors of this study seem confused about symptoms in their subjects and once again invoke **placebo voodoo** as their explanation. An associated editorial in this esteemed journal carries this nonsense further with the byline, "Food Sensitivity or Self-Deception"; the editorial hints darkly that patients with food allergy are dupes. Once again, we are reminded that the mere mention of food allergy invites the most irrational and often prejudiced opinions from some influential members of the medical establishment.

The only conclusion we can reach about provocation tests and this study of it is that you cannot ask subjects to sit in a room for several hours after breakfast or lunch, receiving a variety of injections, with a variety of distractions and suggestions, explicit or implicit, coming from testers and other subjects and make any sense of it! The authors of this study did not seem to realize that any group of subjects sitting in a room will report symptoms, if asked. This is not a mysterious "placebo" effect ; but the "noise" of each person's body which becomes apparent to everyone who sits quietly and does nothing for a few hours. Anyone who has practiced meditation can tell about shifting awareness of body noise; its always there if you pay attention; if it gets very loud then you cannot ignore it.

Cytotoxic Tests

Cytotoxic tests have been offered for definitive "food sensitivity" determination, and have been condemned by the American College of Allergists as ineffective. There is a valid idea behind cytotoxic tests, but commercially applied techniques failed to deliver useful results. The second mechanism of immune-mediated damage is the cytotoxic or cell-killing effect. Cells may also be damaged by direct toxicity of drugs and food-related chemicals. Cytotoxic tests, recently marketed, expose blood cells to food extracts in a chamber, viewed through a microscope; cell counts before and after reveal cell damage.. Automation can be applied to cell counting and evaluation with computer print-outs of test results. While the earlier cytotoxic tests have little to offer, more sophisticated analysis of food antigen and blood interactions is always relevant to our understanding pathogenic mechanisms.

A recent automated variation on this test has been offered as the **ALCAT** diagnostic system[3]. This is more technically satisfying test with interesting possibilities for research not for redesigning your food supply!. The ALCAT brochure repeats our understanding that multiple mechanisms are involved in food allergy and that responses to food antigens by various blood components should be measured in food allergic individuals. The predictive significance of these measurements remains to be discovered.

We doubt if any cytotoxic test will be adequate for the proper design of a safe diet. We will never be certain that, after eating food, blood cells be exposed to the test substances in an identical manner? The idea of developing a valid test of cell response to antigens and toxins remains viable and deserves more work. The practical point is to save the several hundred dollars, usually demanded for cytotoxic testing, and get on with the Core Program to develop your own, custom-fitted Core Diet.

The IgE model of allergy inspired development of antibody-measuring laboratory tests. The idea was to show the affinity of circulating antibodies to different antigens. The hayfever model dominated test ideas; if you had enough IgE directed to June grass pollen, you would sneeze when you inhaled the pollen. The same reasoning was applied to food allergy, and RAST testing was developed to detect IgE antibodies to different food proteins. The RAST has been used instead of, or in addition to, skin scratch tests to assess food allergy. Whenever IgE mechanisms dominate the food allergy problem, RAST may be a useful test. Variations of the RAST idea allow for antigen-specific antibodies to be assayed. The related tests bear the acronyms ELIZA, FAST, and MAST, and others will appear as this testing technology develops. Negative RAST results have been used to deny food allergy and seemed more authoritative, looking official and "scientific" on a computer printout from the lab. This RAST-test denial only demonstrates ignorance of the many mechanisms of food allergy, not related to IgE or not involving the small number of test antigens, selected from the a much larger number of possible antigens in the food supply.

The principles of RAST testing for IgE are now applied to the measurement of other antibody types. The measurement of IgG is of great interest. Current studies suggest frequent IgG responses to food antigens. Recently, new lab tests measuring food-antigen specific IgG have been offered in an impressive computer-reported format. The levels of food-specific IgG are listed, and avoidance of these food is advised. Helpful food lists and food rotation instructions accompany the reports. The results of this evaluation are so convenient, so professional looking, it would appear the problem of food allergy diagnosis is solved. Again, this simplistic approach to food allergy is bound to mislead us; we are not sure what the IgG antibodies to food antigens are doing and, therefore, we do not know what kind of food reactivity this test might hope to predict. While it is likely that avoidance of IgG-positive foods will be helpful, we do not know if that avoidance will really resolve the illness problem. In our limited experience with the IgG test, the predictive value for food reaction is limited.

It is easy to postulate, for example, that the presence of IgG to a food antigen protects you to some extent from the allergic reaction. In pollen allergy, IgG antibodies are thought to block the allergic response, mediated by IgE. It may be that we should eat the IgG positive foods and avoid all the others. This is an unlikely postulate, but illustrates our lack of knowledge of the proper application of these lab results. We are convinced that IgG mechanisms, like IgE mechanisms, do not act alone in producing patients' symptoms and suffering. We need to collect IgE, IgG data, along with other immunological measures before the food allergy complex will be revealed in the laboratory.

IgG RAST Evaluation of IgA and IgM antibodies to food antigens is also of great interest. Studies relating levels of all antibody types to clinical observations are needed before the complexities of food allergy will become apparent.

The measurement of total blood levels of four antibody species (immunoglobin electrophoresis) is of some interest in the complex food allergy patterns. Very often, shifts in the distribution of IgG, IgM, IgA, and IgE manifest immune activity in response to antigen loading through GIT. The most common pattern is an elevation of the IgM with a very low IgE level. Depressed levels of IgM, IgG are seen in patients who have severe or prolonged food allergy; often blood cell counts are also depressed. When IgE levels are low, skin testing and IgE RAST are of little value. Low IgA predisposes to food allergy, and always suggests the diagnosis. Occasionally, elevations in IgA and IgG are seen in the food allergy complex. High IgG is associated with the more serious immune-mediated diseases, and reflects increased antibody production, often against unknown antigens. Normal levels of these antibodies do not rule out the diagnosis of food allergy.

Immune Complex Assays

The detection of circulating immune complexes is an important test of the **IMED** hypothesis. Usually this procedure is reserved for research, and is not routinely employed in patient evaluation. Improvement in techniques and automation is currently making CIC measurement more practical. The most interesting test procedures not only detect CIC's, but also determine what food antigens have complexed with antibody.[4] This demonstration of food-antigen-containing CIC's is gratifying, since the phenomenon of IMED is demonstrated. Unfortunately, we again face the uncertainty principle when we attempt to interpret the test results in terms of dysfunction and disease. We do not know how the type and number of immune complex correlates with disease patterns. Immune complexes differ in their size, shape, and biological significance; some may be very dangerous, others benign. Their dysfunctional results will surely depend on the kind, amount, and frequency of CIC formation. The amount of antigen appearing in the blood, compared with the amount of antibody available, determines the expression of the immunological response. Some CIC's excite reactions, other CIC's increase suppressor effects, others probably do both. The complexities of the immune-network challenge the understanding of even the most knowledgeable experts. Antigens which escape complexing with circulating antibody may be another sort of problem. More research is needed before immune complex assays will be reliable, predicting reactions to foods actually eaten.

Our **conclusions** regarding immunological tests for food allergy can be summarized; no single antibody measurement will predict the immune response to food; and no single type of lab measurement should be used as the only diagnostic test for food allergy. One reason for not pursuing the immunological tests as a basis for practical problem-solving in the Doctor's office is that they will be far too expensive.

Trials of diet revision are practical, effective, and economical. Any government or insurance agency, paying for medical services, should be keenly and devotedly interested in diet revision as a standard diagnostic and treatment method. The adoption of standard DRT could conceivably save billions of health-care dollars per year.

Bizarre Food Sensitivity Tests

Muscle testing is one of the bizarre charades used to demonstrate "food sensitivity". The subject is invited to hold a glass vial containing the test substance and the examiner tests the strength of the other arm which is outstretched. Weakness is interpreted as a food reaction, and the subject is advised to avoid the test substance. Variations on this theme have emerged. A simple resistance meter, dressed up in a fancy box (**Vega meter**), is used to measure skin resistance between a ground plate and an "acupuncture point", usually at the thumb web. A glass vial, containing test substances, is placed somewhere (it doesn't seem to matter where) in the circuit. Meter readings are interpreted as a "positive or negative reactions". The more imaginative Vega meter readers will tell you they can balance levels of certain substances in your body by doing meter readings and prescribing drops. Too good to be true?! There is no biology in these maneuvers. A pseudoscience explanatory system, referring to "oscillations in the electromagnetic field", confuses and misleads the sincere patient.

In any other context, these tests would seem a ludicrous charade. What makes the popularity of these shams a serious matter is the suffering of the patients, who are eager for solutions to their chronic problems and not getting help from qualified physicians. A set of dice with food names on their faces would probably be as successful as muscle testing or Vega meter testing in producing good results; any procedure which leads to diet revision with the exclusion of several foods has a chance of success if several common problematic foods are eliminated from the diet.